Leopoldo F. Montes & J. Thomas Vaughan

ATLAS OF Skin Diseases of the Horse

Diagnosis and Treatment in Equine Dermatology

MUNKSGAARD

North and South America:

W. B. SAUNDERS COMPANY
PHILADELPHIA · LONDON · TORONTO

Atlas of Skin Diseases of the Horse
Diagnosis and Treatment in Equine Dermatology

1st edition

Cover by Lars Thorsen
Composition by Satsform, Åbyhøj
Reproductions by Københavns Kliche & Offset, Copenhagen
Printed in Denmark 1983 by Th. Laursens Bogtrykkeri, Tønder

ISBN 87-16-08586-8

Distributed in North and South America by
W. B. Saunders Company, Philadelphia, Pennsylvania
ISBN 0-7216-6436-9

Library of Congress catalog card No. 82-17009

ATLAS OF
Skin Diseases of the Horse

Acknowledgements

The authors are indebted to many faithful colleagues, students, horse owners and trainers who referred the patients and helped in their management. Special thanks are due to Dr. Walter H. Wilborn for making available his outstanding facilities of the Electron Microscopy Center in Mobile. The entire ultrastructural data included in the Chapter Structure and Function of the Skin was obtained and kindly provided by Dr. Wilborn.

Horatio A. Luro reviewed cases dealing with conditions observed in thoroughbreds and offered valuable suggestions that facilitated their treatment. Virginia Klein and Carolina, Mercedes and Ana Montes generously and tirelessly typed the original manuscript.

Cases dealing with fungal infections were studied with partial support from a grant of The John A. Hartford Foundation.

Brett Day provided supervision and the facilities of the Learning Resources Center, School of Veterinary Medicine, Auburn University, for Gregg Greanoff, medical photographer, to print many of the color photographs used in this Atlas.

This book is dedicated
with great affection
to our loving wives

MERCEDES and ETHEL

vinculum matrimonii in aeternum

Contents

Preface

This is a unique book, in that it is the first one, to our knowledge, fully devoted to the skin of the horse and its diseases.

The two authors, both internationally known in their respective fields, have formed an unusual team characterized by effectiveness, productivity, imagination, hard work, dedication, and an effort to try to make a significant contribution in a rather complicated task. All this should be noted to help the reader to realize that this fantastic accumulation and beautiful display of clinical, histopathological, therapeutic, and research material is not just the result of luck. For as a famous sportsman (Arnold Palmer we believe it was) once said, "The more I practice, the luckier I get." We have witnessed very closely the continuous practice by Leo Montes and Tom Vaughan to gain insight into the great variety of problems dealing with the skin of the horse.

Despite our knowing that this work is the result of a 7-year effort, we must confess that the final manuscript pleasantly surprised us and we feel certain this atlas will also surprise the readers.

It is of interest that, upon completion of their clinical trainings, both Montes and Vaughan chose to enroll in graduate school, learn under basic scientists, and obtain a master's degree. Perhaps this is where the affinity between these two medical scientists of strikingly different backgrounds really lies. If so, it was probably the platform that quickly placed a human dermatologist in a position to understand veterinary medicine and an equine surgeon in a situation to comprehend dermatology.

Pedro C.P. Blaquier, M.D.
President
Haras La Biznaga
Islas, FNG Sarmiento
Provincia de Buenos Aires
Republica Argentina

Walter H. Wilborn, Ph.D.
Professor of Anatomy and Director, Electron Microscopy Center
College of Medicine
University of South Alabama
Mobile, Alabama
USA

Introduction

In the fall of 1973 one of the authors (LFM) sought the advice of Dr. J.E. Greene, then Dean of the School of Veterinary Medicine at Auburn, regarding the establishment of a collaborative effort between that school and the Dermatology Research Unit of the University of Alabama in Birmingham.

Dr. Greene indicated that the forthcoming return from Cornell to Auburn of the other author (JTV) was a timely event, because his great interest in cutaneous diseases of the horse would offer the possibility of a productive association. Thus Dr. Greene undertook to acquaint both authors with each other, and in the winter of 1974 as soon as JTV took charge of the Department of Large Animal Surgery and Medicine, the project began.

In November of 1974 the first Equine Dermatology Clinico-Pathological Seminar was held at Auburn under the direction of both authors and with the attendance of senior students and faculty. The reaction was so enthusiastic that Dr. Greene convinced the authors to continue their work in order to collect enough material for a book.

The clinical material included in this atlas was for the most part obtained at the Large Animal Clinic at Auburn while the biopsy specimens were processed and studied at the Laboratory of Dermatopathology of the Dermatology Research Unit. From the beginning a steady flow of cases produced accumulation of data which led in December of 1976 to the presentation of a scientific exhibit, "Consultations in Equine Dermatology," before the American Academy of Dermatology in Chicago. An expanded version of this exhibit was presented before the American Veterinary Medical Association in Atlanta, July 1977. Both exhibits were very well received.

Meanwhile, at the Annual Meeting of the American Dermatological Association held in Palm Beach in March 1975, a paper was read describing the main cutaneous diseases of the horse that are also observed in humans. Clinical dermatologists were astonished to see the striking similarities in the behavior of the two types of skin and with their comments added more encouragement to the decision to produce this atlas.

Further interest arose from an international survey, carried out by MUNKSGAARD and the authors, which covered the leading countries with activities in equine medicine and revealed the lack of a book devoted fully to skin diseases of the horse.

The grouping of diseases in several different categories was necessary to present the contents in an orderly fashion and also to create some sort of classification for the skin diseases of the horse. It should be kept in mind, however, that not all the diseases that may affect the skin of the horse are in this book because the cases included are only patients that we handled ourselves. We plan in future editions to expand the scope and contents of the book adding new patients with other diseases so a more complete coverage of equine dermatology can be presented.

A very stimulating aspect of our work was the gradual and increasing realization that many diseases affect equally human and equine skin. Thus we found ourselves dealing with truly applied comparative dermatology. An important result of this was a better and deeper understanding of those diseases and their treatment, which often resulted in better management of humans and horses. We hope that, likewise, the readers will find this atlas useful in this regard.

Although it was not designed as a textbook or a treatise of equine dermatology, the great need for this type of publication by students, practitioners, horse trainers and horse owners was another important motive to prepare this atlas.

We realize that our work is far from perfect, but we trust it can be the right step towards a better understanding of the skin of the horse and its diseases.

Leopoldo F. Montes *J. Thomas Vaughan*

Structure and Function of the Skin

The skin is the largest organ of the horse's body. It is a most important part with a remarkable ability to adapt to the environment, preventing the body from desiccation while maintaining it in constant communication with the outside (MONTAGNA and PARAKKAL 1974).

A large and varied number of functions are played by the skin: thermoregulation, perception of pain and itching, excretion, mineral and vitamin metabolism, water and electrolytes regulation, protein synthesis, lipid and carbohydrate metabolism, oxygen uptake and carbon dioxide delivery (URBACH 1946, ROTHMAN 1954). In addition, the skin is an ecosystem (MARPLES 1965) because it is in itself an environment normally or abnormally inhabited by the living organisms (bacteria, fungi, viruses, parasites, insects) which comprise the cutaneous flora and fauna.

The following pages depict the main components of the skin of the horse as demonstrated by correlated light and scanning electron microscopy. A brief explanation of the main function of each part of the skin is also included. In the diseases described later in this book, according to the nature of each one of them, these parts of the skin may suffer alterations of major or minor degree or they may be spared.

Normal Epidermis and Dermis

A low magnification microphotograph (Fig. A) shows a panoramic view of normal skin of the thigh of the horse. Epidermis (1), hairs in different stages of the growth cycle (2), sebaceous glands (3), sweat glands (4), blood vessels (5) are outstanding features.

Figure B demonstrates at higher magnification one of the hairs in Figure A. Notice the complexity of the hair root which includes the dermal papilla (1), the onion-shaped bulb (2), and the multilayered keratogenous zone (3). A lobule of a sebaceous gland (4) and capillaries (5) are in the vicinity of the hair.

The arrectores pilorum muscle (Fig. C) shown in an oblique section attaches itself to the wall of the hair follicle on one end and interweaves with the collagenous fibers (c) of the upper dermis on the other end (TALUDKAR 1972). It is formed by thin smooth muscle fibrils (f) and has a good capillary supply (b). RACKOW (1898) believed that the arrectores pilorum muscles were responsible for the bristly and erect hairs of the winter coat. Guyton (1956) feels that the pilomotor response (Coon and Rothman 1940) in hairy animals allows the hairs to stand up in cold weather entrapping a thick layer of insulator air next to the skin so the transfer of heat to the environment is greatly diminished.

A

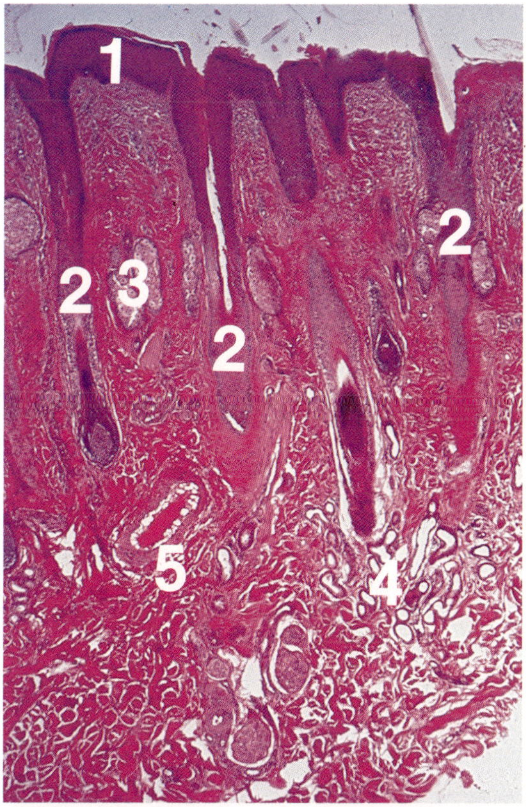

B

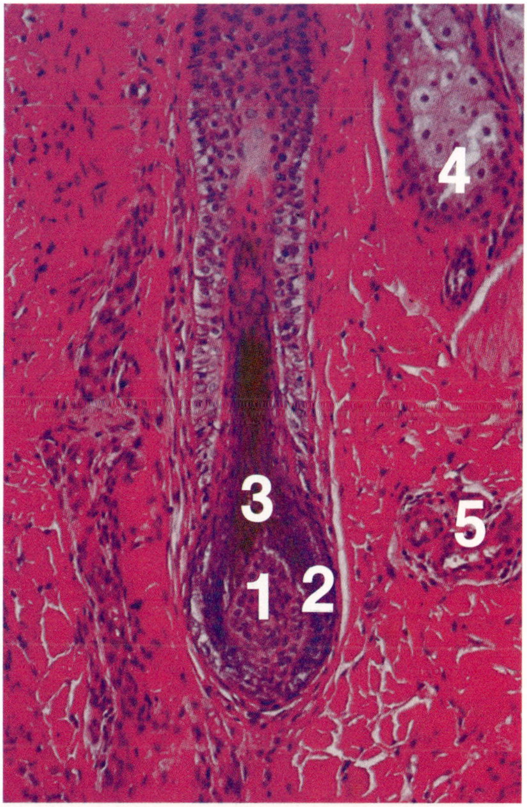

C

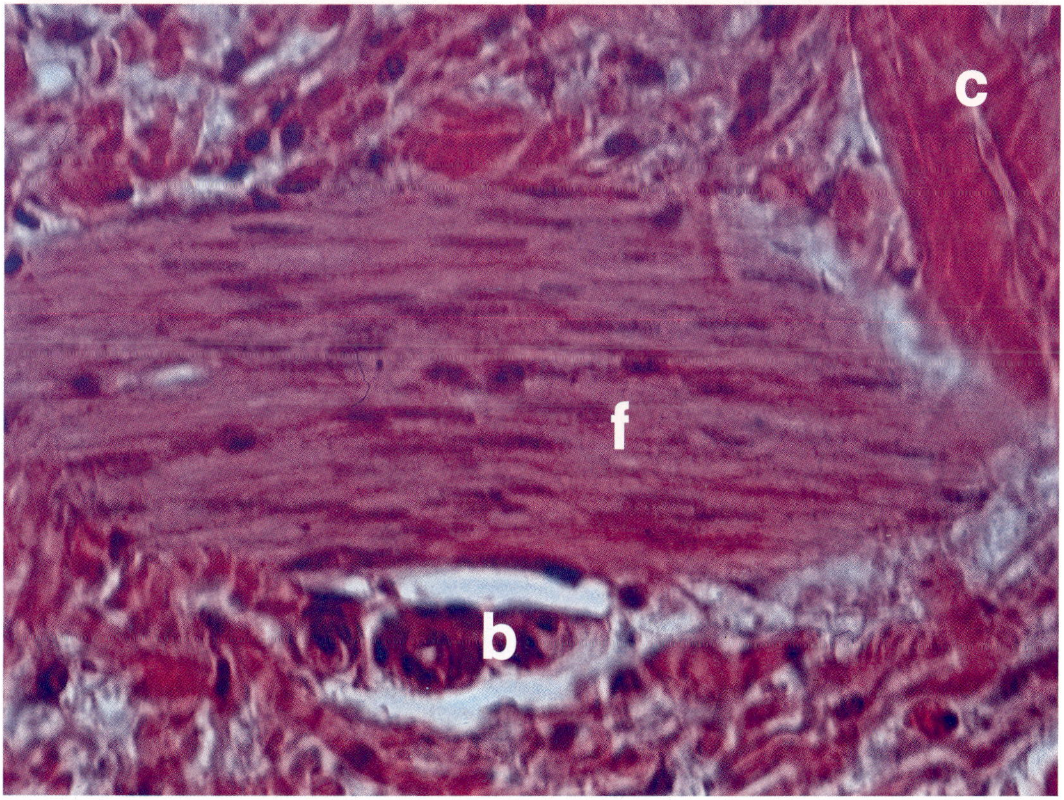

Layers of the Skin

The skin surface (S) is formed by the outer layer of the stratum corneum (SC). Notice the loose scales and the undulating appearance of the surface where depressions alternate with elevations.

The stratum corneum slows down water loss by the body and prevents penetration of harmful substances thus acting as a barrier. The stratum spinosum (SS) or stratum Malpighii is formed by cells which divide and migrate towards the surface (keratinocytes) while they synthesize keratin and by other cells which synthesize melanin pigment (melanocytes).

The dermis (D) lies between the epidermis and the subcutaneous tissue and is composed of fibers, cells and ground substance. The dermis protects the body from external injury through the integrated action of its various components: a) fibers (collagen, reticulin and elastin); b) cells (fibroblasts and mast cells) and c) ground substance (mucopolysacharides, water, inorganic material, proteins).

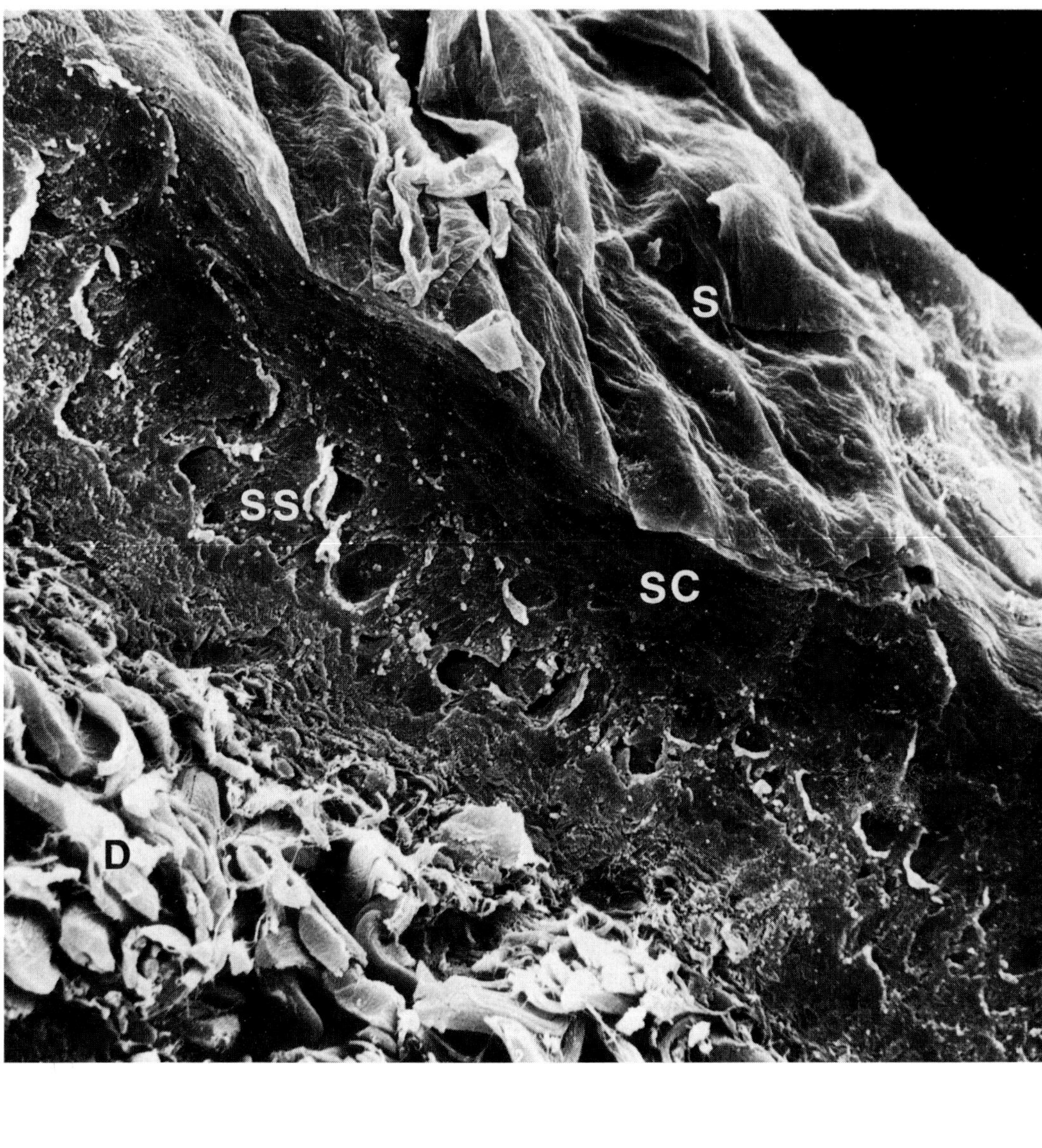

Thickness of the Skin

The skin of the horse has substantial thickness. This is a biopsy specimen obtained from the medial femoral region, an area where measurements by TALUDKAR et al (1972) showed 2.9–4.1 mm of total cutaneous thickness (50–75 mu for the epidermis and 2.8–4.0 mm for the dermis.)

This investigator also found that in comparison with other domestic animals, the skin of the horse is thicker than that of swine, goat and sheep. On the other hand it is thinner than the skin of Hereford and Angus cattle. The photograph below obtained by SEM at relatively low magnification provides a view of most of the cutaneous thickness from the superficial to the deeper layers.

Large number of hairs (H) emerge from the skin surface. The collagen bundles (C) seem to adopt a parallel course in an horizontal fashion in the mid-dermis. A large arteriole (A) is seen in the deep dermis at the lower right corner of the picture.

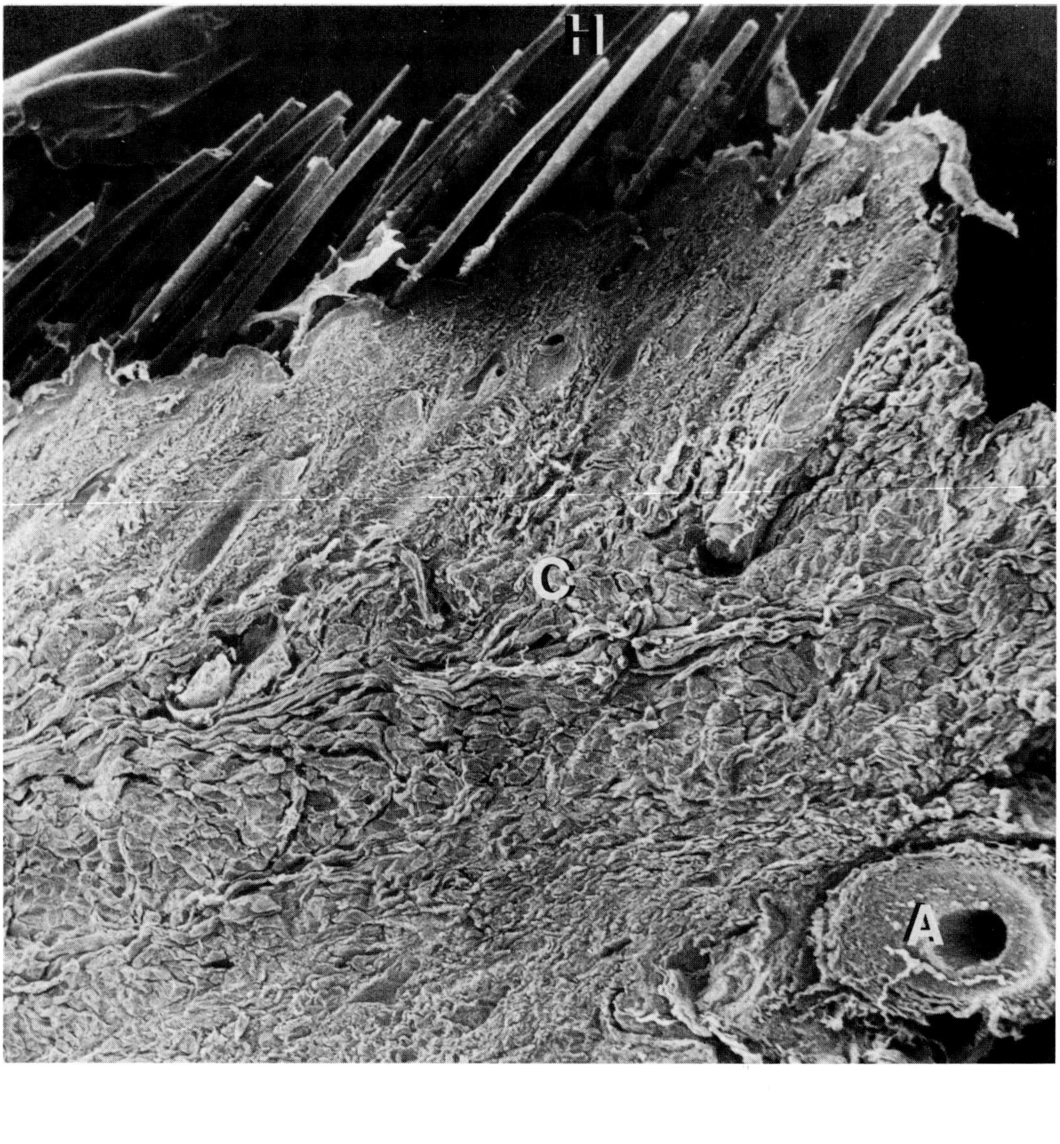

Blood Supply

The same arteriole shown in the previous photograph is seen here at higher magnification. Notice the thickness of the sectioned wall (W) and the appearance of the endothelial surface (E) surrounding the lumen (L). Arterioles such as this one are part of a rich vascular system which provides the skin with a continuous and significant blood supply.

This vascular system plays an important role in the control of body temperature (BURTON 1961), in the access of nutrients to the skin, in the absorption of topically applied medications, in the delivery to the skin of systemically administered drugs, in the cutaneous reaction against infectious and traumatic agents, in the healing of ulcers and wounds, and in the degree of redness and paleness.

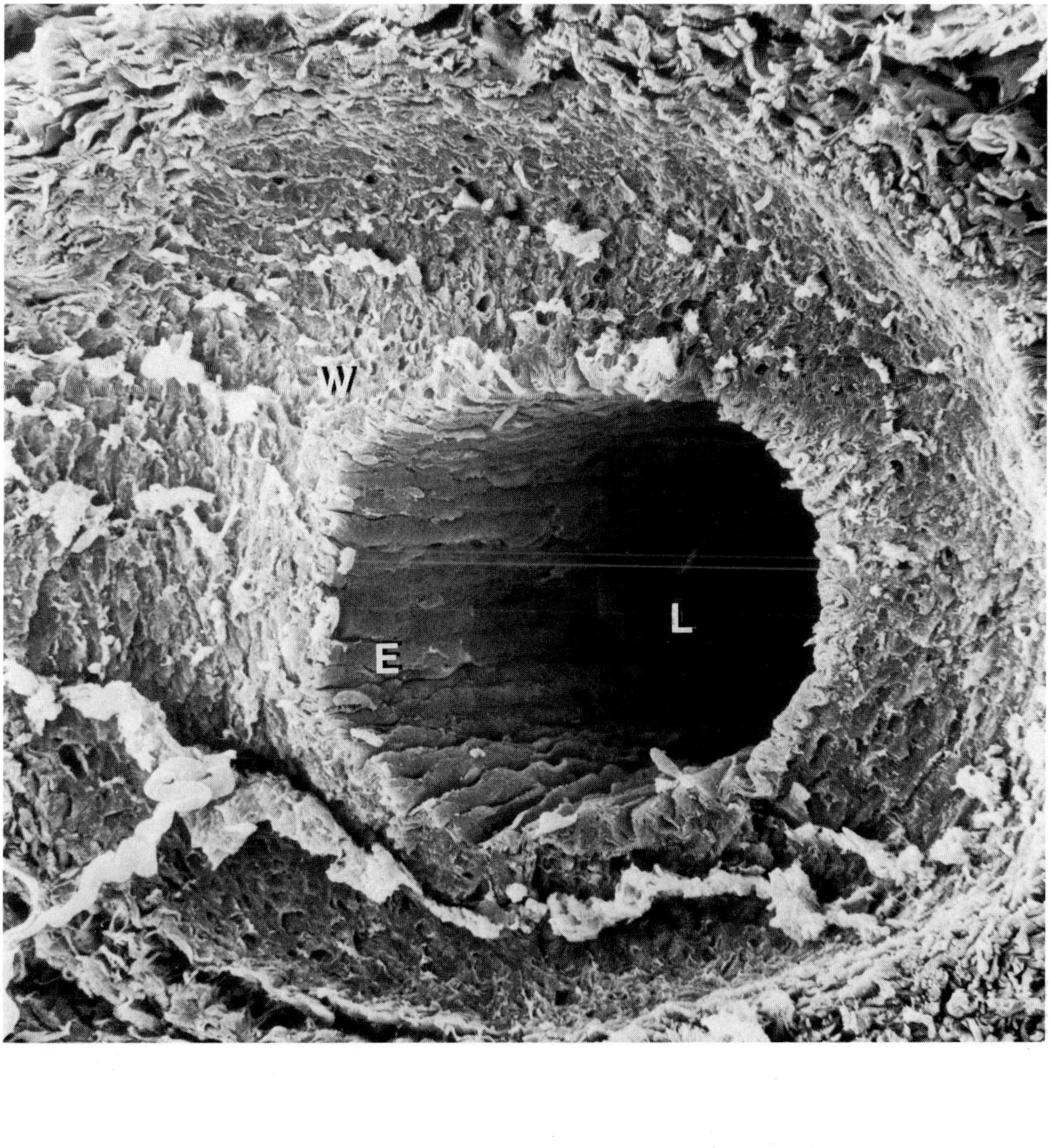

Dermis

This is a view of the mid-dermis where collagen fibers (C) group themselves to form thick bundles. The fibers are seen after sectioning in different angles. The apparently empty spaces between the fibers are occupied by the structureless part of the dermis known as the ground substance (GS). The cellular components of the dermis (fibroblasts and mast cells) are not seen in this field.

The dermis provides support and a substrate for the epidermis (VAN SCOTT and FLAXMAN 1968), is an important site for collagen synthesis, is a barrier to infection from both external and internal sources, contains enzymes, is a target for hormone action including corticosteroids, and participates in the immune response.

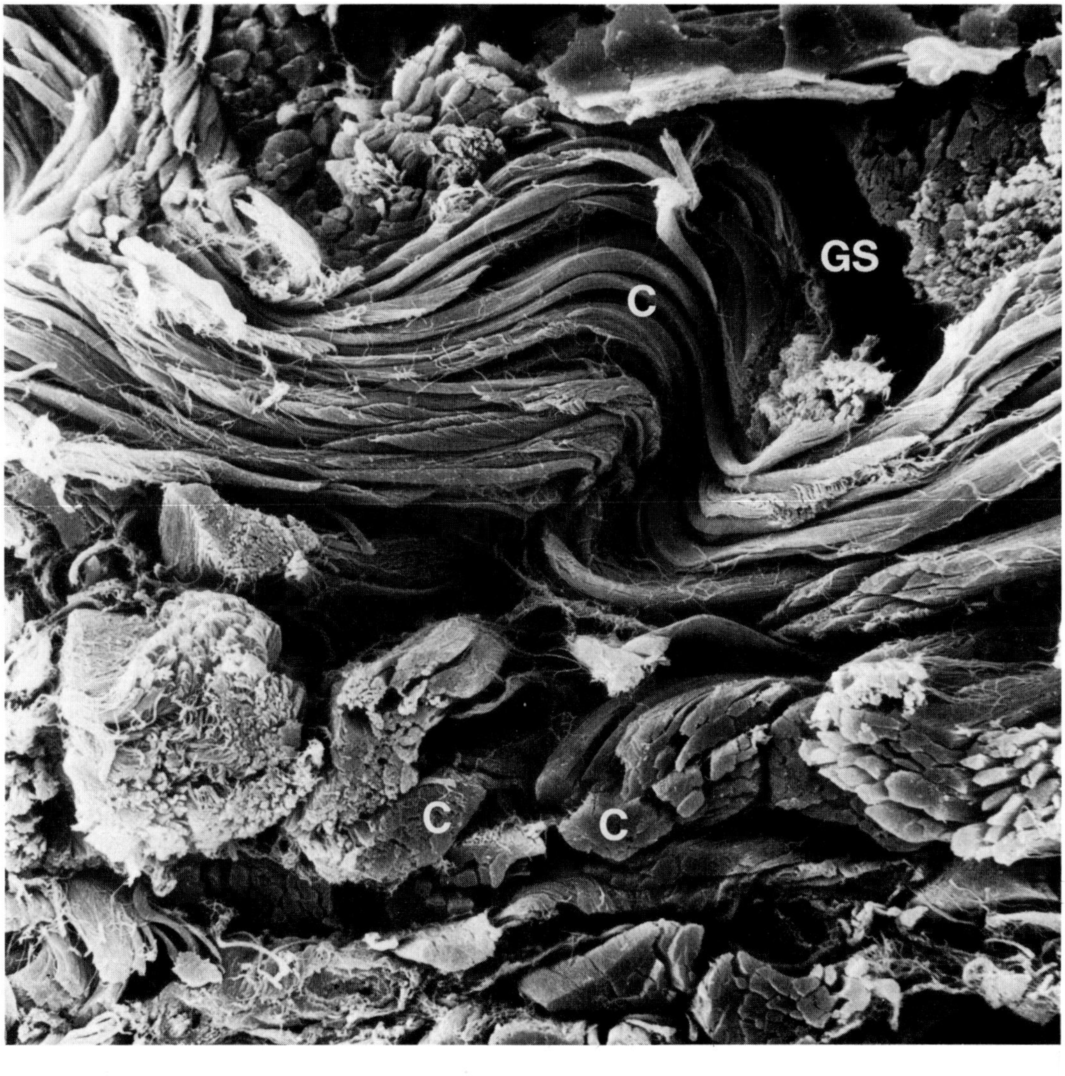

Sebaceous Glands

Sebaceous glands are composed of multiple acini such as the one partially shown in this picture. The secretion is a centripetal process. The peripheral cells are more immature and as they move centripetally towards the lumen (L), they undergo fragmentation with release of many rounded lipid droplets of sebum. Sebaceous glands are found everywhere in the skin of the horse and they open into the hair follicle.

Sebaceous secretion is influenced by hormones, atmospheric temperature and the nervous system. In humans a great increase in sebaceous gland activity and volume is one of the signs of puberty.

According to ROTHMAN (1954), sebum is liquid inside the duct and hair follicle and after reaching the skin surface it diffuses all over the skin and penetrates the stratum corneum where it functions as an emollient (MONTAGNA 1974).

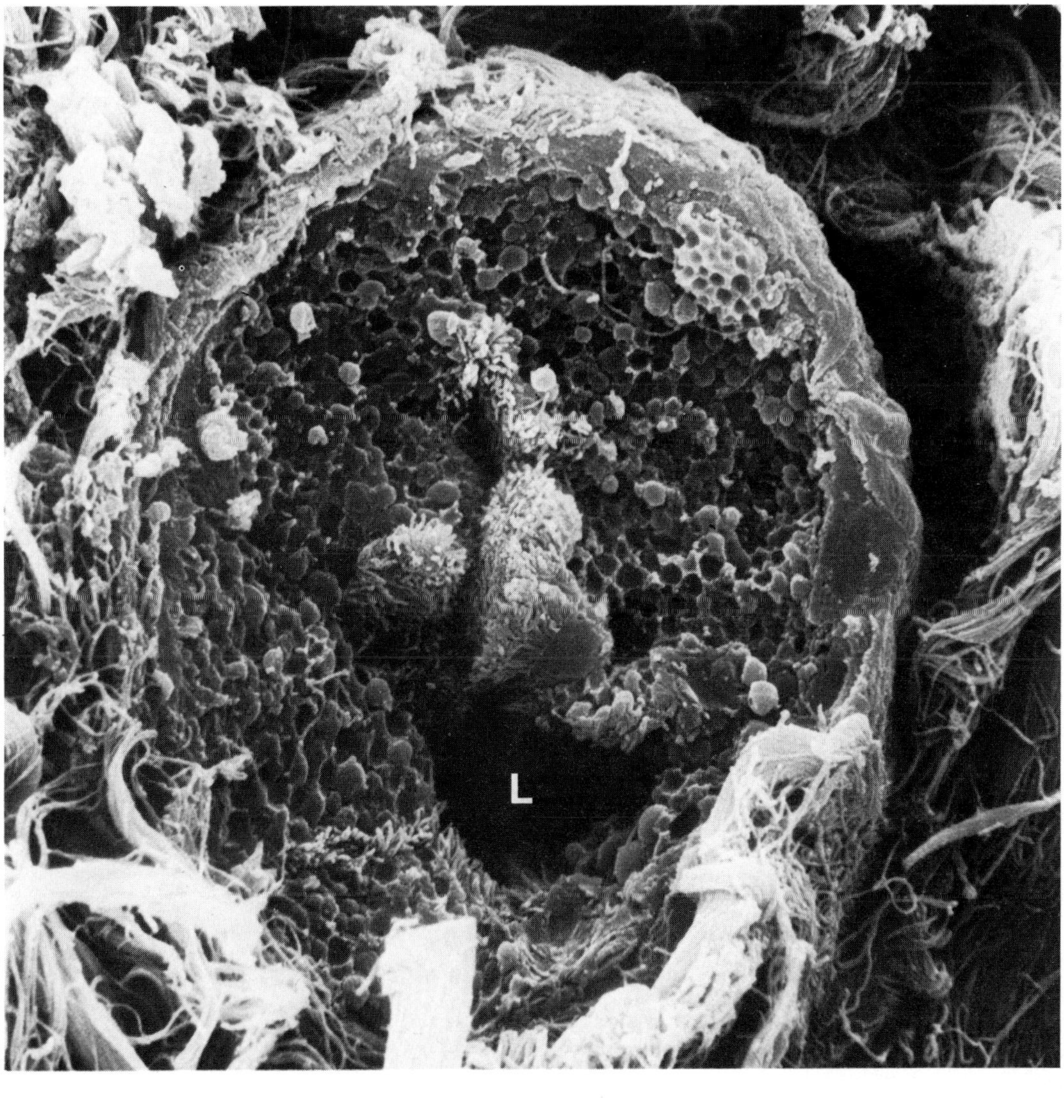

Hairs

Shafts of hairs (H) are present throughout the skin of the horse. They are seen in this section emerging at the surface among scales (upper part of the photograph) and also through the follicular openings. Other hairs have been sectioned at the level of the mid-dermis (central part of the photograph).

Hairs play a role as sensory organs because they are surrounded by nerves which react to pressure on the hair shaft (MONTAGNA and PARAKKAL 1974). According to ROTHMAN (1954) hairs have vital importance in thermoregulation allowing the exposed areas to have a special environment and almost maintain a "private climate" similar to clothed areas. This being the case in humans, one can understand the important thermoregulatory function of hairs in the horse particularly the thick hairs of the winter coat. Hairs provide protection against ultraviolet and heat rays and promote evaporation of sweat and water.

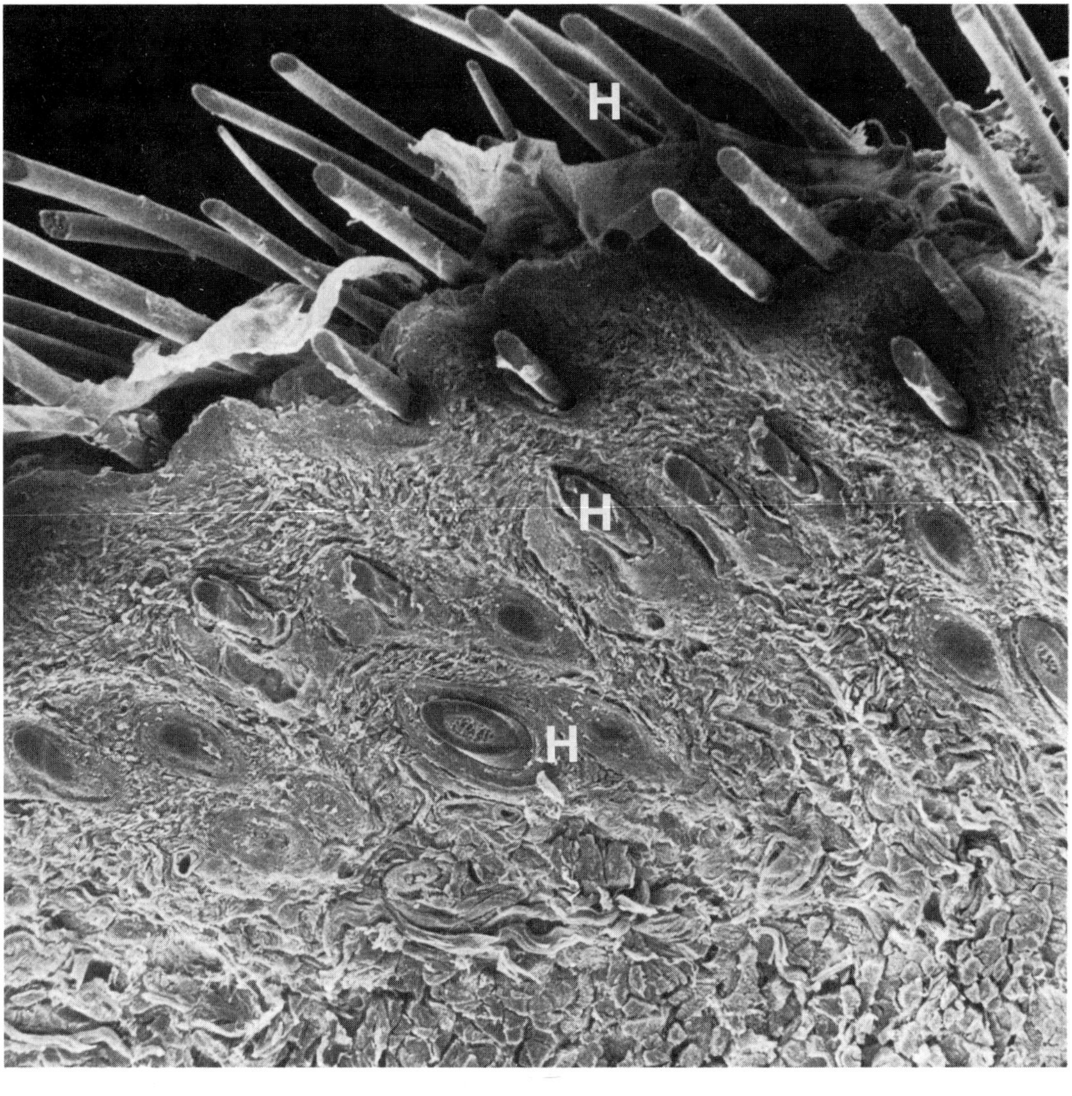

Hairs

This is a view of the shafts of four different hairs (H) as seen at different levels of focus outside the skin surface. The proximal parts of these hairs are at the lower part of the photograph. The free edges of the imbricated cuticle cells are slightly dentate and face the distal end of the hairs. Particles of sebum are attached to the surface of the cuticle cells.

Hairs have an important excretory function particularly of minerals. Keratin of hairs has a special affinity for arsenic and takes up more arsenic following oral or systemic administration than other tissues (SMITH and HENDRY 1934). Copper, iron, sulfur, zinc, lead, selenium and mercury are also excreted in hair.

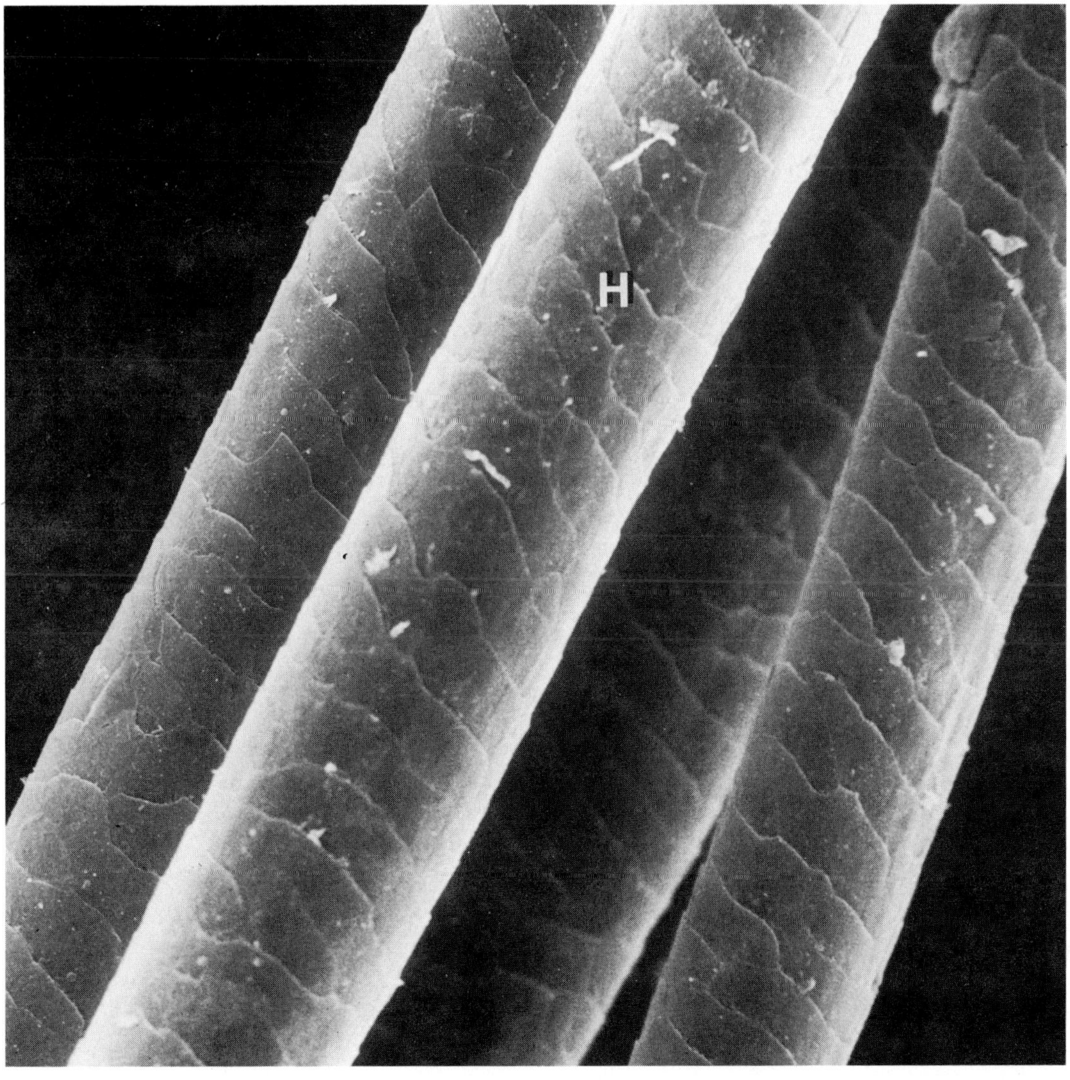

Hair

This is a portion of a growing (anagen) hair at the level of the upper dermis which has been longitudinally sectioned to present a view of the medulla (1), the cortex (2) and the cuticle (3).

The *medulla* originates from the matrix cells of the hair papilla and is composed mainly of an amorphous protein with a low cystine and high glutamic acid and glutamine content. It also contains citrulline (MONTAGNA and PARAKKAL 1974).

The *cortex* is made up of keratin as shown by ORFANOS and RUSKA (1970) in their transmission electron microscopic studies which revealed characteristic filaments surrounded by a dense matrix. The proteins of the cortex contain sulfur.

The *cuticle* adheres to the cortex with its cells forming an imbricated pattern. Cystine is an important component of the cuticle. Cuticular proteins are amorphous and have only few filaments.

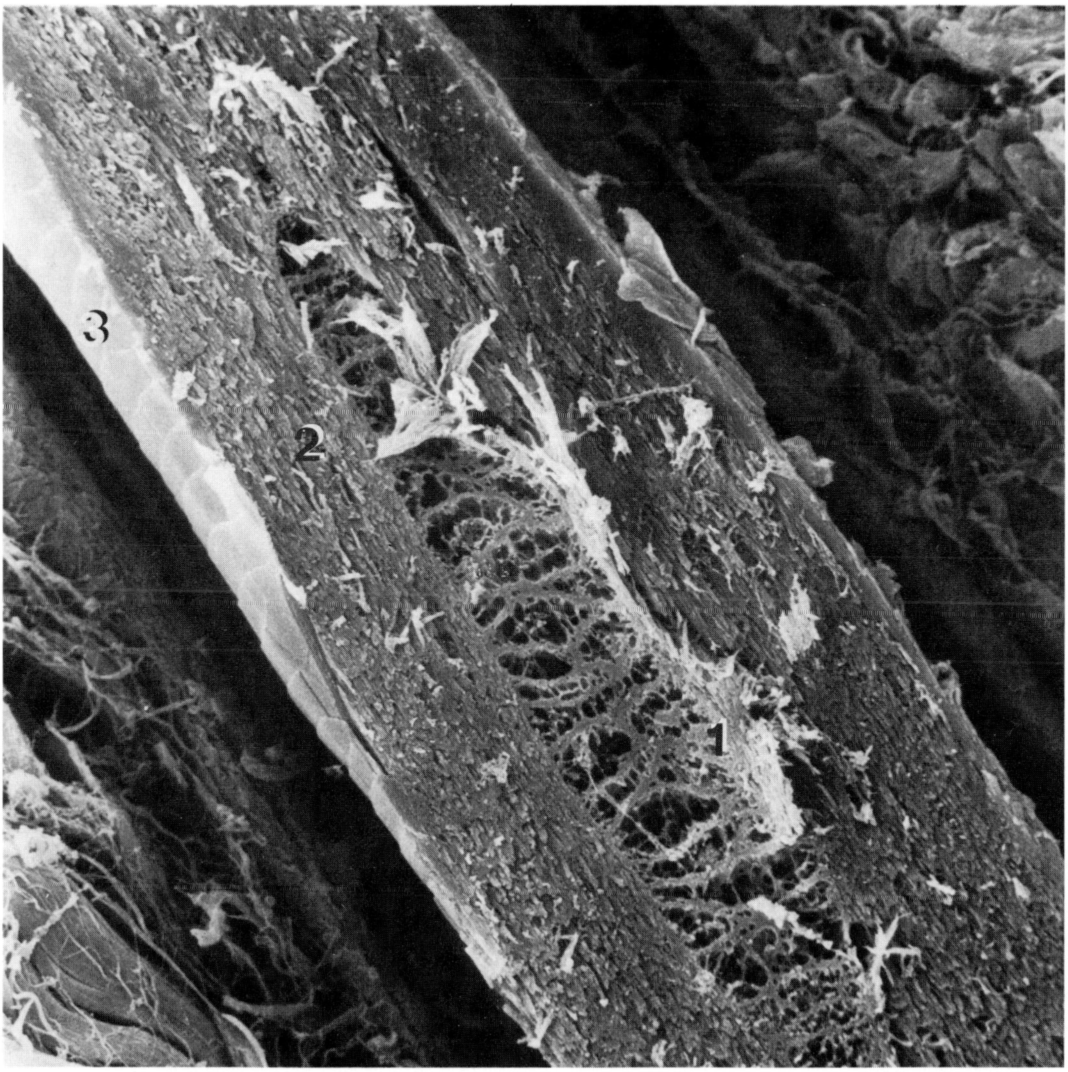

Sweat Glands

Sweat glands are well developed in most areas of the horse's skin (TALUDKAR 1970). Normal sweat gland function is essential to the good health of every horse.

The secretory coils of the sweat glands are surrounded by a network of fine nerve fibers that end up in the myoepithelial cells, the contractile organ which releases the sweat onto the skin surface (JENKINSON and BLACKBURN 1968), (JIRKA and KOTAS 1959). Sympathectomy results in hypersensitivity of the glands to their normal stimuli, namely exercise and epinephrine. The glands respond to sympathetic and parasympathetic drugs. The sweat in the horse is proteinaceous with albumin as the main protein.

The introduction of dinoprost tromethamine (tromethamine salt of the naturally occurring prostaglandin F2 alpha) for clinical use in mares led to the observation of profuse sweating following administration of a single intramuscular injection. It is observed after injecting 1–2 ml (5.0 mg/ml), usually starting about 15 minutes later (Fig. A), and is accompanied by a decrease in rectal temperature.

Unstimulated secretory tubules of sweat glands show their cells in the process of synthesis of the secretion. They appear large and tall, have prominent nuclei, a luminal border with evidence of decapitation or a brush appearance, a thick basement membrane closely attached to the myoepithelial cells and a good capillary network which insures continuous blood supply (Fig. B).

A

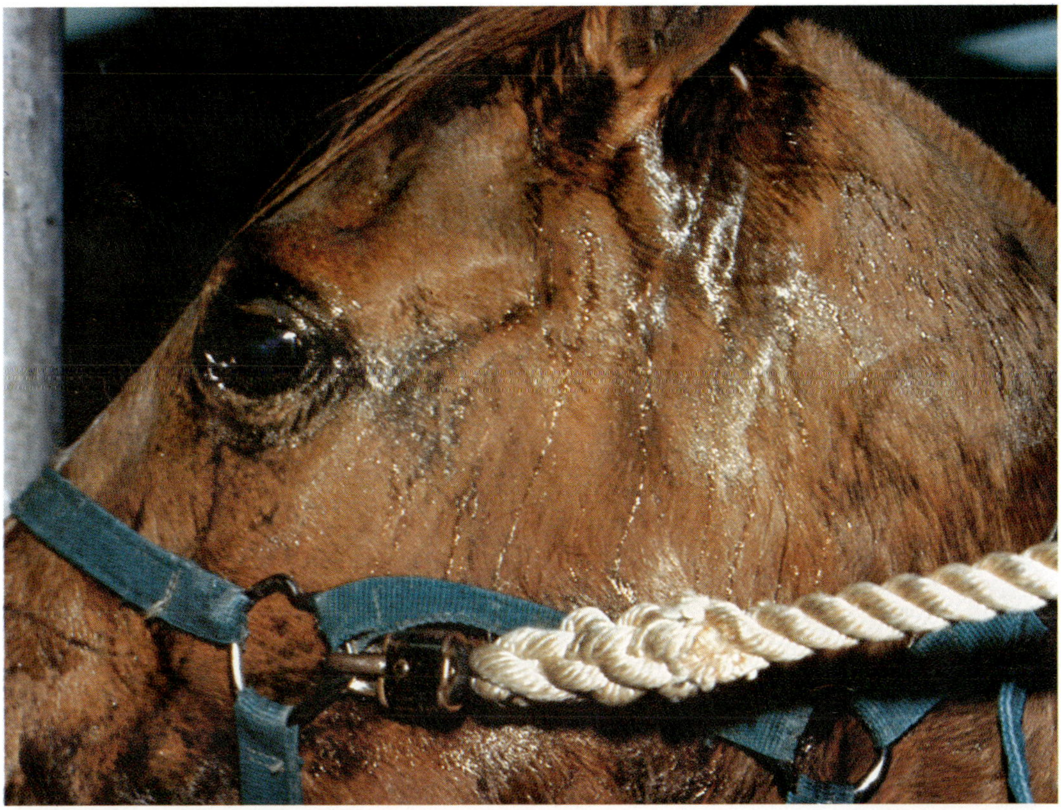

B

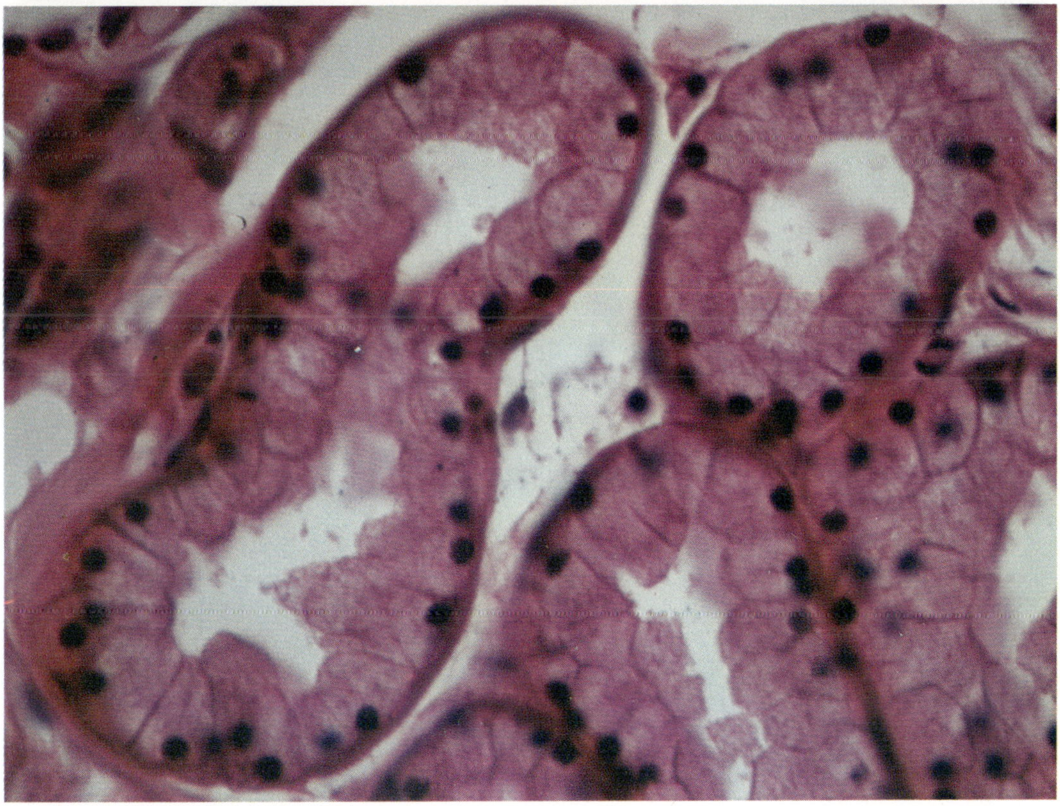

Sweat Glands

The secretory tubules of the sweat glands (SG) are located in the deep dermis and surrounded by connective tissue (CT). The lumen of the tubules contains secretory products. The sweat gland of the horse is considered an intermediate form of gland between eccrine and apocrine glands (EVANS et al 1957). Some glands contain an irregular luminal surface and show an uneven projection or a pinched-off apical end of the cells as in man (MONTES et al 1960).

A study of thirty-five areas of the skin in adult horses (TALUDKAR et al 1970) showed numerous glands in most areas. The glands appeared less developed on the middle of the back and on the limbs.

Although it is generally agreed that sweat glands are essential to temperature regulation and electrolyte balance, a great deal of research is needed to understand well their function in normal and abnormal conditions. In general, the glands are cytologically similar to the apocrine sweat glands of human axillary skin (BIEMPICA and MONTES, 1965).

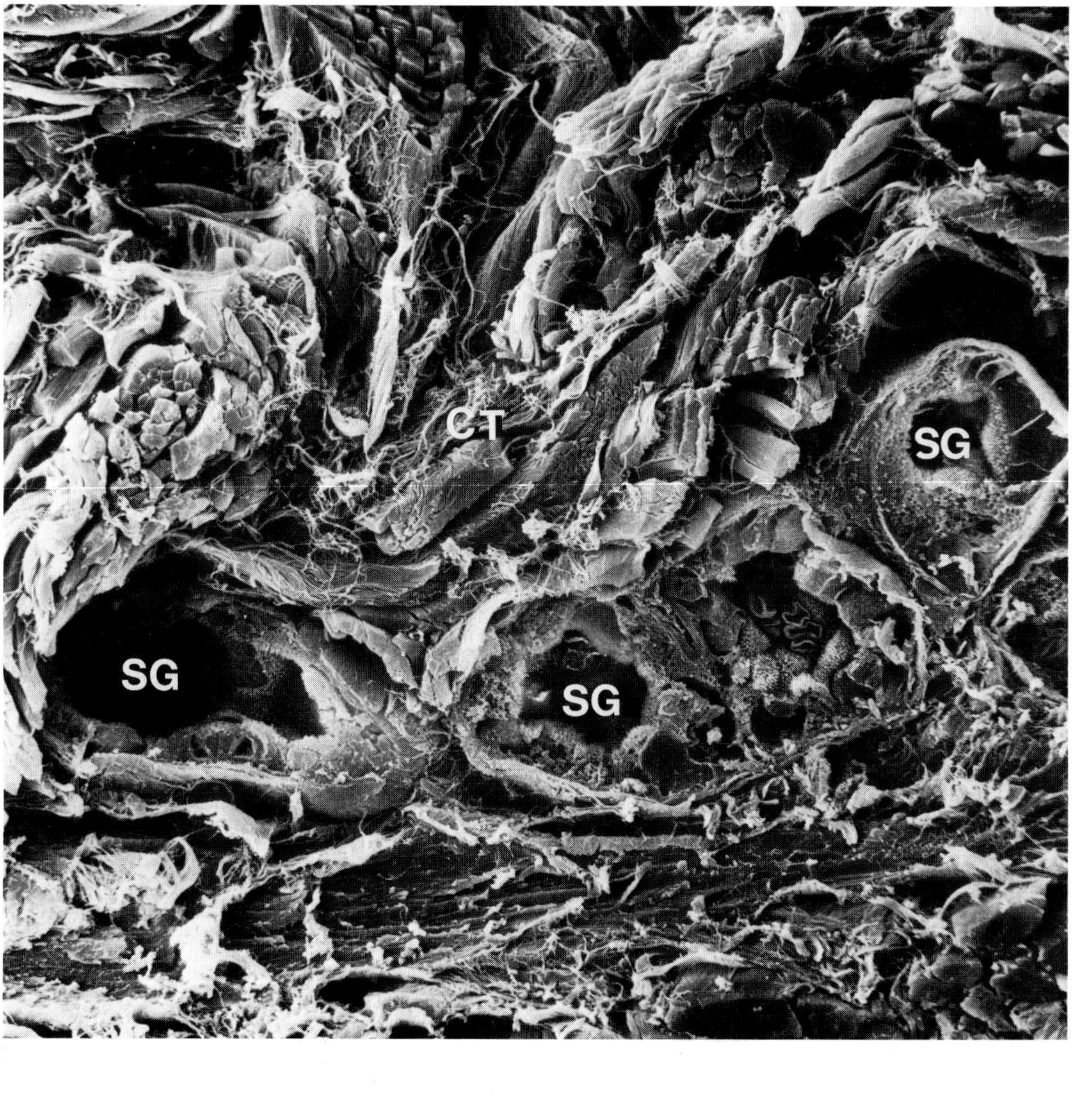

BIEMPICA, L. and MONTES, L.F.
Secretory Epithelium of the Large Axillary Sweat Glands. A Cytochemical and Electron Microscopic Study. American Journal of Anatomy 117:47, 1965.
BURTON, A.C.
Special Features of the Circulation of the Skin. In Advances in Biology of the Skin. Blood Vessels and Circulation. (W. Montagna and R.A. Ellis Editors). Vol. 2, p. 117. Pergamon. Oxford 1961.
COON, J.M. and ROTHMAN, S.
The Nature of the Pilomotor Response to Acetylcholine. Some Observations on the Pharmacodynamics of the Skin. Journal of Pharmacology and Experimental Therapeutics 68:301–11, 1940.
EVANS, C.L., NISBET, A.M. and ROSS, K.A.
A Histological Study of the Sweat Gland of Normal and Dry-Coated Horses. Journal of Comparative Pathology and Therapy. 67:397, 1957.
GUYTON, A.C.
Textbook of Medical Physiology. W.B. Saunders. Philadelphia 1956.
JENKINSON, D.M. and BLACKBURN, P.S.
The Distribution of Nerves. Monoamine Oxidase and Cholinesterase in the Skin of the Horse. Research Veterinary Science. 9:165, 1968.
JIRKA, M. and KOTAS, J.
Some Observations on the Chemical Composition of Horse Sweat. Journal of Physiology 147:74, 1959.
MARPLES, M.J.
The Ecology of Human Skin. Charles C. Thomas. Springfield, Illinois 1965.
MONTAGNA, W. and PARAKKAL, P.F.
The Structure and Function of the Skin. Academic Press, New York, 1974.
MONTES, L.F., BAKER, B.L. and CURTIS, A.C.
The Cytology of the Large Axillary Sweat Glands in Man. Journal of Investigative Dermatology 35:273, 1960.
ORFANOS, C.E. and RUSKA, H.
Die Keratine der Haut und des Haares. Hautarzt 21:343, 1970.
RACKOW, J.
Beitrag zur Histologie und Physiologie des glatten Hautmuskels des Pferdes. Arch. Tierheilk 24:273, 1898.
ROTHMAN, S.
Physiology and Biochemistry of the Skin. The University of Chicago Press. Chicago 1954.
SMITH, S. and HENDRY, E.B.
Arsenic and its Relation to Keratin Tissue. British Medical Journal 2:675, 1934.
TALUDKAR, A.H., CALHOUN, M.L. and STINSON, A.W.
Sweat Glands of the Horse: A Histologic Study. American Journal of Veterinary Research 31:1751, 1970.
TALUDKAR, A.H., CALHOUN, M.L. and STINSON, A.W.
Microscopic Anatomy of the Skin of the Horse. American Journal of Veterinary Research 33:2365, 1972.
URBACH, E.
Skin Diseases. Nutrition and Metabolism. Grune and Stratton. New York 1946.
VAN SCOTT, E.J. and FLAXMAN, B.A.
Environmental Control of Epithelial Cells "in vivo" and "in vitro". In Epithelial-Mesenchymal Interactions. (R. Fleischmajer and R.E. Billingham Editors). p. 280. Williams and Wilkins Co. Baltimore, 1968.

Regional Dermatology

As one gradually realizes how wide the variety of equine skin diseases is, an awareness of the need to know the topography of the horse develops.

From an anatomic viewpoint STEDMAN's (1972) defines topography as "the description of any part of the body, especially in relation to a definite and limited area of the surface". Thus the names used in cutaneous anatomy of the horse to designate the different regions should be properly known and employed in managing equine dermatoses. Because as ORMSBY and MONTGOMERY (1954) wisely emphasized "diseases select particular areas and not infrequently the nature of the disease is intimated by the region in which it occurs".

This basic principle which is so generally used now in human dermatology and in small animal dermatology (MULLER and KIRK 1976) will likely be employed later in equine dermatology also as knowledge accumulates. Equine dermatology is still a young specialty with relatively few people managing the dermatoses of the horse. But as knowledge and experience increase, like is happening to ourselves, the tendency for some diseases to have a regional predilection will become apparent as shown in certain cases throughout the book.

The diagram on the opposite page* has been particularly useful to us in our diagnostic work thus it is reproduced here to facilitate the work of those involved in equine dermatology.

* This diagram was part of JANE KIDD's chapter Horse and Pony Breeding published in The Colorful World of Horses.
It is reproduced here through the courtesy and with permission of Longmeadow Press, Norwalk, Connecticut; Hennerwood Publications Limited and Mandarin Publishers Limited, Hong Kong.

STEDMAN's MEDICAL DICTIONARY
The Williams and Wilkins Company Baltimore, 1972.
ORMSBY, O.S. and MONTGOMERY, H.
Diseases of the Skin. p. 120 Lea and Febiger, Philadelphia, 1954.
MULLER, G.H. and KIRK, R.W.
Small Animal Dermatology. p. 96, W.B. Saunders Company, 1976.

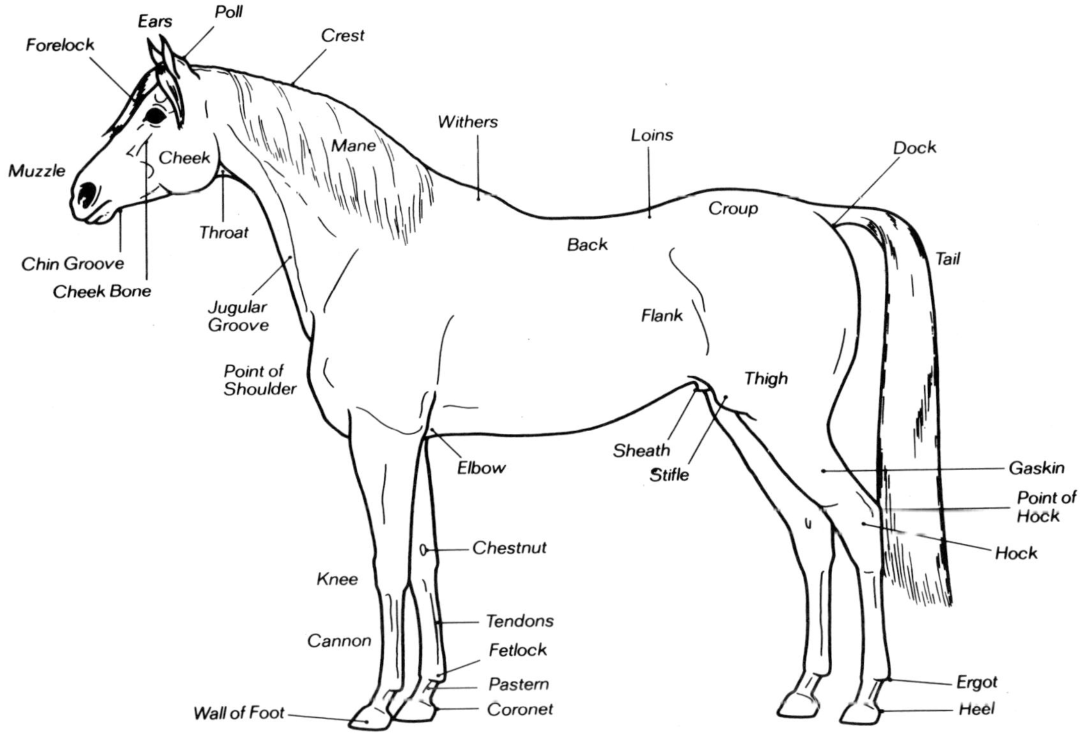
Ears
Poll
Forelock
Crest
Withers
Loins
Dock
Mane
Cheek
Muzzle
Croup
Throat
Back
Tail
Chin Groove
Cheek Bone
Jugular
Groove
Flank
Point of
Shoulder
Thigh
Sheath
Stifle
Elbow
Gaskin
Point of
Hock
Chestnut
Hock
Knee
Tendons
Cannon
Fetlock
Pastern
Ergot
Wall of Foot
Coronet
Heel

Gross Dermatology

Proper evaluation of the skin requires close inspection and careful description of the cutaneous changes. The latter is accomplished mainly through the use of words which have a specific meaning. This chapter was written to present a definition of many such words. In a few instances, the same term is used to describe a microscopic change.

Abscess:
A circumscribed accumulation of pus.

Atrophy:
The skin is thinner than normal often as a result of loss of connective tissue. The surface of the atrophic area may show depressions.

Bulla:
A cavity of appreciable size containing fluid.

Depigmentation:
A lack of melanin resulting in skin of lighter color than normal.

Edema:
Accumulation of fluid in the skin which appears distended.

Erosion:
A superficial loss of skin including a portion of the epidermis in a circumscribed area.

Erythema:
Red color of the skin, usually as a result of inflammation.

Excoriation:
A circumscribed loss of epidermis.

Exfoliation:
Scales are shed in a large area of the skin surface, sometimes the entire skin.

Fistula:
An abnormal passage leading from an abscess or a hollow organ to the surface.

Hyperpigmentation:
Darker color of the skin, usually from an overproduction of melanin.

Hypopigmentation:
Lighter color of the skin, usually from a decrease in melanin synthesis.

Koebner Phenomenon:
The development of lesions in areas that have been irritated by mechanical, physical or chemical agents.

Laceration:
A tear or torn wound.

Lichenification:
Thickening of the skin due to prolonged scratching or rubbing.

Macule:
A circumscribed change in the normal skin color without elevation of the skin.

Nodule:
An elevation of the skin ranging in size between a papule and a tumor.

Papillomatosis:
The development of numerous papillomas.

Papule:
An elevation of the skin of small size.

Plaque:
An elevation of the skin in an area of appreciable shape and distinct size.

Pustule:
An elevation of the skin of small size containing one or several kinds of materials (fluid, leukocytes, microorganisms, keratinized cells, sebum).

Scales:
An accumulation of keratinized cells which are shed at a faster than normal rate.

Sinus:
A fistula or tract leading to a suppurating cavity.

Telangiectasia:
A dilated blood vessel.

Tumor:
An elevation of the skin of large size.

Ulcer:
A loss of skin including a portion of epidermis and dermis in a circumscribed area.

Vesicle:
A small cavity containing fluid.

DEGOS, R.
Dermatologie. Editions Medicales Flammarion. Paris, 1953.
MAZZINI, M.A.
Dermatologia Clinica. Lopez Libreros Editores. Buenos Aires, 1977.
STEDMAN's MEDICAL DICTIONARY
The William and Wilkins Company Baltimore, 1972.

Microscopic Dermatology

In the description of microscopic changes throughout this atlas, it has been necessary to use terms which have definite meaning for those versed in dermatopathology. This chapter is presented in order to define those terms for the readers who are not acquainted with microscopic pathology of the skin and to facilitate an understanding of the histopathological material in the book.

Acantholysis:
The cells in the stratum spinosum become loose from each other due to weakened intercellular attachment, a process which leads to formation of intraepidermal blisters.

Acanthosis:
The stratum corneum increases its thickness.

Alteration cavitaire:
Fluid accumulates within epidermal cells in small amounts.

Bulla:
Fluid and/or inflammatory cells accumulate in one of three locations: under the stratum corneum (subcorneal bulla); in the stratum spinosum (intraepidermal bulla); or underneath the stratum spinosum (subepidermal bulla).

Crust:
Fluid coagulates on the surface of the skin, usually trapping inflammatory cells in the process.

Dyskeratosis:
The keratinocytes undergo an abnormal maturation and appear deformed.

Erosion:
The epidermis is destroyed in a limited area.

Exocytosis:
Inflammatory cells penetrate the epidermis.

Granulation tissue:
Fibroblasts accumulate with production of new collagen and formation of capillaries in healing ulcers and wounds.

Granuloma:
Inflammatory cells accumulate in chronic fashion together with giant cells as a result of invasion of the dermis by different agents (fungi, bacteria, foreign body, metals, dyes).

Hydropic degeneration:
Cells of the basal layer appear vacuolated (this process is also known as liquefaction degeneration).

Hyperkeratosis:
The stratum corneum increases in thickness.

Hypergranulosis:
Keratohyalin increases over the amount normally found in the granular layer.

Hyperplasia:
Cells in a tissue increase in number without tumor formation.

Hypertrophy:
An organ increases in size without tumor formation.

Incontinence of pigment:
Melanocytes lose their melanin which drops into the upper dermis where it may become phagocytized by macrophages.

Metachromasia:
Tissues react to a dye with a different color than the one used.

Microabscess:
Inflammatory cells accumulate and concentrate in one place.

Papillomatosis:
The dermal papillae proliferate towards the surface of the skin.

Parakeratosis:
The stratum corneum increases in thickness and at the same time shows a retention of nuclei.

Pleomorphism:
The nuclei show an abnormal shape.

Pseudoepitheliomatous hyperplasia:
Cells of the stratum spinosum increase in number in a marked degree which resembles carcinoma; growth remains limited and noninvasive, however.

Pustule:
Polymorphonuclear leukocytes, usually neutrophils, concentrate and accumulate in one place.

Reticular degeneration:
Fluid accumulates in large amounts within epidermal cells leading to their rupture and formation of intraepidermal bullae.

Spongiosis:
The intercellular space in the stratum spinosum becomes dilated as a result of accumulation of fluid.

Ulcer:
The epidermis and the dermis are destroyed.

CIVATTE, J.
Histopathologie Cutanee. Editions Medicales Flammarion. Paris, 1967.
LEVER, W. F.
Histopathology of the Skin. J. B. Lippincott Company, Philadelphia, 1975.
PINKUS, H. and MEHREGAN, A.
A Guide to Dermatohistopathology. Appleton Century Crofts. New York, 1981.

Skin Biopsy

Surgical Instruments

Like in small animal dermatology (MULLER and KIRK 1976), the importance of biopsies is continually increasing together with the new knowledge and understanding of microscopic equine dermatology.

The surgical instruments required for a skin biopsy are shown in Plate 3 on the opposite page.

Figure A illustrates our complete biopsy tray including instruments for excisional biopsies and for punch biopsies. The scalpel blades are not included. Our preference is for Bard-Parker blades sizes 15 (smaller biopsies) or 10 (larger biopsies). Disposable sterile scalpels with blades like the one being employed in Plate 4 C are also useful. A bottle for the specimen (upper right) must be large enough to contain at least 15 cm^3 of the fixative, usually formalin for light microscopy or glutaraldehyde for electron microscopy.

Figure B illustrates biopsy punches of 3 different sizes: 4 mm, 6 mm and 8 mm (from left to right). These are examples of the KEYES punch (SUTTON and WAISMAN 1975).

Figures C, D and E show a close-up view of an 8 mm punch. The acute sharpness of the edge is a great advantage to insure a smooth, artifact-free border in the skin specimen. Punches like this one require meticulous cleansing and care to avoid damage of the edge such as the small indentation shown in Fig. E.
Disposable punches already sterile are commercially available. High speed, motor driven, rotatory punches (HURLEY 1977) have been known for many years but are not widely employed.

HURLEY, H. J.
Skin Surgery. p. 235 Charles C. Thomas. Springfield, Illinois, 1977.
MULLER, G. and KIRK, R. W.
Small Animal Dermatology. p. 160 W. B. Saunders Co., Philadelphia, 1976.
SUTTON, Jr. R. L. and WAISMAN, M.
The Practitioners' Dermatology. p. 63. Yorke Medical Books. New York, 1975.

A

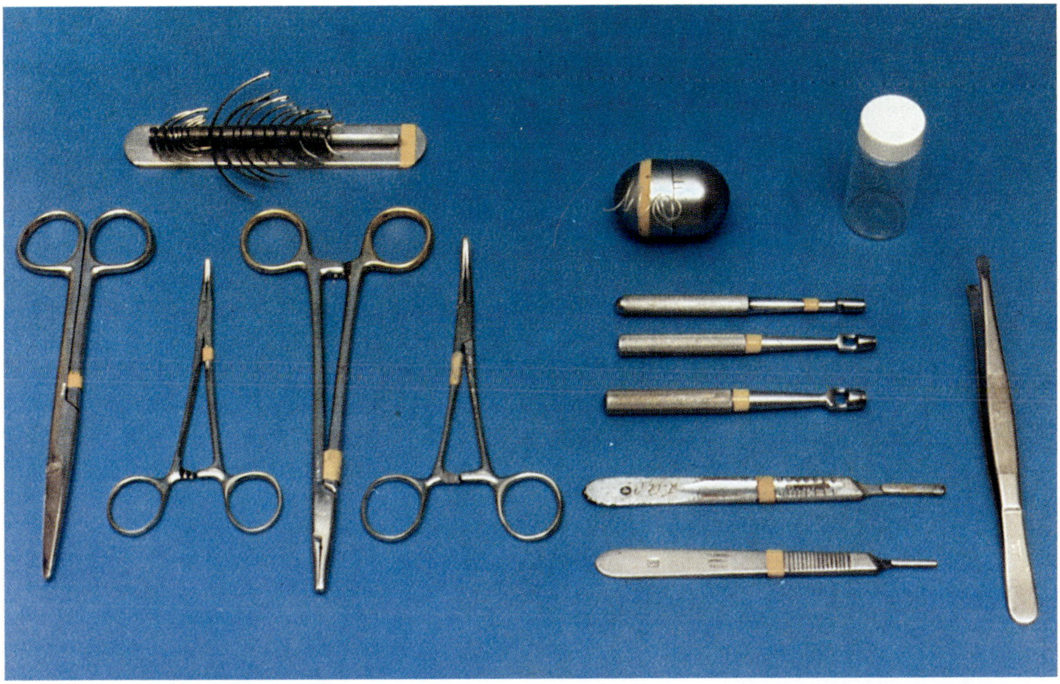

C

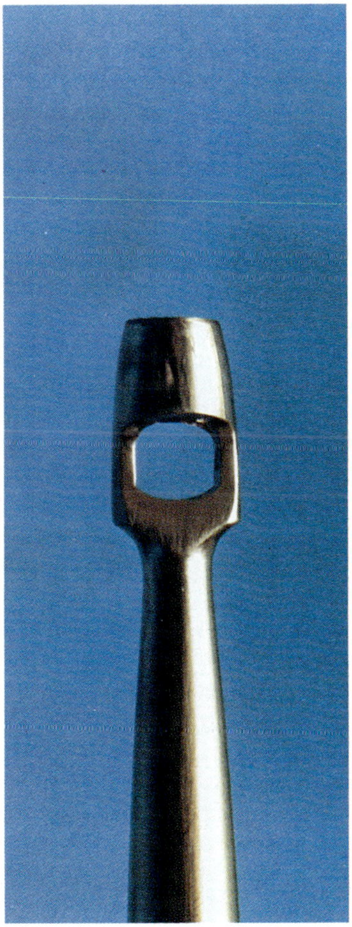

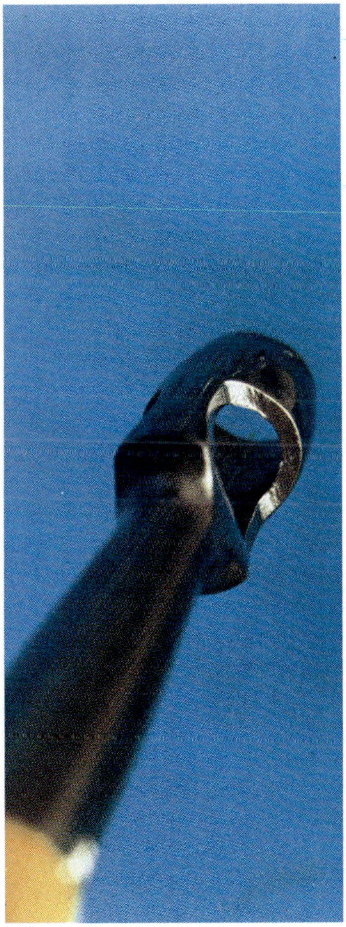

B

D

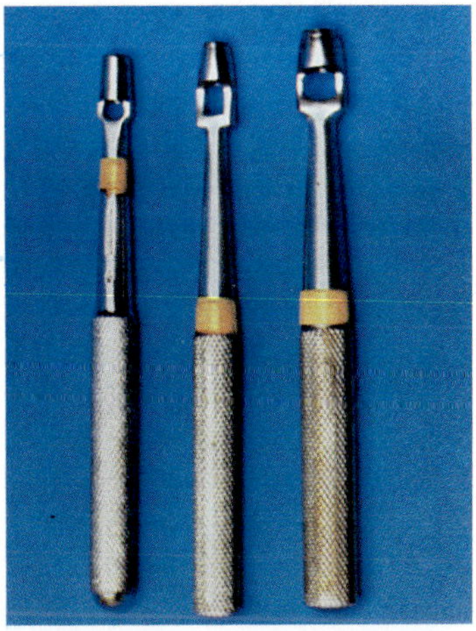

E

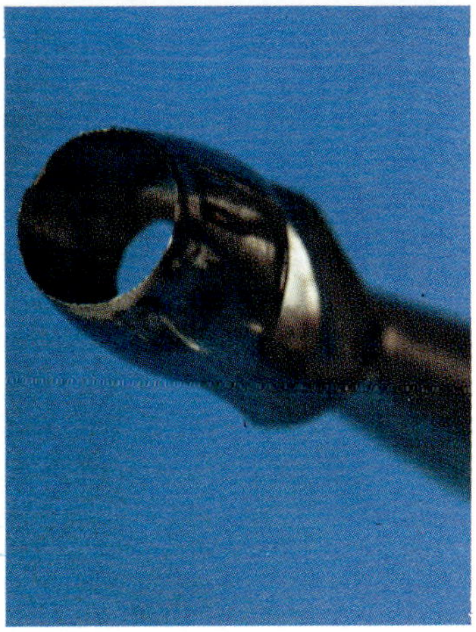

Skin Biopsy

Procedures

1. **Preparation of the Patient**
Biopsy of the skin usually requires only that the patient be held at the halter or cross-tied in stocks (Fig 4A) with at least one attendant at the horse's head to divert its attention from the work in progress and a second attendant to restrain the part (leg, tail, etc.) or assist with equipment.

2. **Anesthesia**
Local infiltration of the biopsy site with 2% lidocaine or mepivacaine HC1 is sufficient for the majority of cases. For the exception, remote perineural injection or peripheral field blocks can be used. Tranquilizers, sedatives, myoneural blocking agents, and general anesthetics are indicated more for restraint than analgesia. For further description, the references by LUMB and JONES (1973) or SOMA (1971) may be used.

3. **Local Care of the Biopsy Site**
Preparation of the site parallels that done for any minor surgical procedure and should make allowance for the desirability of closure under suture with the expectation of primary healing. This necessitates removal of hair, scrubbing with a surgical soap, disinfection with topical antiseptics, and isolation from secondary contamination, as with drapes.

4. **Surgical Technique**
Twenty-five years ago when PILLSBURY, SHELLEY and KLIGMAN (1956) presented a careful description and analysis of the main points to be considered in a skin biopsy procedure, we learned their recommendations which today we still follow. If the lesions are sufficiently small, they should be removed "in toto" thus achieving a therapeutic result and at the same time providing the entire lesion for a complete analysis. According to the characteristics of each patient we perform either a punch biopsy or an excisional biopsy.

a. Punch Biopsy. (Fig. B)
We have been using for many years the method proposed by WHYTE and PERRY (1960). Their main steps are as follows: 1) the lines of maximal tension are determined for the area where the lesion is located; 2) lateral stretch is firmly applied with the fingers away from and on either side of the lesion; 3) this stretch is better performed by an assistant; 4) tension is maintained while the lesion is punched out; 5) when the tension is released the previous circular defect becomes elliptic; 6) hemostasis if needed is carried out; 7) vertical mattress sutures using silk or monofilament synthetic are applied to close the wound. (MONTES and PARKER 1975).

b. Excisional Biopsy. (Fig. C)
The excisional biopsy is performed using a scalpel. It has the advantage over the punch biopsy in that the shape, size and depth of the specimen can be decided according to the individual disease. If the biopsy is deep and bleeding vessels are found, electrocoagulation and/or absorbable buried sutures may be necessary before the final closing sutures are applied.

5. **Postoperative Care**
Immediately after completion of the surgical procedure, the suture line is treated with a small amount of a topical antibiotic. We prefer an ointment base because it lubricates the suture holes thus minimizing suture marks and it protects the wound from external contamination. One of the triple combinations such as neomycin-bacitracin-polymyxin B is usually employed. A nonocclusive, nonadhesive dressing is finally applied and should be changed daily with additional antibiotic ointment until the sutures are removed.

MONTES, L.F. and PARKER, J.M.
Punch Excision Technique for Removing Basal Cell Epithelioma. Geriatrics: 65, 1975.
PILLSBURY, D.M., SHELLEY, W.B. and KLIGMAN, A.M.
Dermatology. p. 265. W.B. SAUNDERS Company, Philadelphia, 1956.
WHYTE, H.J. and PERRY, H.O.
A simple Method to Minimize Scarring Following Large Punch Biopsies. Archives of Dermatology, 81: 520, 1960.
LUMB, W.V. and JONES, E.W.
Veterinary Anesthesia. Lea & Febiger, Philadelphia, 1973.
SOMA, L.R.
Textbook of Veterinary Anesthesia. The Williams & Wilkins Company, Baltimore, 1971.

A

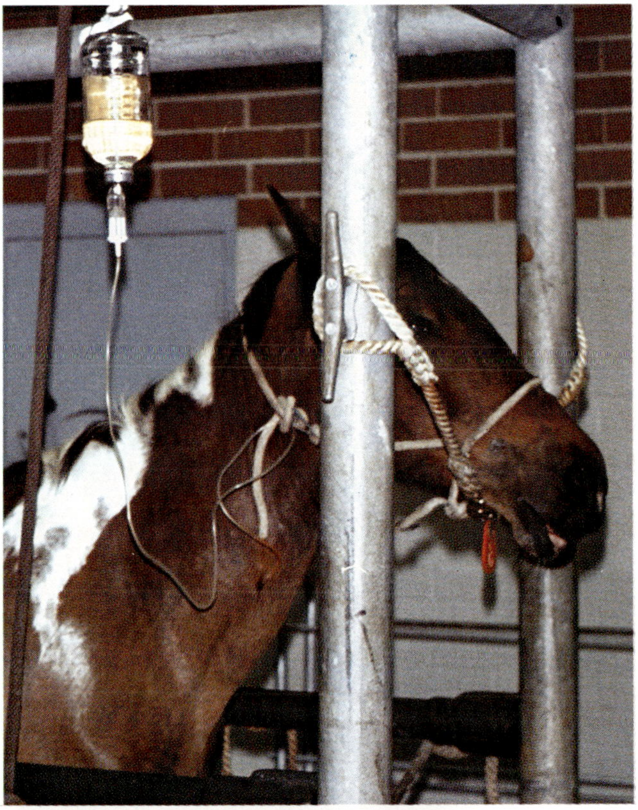

C

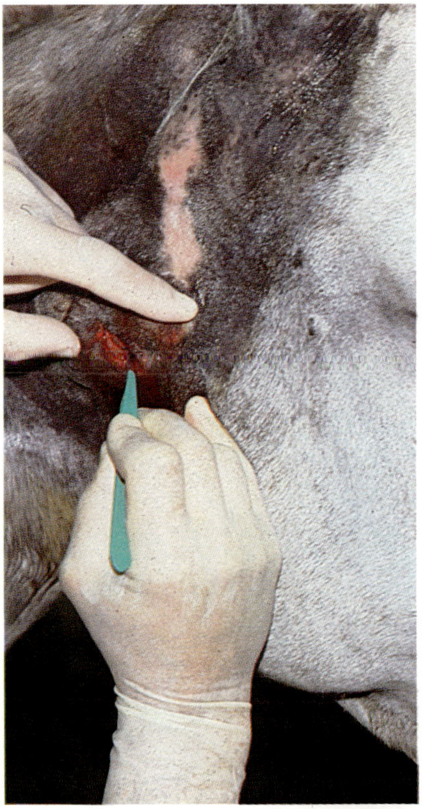

B

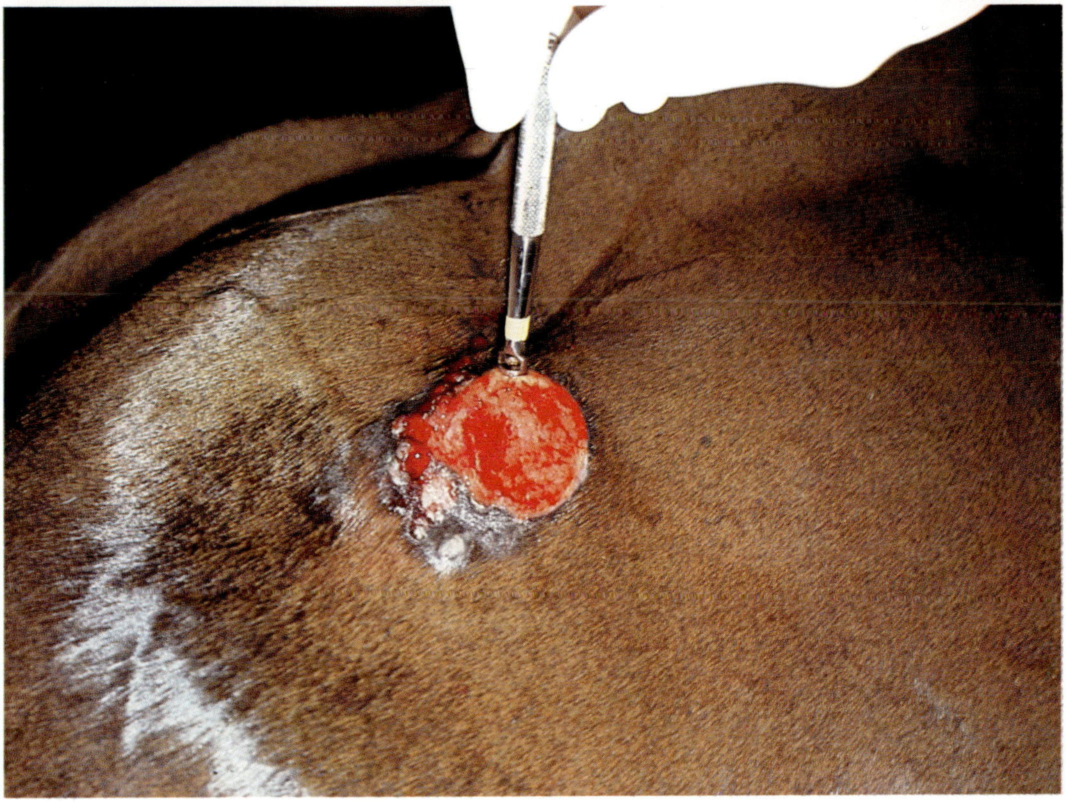

Pododermatoses

The pododerm (greek pous (POD), foot, + derma, skin) is defined as the portion of the skin in *ungulata* that lies beneath thc hoof and secretes the horny structure (STEDMAN's 1972).

This chapter describes nine selected cases of diseases affecting the pododerm. Their causes are varied and often multiple.

The main significance of pododermatoses lies in the variable degree of lameness which may occur in addition to the esthetic problem.

STEDMAN's Medical Dictionary
The Williams and Wilkins Company, Baltimore, 1972.

Eczematoid Dermatitis

(Scratches)

A 6-year-old male Paint Horse was examined because of a bilateral symmetrical rash noticed about two weeks earlier on both hind feet.

Clinically, the posterior surface of both hind pasterns displayed a subacute dermatitis consisting of erythema, fine scales and dried-out vesicles. Yellowish crusts on the deeper fold partially covered by hair, were also prominent (Fig. A).

Histopathologically, two 6 mm punch biopsies were taken. One was from the zone of yellowish crusts (upper part of lesion in Fig. A); the other was from the zone of scaly erythema (lower part of lesion in Fig. A). The microscopic features were different in each one of the specimens. The first specimen showed crusts composed of fibrin, leukocytes, keratinized cells and gram positive bacteria (Brown and Brenn stain). The bacteria were more numerous in the openings of hair follicles. The crusts were overlying a stratum spinosum that was somewhat acanthotic. There was a large accumulation of erythrocytes in the papillary dermis (Fig. B). The second specimen demonstrated parakeratosis, vacuolated cells in the stratum spinosum and a chronic inflammatory infiltrate in the upper dermis (Fig. C).

Treatment consisted of daily cleansing of the lesions with povidone-iodine surgical soap, followed by topical applications twice daily of a 0.025% betamethasone gel. Complete clearing of the rash was achieved after two weeks on this program. One gram of this gel (Physicians Desk Reference 1979) contains 0.25 mg of betamethasone benzoate in a base consisting of 13.8% (w/w) alcohol, carboxy vinyl polymer, propylene glycol, disodium edetate, diisopropanolamine and purified water. This preparation is self-liquefying, clear, greaseless and nonstaining. The active steroid is completely solubilized and the gel rapidly disappears into the skin after gentle rubbing.

It seems unlikely that, although they were present on the surface, bacteria could have played a primary role in this condition. Nevertheless the fact that the local preparation contained alcohol must have acted as an antiseptic. McBride et al (1968) established that antibacterial activity of antiseptics can be demonstrated in the deeper layers of the stratum corneum and that it persists for many hours. The finding of a larger number of bacteria in the follicular openings cannot be interpreted as pathologic because of their natural predilection for that anatomical site (WILBORN and MONTES, 1970).

Understandably, punch biopsies need not be routinely used in locations such as this one; however it was justified here for purposes of characterization of the histopathology in this common malady.

McBRIDE, M.E., MONTES, L.F. and KNOX, J.M.
The Persistence and Penetration of Antiseptic Activity. Surgery, Gynecology and Obstetrics 127:270, 1968.
MONTES, L.F. and WILBORN, W.H.
Anatomical Location of Normal Skin Flora. Archives of Dermatology 101:145, 1970.
PHYSICIANS' DESK REFERENCE
Page 1811. Medical Economics Company, Oradell, New Jersey, 1979.

A

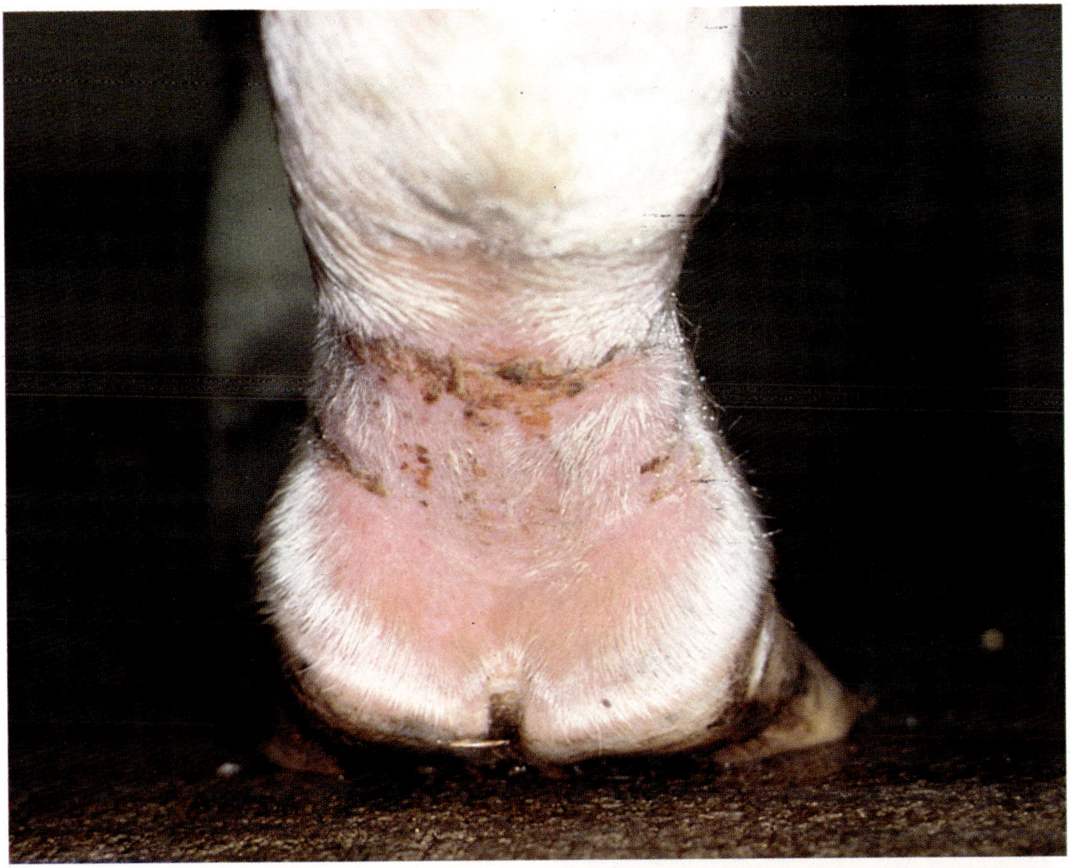

B

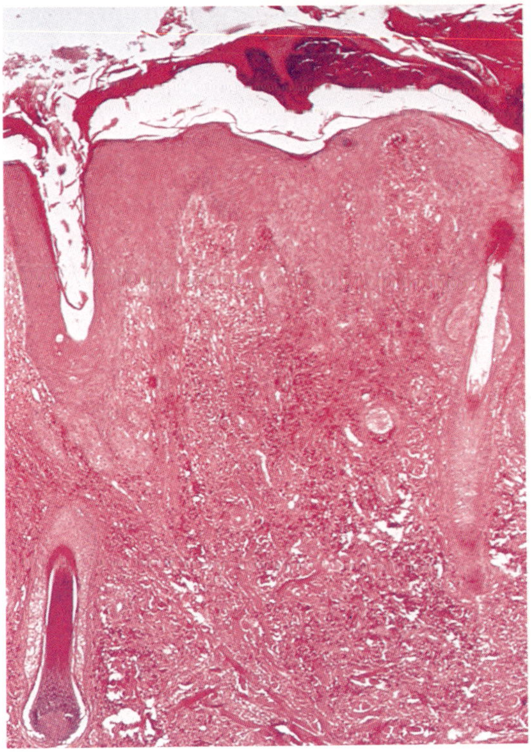

C

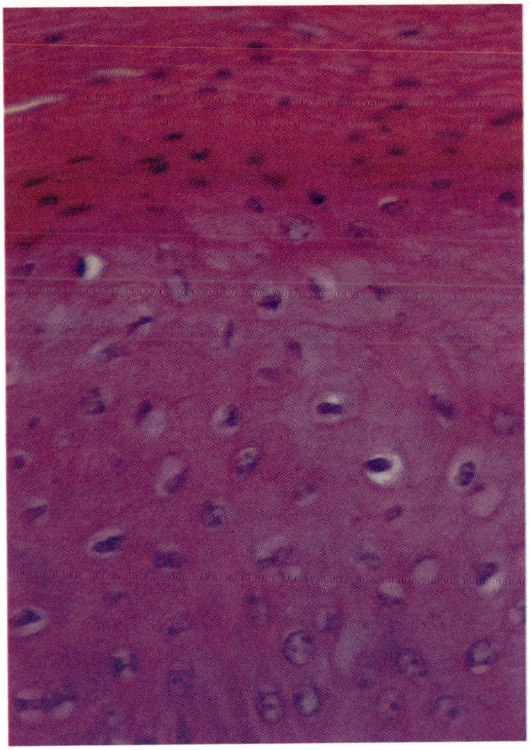

Eczematoid Dermatitis

(Scratches)

A 7-year-old male Tennessee Walking Horse required dermatological care because of a bilateral condition of three weeks duration on both hind feet. The problem had been treated locally with a variety of home medications, among them copper sulfate solution.

Clinically, the heels of both hind feet were involved by an acute moist dermatitis manifested by very intense erythema, clear to whitish exudate and mild edema. The affected area was surrounded by a wide border of green stained skin where hairs had partially fallen out. (Fig. A).

Histopathologically, the condition showed parakeratosis, numerous polymorphonuclear leukocytes in the stratum corneum and migrating acanthosis, spongiosis, focal disorganization of the epidermodermal junction and a subacute inflammatory infiltrate in the upper dermis. (Figs. B and C).

Treatment was carried out first by cleansing of the affected areas as described in the previous case. Afterwards, the patient was placed on local fluocinonide 0.05% in a gel base consisting of propylene glycol, propyl gallate, disodium edetate and carboxypolymethylene with NaOH or HC1 added to adjust the pH. This clear and greaseless formulation (Physicians' Desk Reference 1979), with the steroid in complete solution, is especially suitable and very well tolerated in acute dermatitis where we prefer to avoid greasy vehicles. This preparation was applied twice daily for four weeks. At this point the condition had experienced about 90% clearing. The owner of the horse was instructed to continue treatment for another two weeks but reducing the frequency of the applications to once/daily. Complete clearing was obtained.

In human dermatology (DOMONKOS 1971) the term infectious eczematoid dermatitis is used to describe a condition where large weeping patches with a combination of moist and crusted lesions are outstanding features. Histopathological changes (ORMSBY and MONTGOMERY 1954) resemble those found in this patient and demonstrate that the pathological process is rather superficial in location. The intense redness of the involved area is highly suggestive of superimposed irritation due to excessive treatment (perhaps from copper sulfate in this patient). It is easy for anyone under the anxiety to obtain rapid cure of such an annoying problem to produce what is known as overtreatment leading often to autosensitization.

DOMONKOS, A.N.
Infectious Eczematoid Dermatitis. Andrew's Diseases of the Skin, p. 132. W.B. Saunders Co., Philadelphia, 1971.
ORMSBY, O. and MONTGOMERY, H.
Diseases of the Skin. p. 302. Lea and Febiger, 1954.
PHYSICIANS' DESK REFERENCE.
Page 1715. Medical Economics Company. Oradell, New Jersey, 1979.

A

C

B

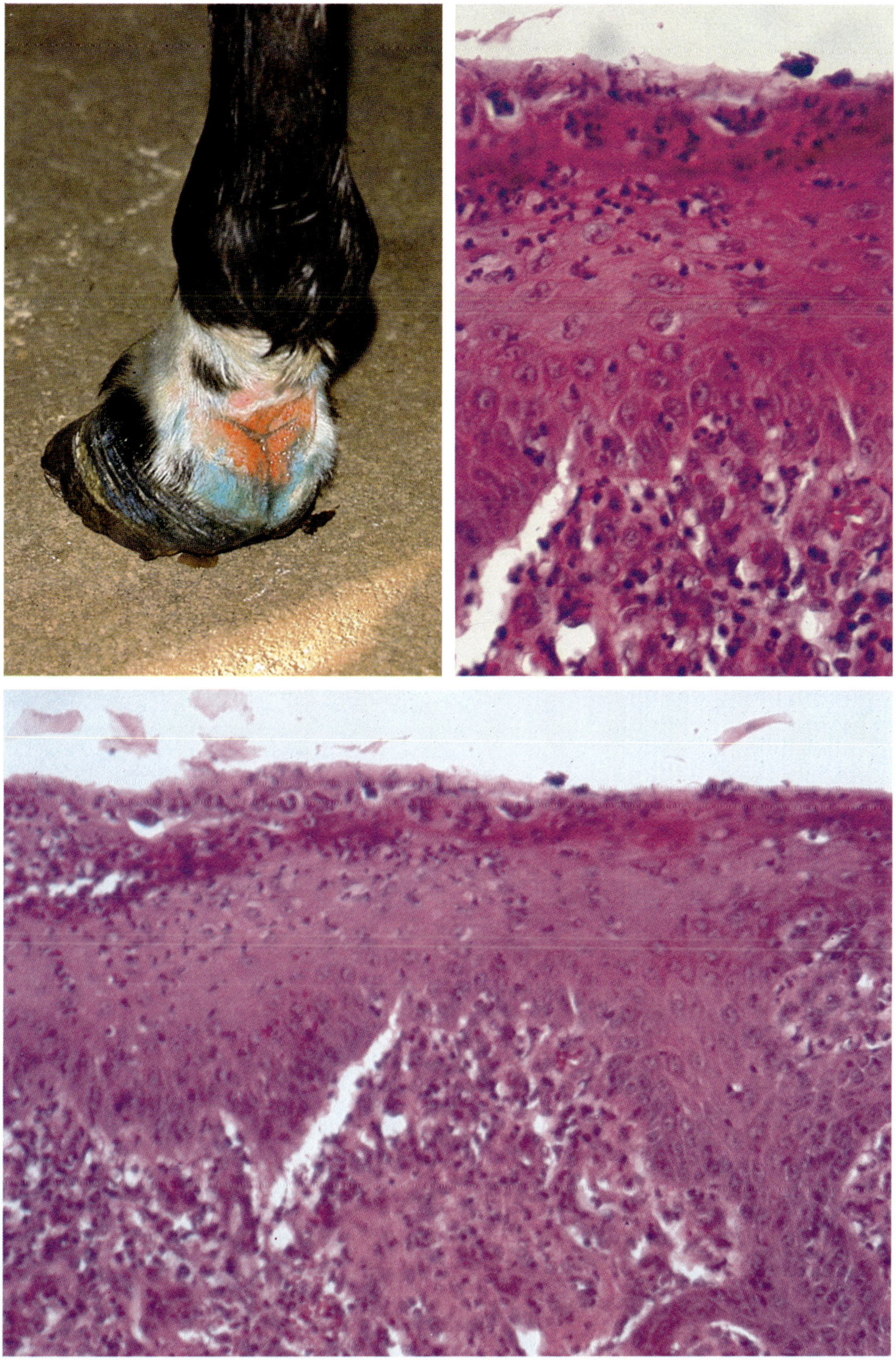

Verrucous Pododermatitis

(Grease Heel)

A 7-year-old Chesnut Tennessee Walking Horse gelding was admitted for evaluation and management of a chronic, refractory sore on the pastern of the right hind leg.

Clinically, the lower part of the affected region showed a verrucous greyish skin while the upper part was erythematous, partially denuded, exudative in some places and crusty in other places (Fig. A).

Histopathologically, two punch biopsies were obtained. One, from the lower part, displayed hyperkeratosis alternating with parakeratosis. The keratinized cells were loose in some areas and compact in other areas, the deeper levels of the stratum corneum interdigitating with the underlying stratum spinosum (Fig. B). The latter was acanthotic including some pseudoepitheliomatous hyperplasia. The dermis contained a chronic inflammatory infiltrate. The second specimen was from the upper part and included features of a more acute dermatitis. The stratum corneum was invaded by leukocytes and Gram positive bacteria. The stratum spinosum showed spongiosis and displayed exocytosis, The upper dermis demonstrated dilated capillaries and a subacute inflammatory infiltrate.

Treatment involved a combination of surgery and medicine. Following thorough cleansing and preparation for surgery under local anesthesia the verrucous folds of granulomatous and hyperkeratotic tissue were carefully excised in successive planes down to the normal contours of the pastern, but not beyond grossly visible islands of epidermis. In order to make this distinction, it is essential that dissection be done in a bloodless field as provided by an Esmarch tourniquet. Otherwise, the epidermal boundaries may be removed inadvertently by overzealous and undiscriminating dissection, sacrificing the very important advantage of having multifocal sites of resident skin remaining to provide for early epithelialization of the defect. The temperament of the patient may necessitate restraint in lateral recumbency under general anesthesia, which is completely justified by the need for careful dissection.

Another consideration is the proximity of the digital tendon sheath and neurovascular bundles (medial and lateral) to the skin surface. When normal architecture is obscured by pathologic changes and tissue planes are almost impossible to recognize, the need is even greater for dissection under hemostasis.

The pastern was placed under sterile dressings and a snug, absorbent bandage prior to release of the tourniquet. Expected hemorrhage into the bandage necessitated its change in 24 hours, after which redressings were determined by need to control superficial skin infection (present at the time of surgery) and to maintain a fresh dressing. Medication consisted of parenteral penicillin and streptomycin I.M., B.I.D. for 5 days and topical neomycin-hydrocortisone cream under a nonadhering gauze strip. Continuation of treatment under bandage is required to expedite healing and to control exuberant granulation.

A

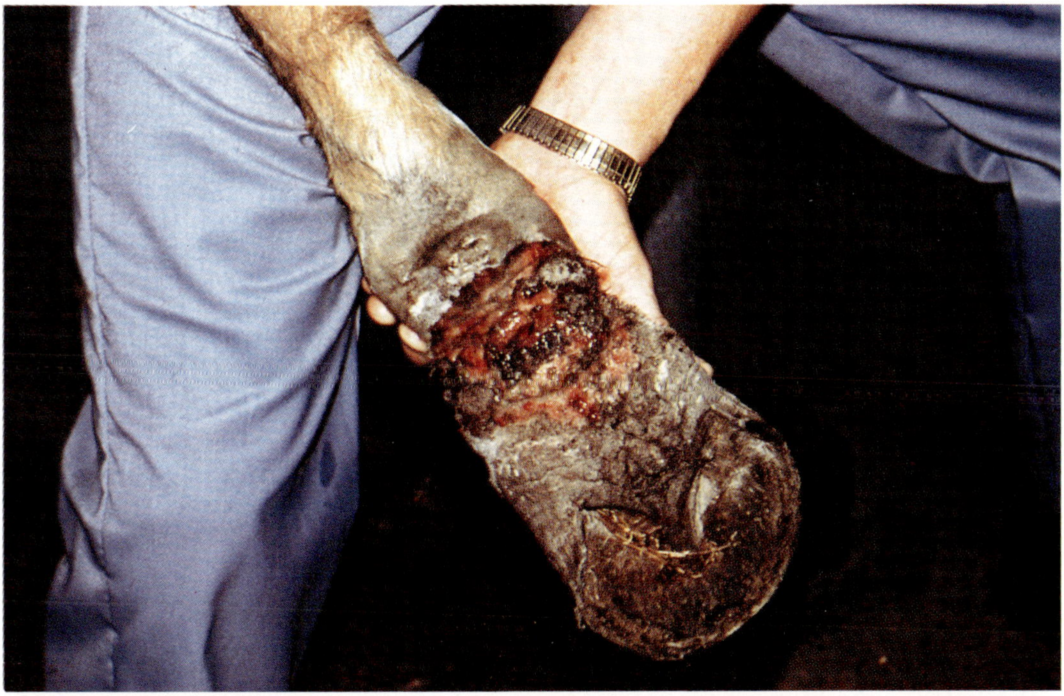

B

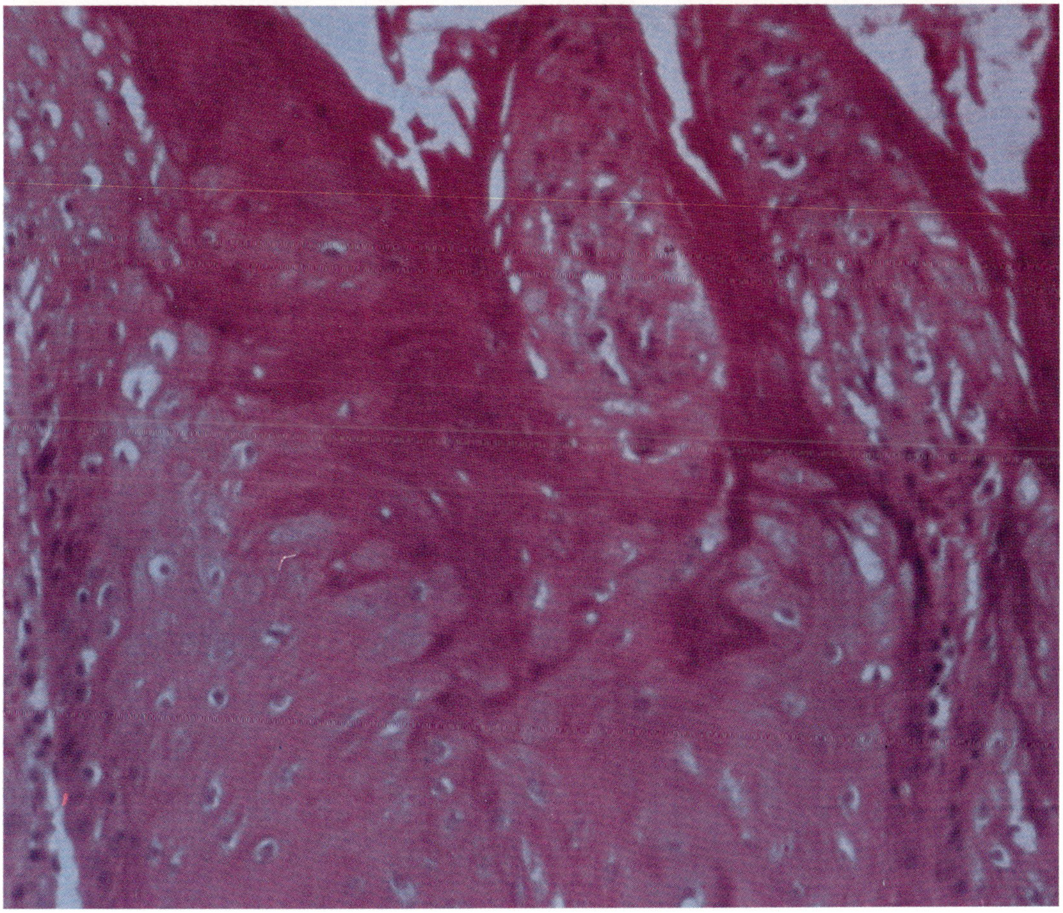

Verrucous Pododermatitis

(Grease Heel)

A 5-year-old bay Tennessee Walking Horse gelding was admitted with the complaint of a productive sore on the pastern of the right foreleg.

Clinically, the entire posterior surface of the pastern was involved by a process characterized by pronounced thickening of the skin with formation of numerous verrucous papules and nodules, many of them confluent to form plaques. The surface of the individual lesions was fairly glossy and pink to yellow-brown in color (Fig. A). A greasy, malodorous exudate covered the lesion initially, but was removed by cleansing in preparation for surgery. The patient was quite tender to manual inspection of the leg.

The term dermatitis verrucosa has been generally used to define this condition (FRANK 1964). We have slightly modified this designation because dermatitis verrucosa is also a synonym for chromoblastomycosis, one of the deep mycoses (CONANT et al 1971). When verrucous pododermatitis becomes fully developed, clusters of nodular growths as shown in Fig. A are formed on the involved area, which is often referred to as "grapes."

Histopathologically, the stratum corneum displayed tremendous thickness (Fig. B), showing both hyperkeratosis and parakeratosis. There were white cells and red cells between the keratinized cells. Brown and Brenn stained sections demonstrated Gram positive bacteria. PAS stained sections did not reveal fungi. There was marked acanthosis and intact epidermodermal junction and a chronic upper dermal inflammatory infiltrate.

Treatment consisted of surgical removal of the warty outgrowths, under general anesthesia according to the technique described in the preceding case 7. Initial postoperative medication was iodoform and bismuth formic iodide applied as a topical powder under bandage for antiseptic and astringent effects and phenylbutazone 2 gm q.d. per os to reduce local inflammation. During the 30-day course of treatment, nitrofurantoin and prednisolone in a creme base were used the last 2 weeks. Podophyllin in benzoin was used briefly to control exuberant granulation tissue. The patient was greatly improved upon discharge, but still required a bandage.

Etiology is varied and has been associated with damp, filthy stables, as well as use of irritants (e.g., oil of mustard) and chain devices to exaggerate the gait. It has also been attributed to neglected or mismanaged cases of scratches (FRANK 1964), as described in case 5.

FN Grateful acknowledgement to Dr. J. M. Humburg, School of Veterinary Medicine, Auburn University, AL 36849.

CONANT, N.F., SMITH, D.T., BAKER, R.D. and CALLAWAY, J.L.
Manual of Clinical Mycology, p. 417. W. B. Saunders Co., Philadelphia, Pennsylvania 1971.
FRANK E.R.
Veterinary Surgery, P. 209. Burgess Publishing Company, Minneapolis, Minnesota 1964.

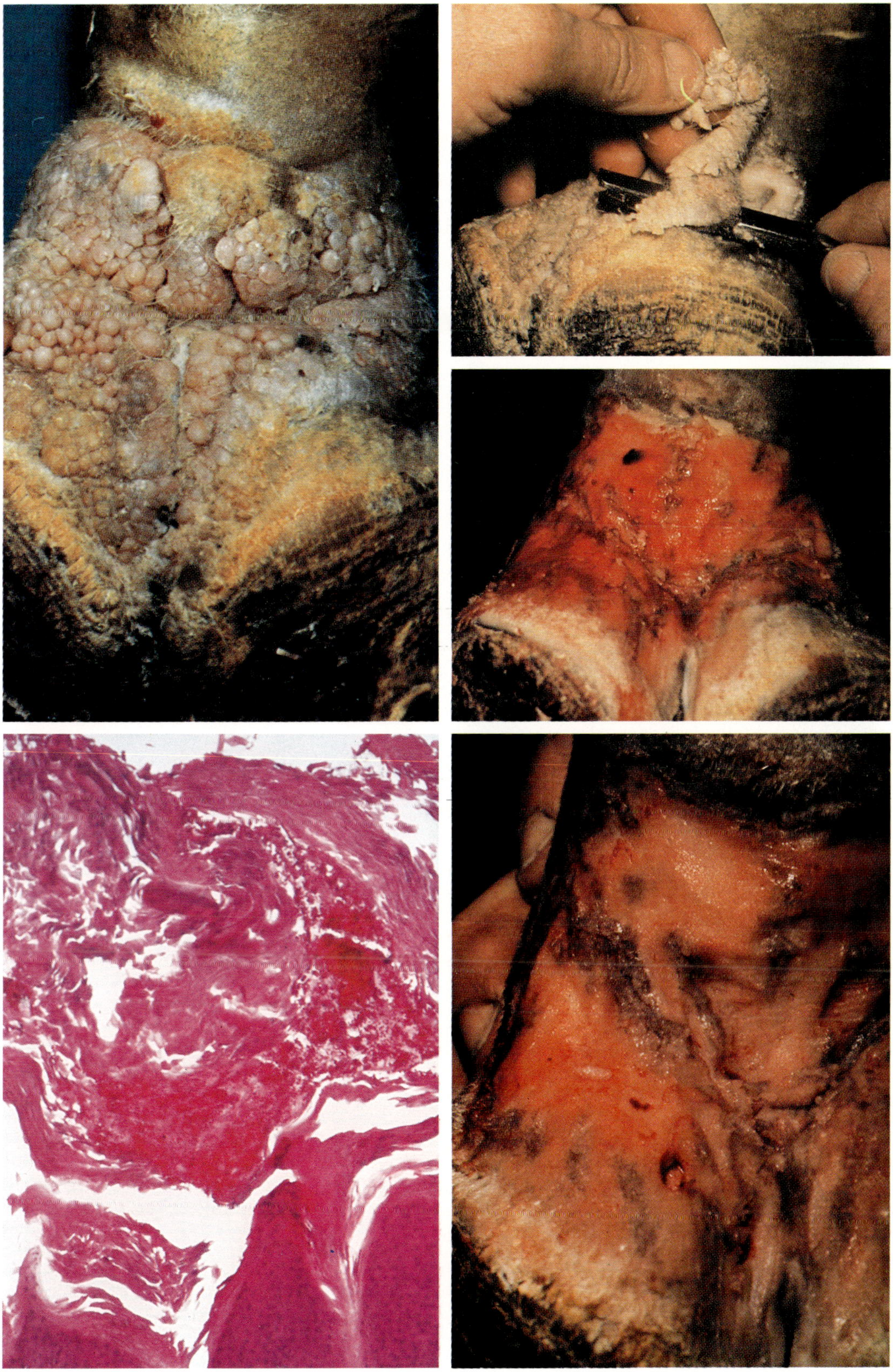
A
B
C
D
E

Coronitis

A 5-year old Chestnut Quarterhorse mare was affected by a dermatosis of the left hind foot of several weeks duration. Gentian violet had been applied locally without much effect prior to the dermatologic consultation.

Clinically, the skin above the coronary band was thickened, scaly and swollen. The periople was separated from the perioplic corium around the circumference of the coronary band.

Histopathologically, a 4 mm punch biopsy – reaching the deeper levels of the epidermis and only a very minimal amount of the dermis, namely the papillary tips between the rete pegs – was obtained. There was parakeratosis and marked acanthosis. Serial sections stained with PAS in an attempt to detect fungi failed to show fungal cells but, interestingly, provided the view of an increased accumulation of glycogen in the stratum spinosum. The epidermodermal junction was intact. The capillaries in the dermal papillae were dilated (Figs. B and C). The coronary band is formed by the perioplic corium, the coronary corium and the coronary cushion. As emphasized by ADAMS (1974) it is the primary growth and nutritional source for the hoof wall. Injuries to the coronary band may leave a permanent defect on the hoof wall. Because of this, a large and deep biopsy in this patient was avoided; thus the entire histopathological process could not be observed.

Treatment consisted of removal of hair, crusts, and debris overlying the coronary band to provide exposure to air and to allow direct contact with a topical medication combining nystatin, neomycin sulfate, gramicidin and triamcinolone acetonide in an aqueous cream base (PHYSICIANS' DESK REFERENCE, 1980). The stall was kept clean and dry, and the foot was treated daily. Inasmuch as the condition was in an early stage of convalescence at the time of admittance, progress was rapid, and local treatment could be discontinued after 10 days. However, stable hygiene and good management practices were prescribed indefinitely.

In old descriptions, "specific coronitis" (REEKS, 1906) is ascribed a common etiology with canker (unguilysis) and alternative treatment methods may include some of those recommended for canker (see Case 21).

ADAMS, O.R.
Lameness in the Horse. Lea and Febiger, Philadelphia 1974

PHYSICIANS' DESK REFERENCE, p. 1661, 1980
Medical economics Co., Litton Industries, Inc. Oradell, N.J. 07649

REEKS, H.C.
Diseases of the Horse's Foot, p. 324-7. Alex. Eger, Chicago, 1906.

A B

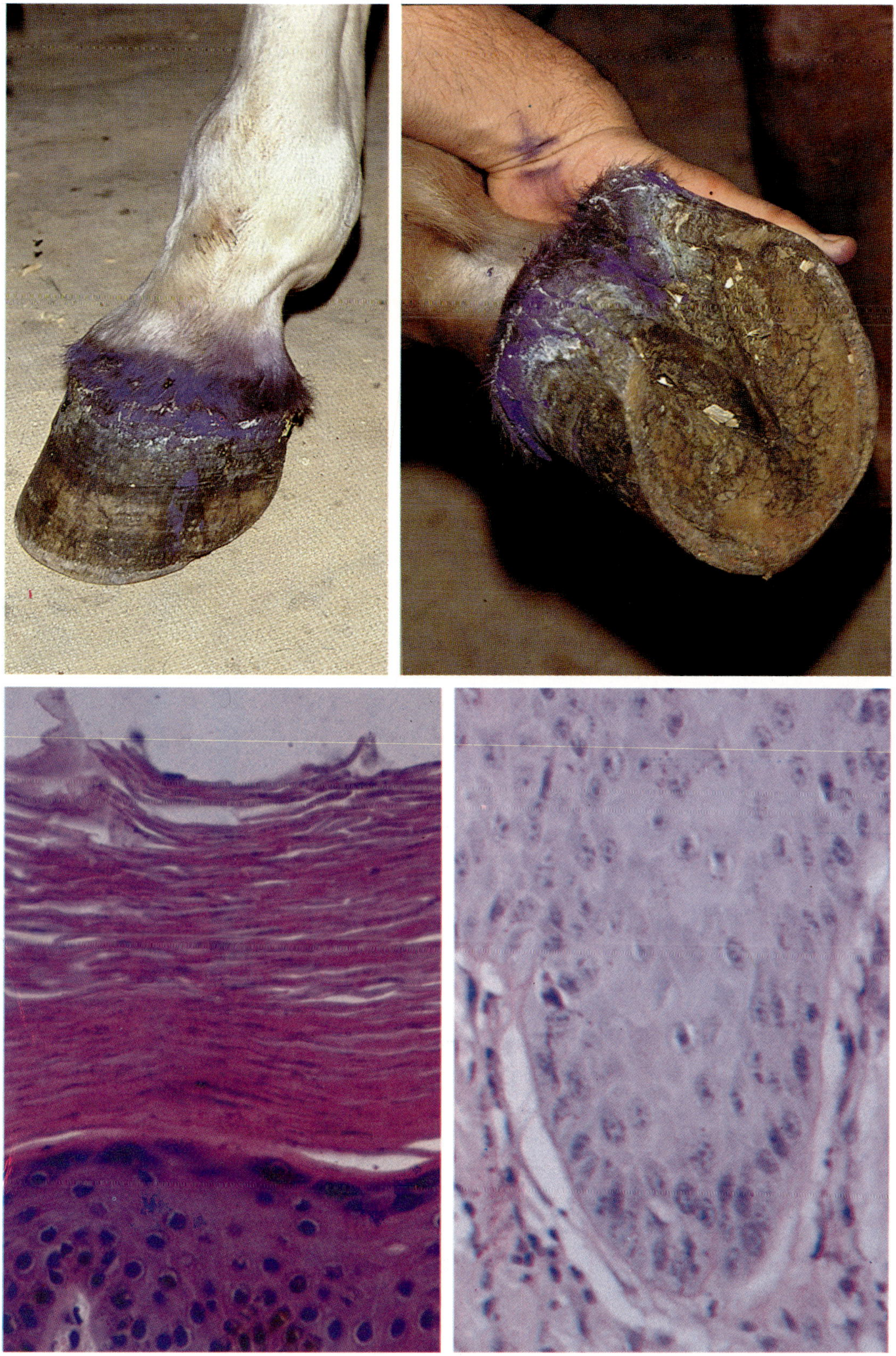

C D

Prurigo Nodularis

(Chain Calluses)

A 13-year-old gelding Tennessee Walking Horse was admitted to the hospital because of a bilateral, symmetrical dermatosis which had developed about 6 months earlier during a period of active training before the show season.

Clinically, there were several hard, well demarcated hyperkeratotic excrescences ranging in size from nodules to tumors. Some of the lesions were confluent. There was no visible hair growing in the affected sites. These were the same areas where the horse had been subjected to daily periods of chain friction and irritation sometimes employed in training Tennessee Walking Horses.

Histopathologically, the stratum corneum was tremendously increased in thickness but quite compact and with focal parakeratosis. There was also follicular plugging in most of the hair follicles throughout the sections. The stratum spinosum showed marked acanthosis in some places and pseudoepitheliomatous hyperplasia in other places. The epidermodermal junction was intact. The papillary capillaries were dilated and contained large numbers of red blood cells. There was a chronic inflammatory infiltrate in the dermis, more prominent around nerves and blood vessels which were generally dilated. Foreign body giant cells were found in the deeper part of the papillary dermis surrounding an eosinophilic amorphous material (Figs. C and D).

Treatment consisted of excision of progressive serial sections of the calluses down to the level of normal adjacent skin, after the technique described in Case 7. Neomycin-hydrocortisone cream under sterile, absorbent bandage was used to control superficial infection and exuberant granulation. Healing of tissue beds under such mature and organized fibrous tissue as exists in chain calluses is slow and imperfect. The objective is to reduce the scarring and return the horse to work rather than to achieve a completely cosmetic result. Long periods of treatment under bandage should be expected and secondary surgical excision is not unusual.

The clinical and histopathological features of this patient were very similar to prurigo nodularis, a dermatosis in humans resulting also from frequent rubbing of the skin. A less severe cutaneous reaction to the same stimulus of milder degree is called lichen simplex chronicus (SHAFFER and BEERMAN 1951) or localized neurodermatitis. The clinicopathological correlation of these lesions indicates that that there was no damage of the epidermodermal junction and therefore this patient could have healed in the earlier stages of disease by strict avoidance of intentional irritation and vigorous topical treatment using steroids under occlusion.

Because this regime could not be instituted it was advisable to proceed with cutaneous surgery. Other practical ways to achieve removal of the hypertrophic epidermis is the use of wire brush surgery or dermoabrasion (BURKS, 1956) or cryosurgery (ZACARIAN 1969).

BURKS, J.W. Jr.
Wire Brush Surgery. Charles C. Thomas, Springfield, Illinois, 1956

SHAFFER, B. and BEERMAN, H.
Lichen Simplex Chronicus and Its Variants. Archives of Dermatology 64:340, 1951.

ZACARIAN, S.A.
Cryosurgery of Skin Cancer and Cryogenic Techniques in Dermatology. Charles C. Thomas, Springfield, Illinois, 1969.

A

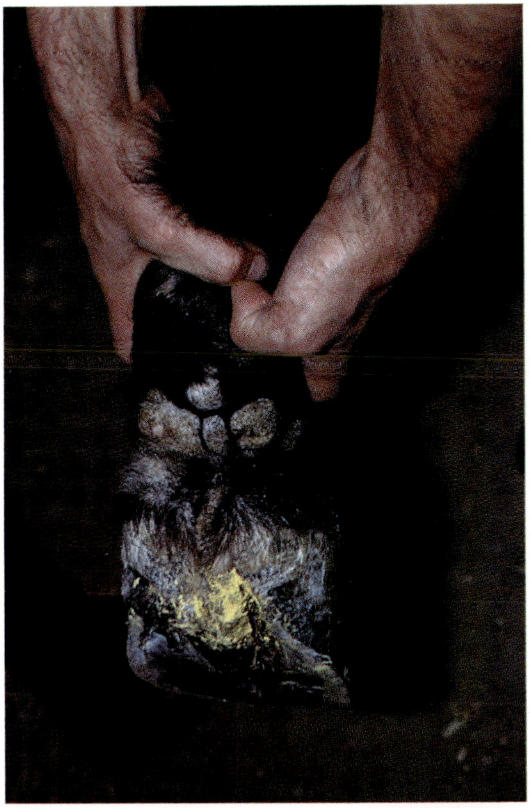

B

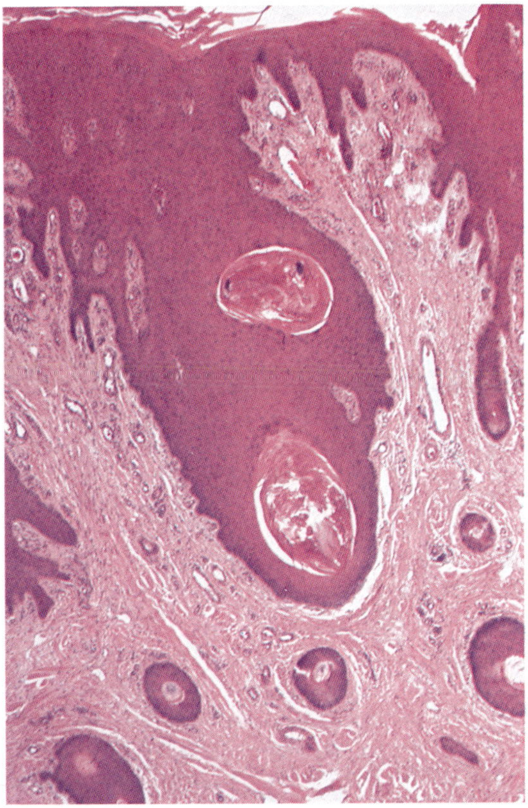

C

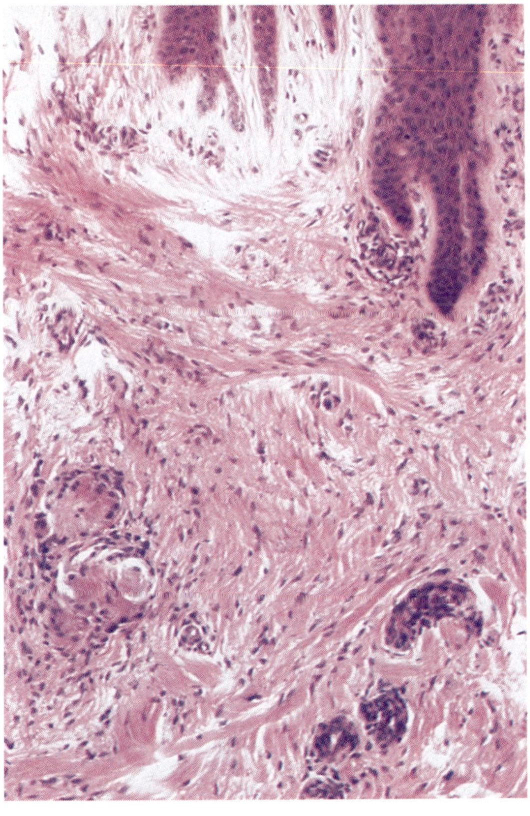

D

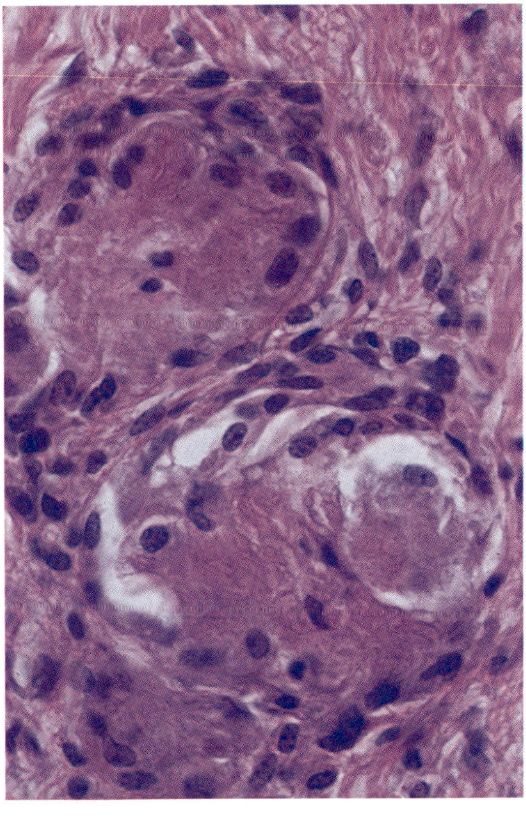

Prurigo Nodularis

(Chain Calluses)

A 9-year-old Tennessee Walking Horse presented a bilateral symmetrical dermatosis involving the anterior aspect of both feet. The condition had developed after 1 year of intensive training.

Clinically, the patient had large hyperkeratotic plaques of markedly thickened skin. The plaques were made up of individual nodules that had undergone coalescence.

The surface showed some smooth areas, alternating with lichenified places, excoriations, crusts and some small violaceous nodules (Fig. A). There was general lack of hair over the affected skin.

Histopathologically, the main features were very pronounced hyperkeratosis with focal parakeratosis and irregular marked acanthosis with sites of pseudoepitheliomatous hyperplasia. The epidermodermal junction was intact. The papillary dermis and the mid-dermis showed dilated capillaries and a chronic inflammatory infiltrate (Figs. B and C).

Treatment was confined to surgically planing the most exaggerated areas of hyperkeratosis to reduce the dimensions of the scarring and subsequent treatment under bandage with a combination antibiotic-hydrocortisone cream under a nonadhering gauze dressing. Skin grafting of such areas has been attempted with largely disappointing results, attributed to the lack of receptivity of the dense, scar tissue bed, the relatively inelastic tissue planes and adjacent skin areas, and the difficulty in immobilization of the part during the critical early stages after grafting. Pinch grafts have been employed with uneven results and the cosmetic effect leaves something to be desired.

As an alternative to surgery or after healing following surgery, the use of one of the stronger topical fluorinated steroids such as 0.1% halcinonide cream under polyethylene film occlusion can be suggested. If used for a rather prolonged period of time – 12 to 18 months – partial or even complete involution may be achieved. After washing with an antiseptic soap the steroid must be rubbed on the surface of the lesion until it disappears into the skin. Then a small amount should be left on the surface and the lesion must be covered with polyethylene film the edges of which should be secured with adhesive nonirritant plastic tape. The area is finally covered with a bandage which should be left on for 12 hours each day. Many years ago (BAKER and WHITAKER 1948) (BAKER and MONTES 1961) it became apparent that prolonged local application of natural adrenal corticosteroids results in thinning of epidermis and compaction of collagenous bundles. This action is much stronger for the newer synthetic steroids. In prurigo nodularis of human skin (which interestingly develops also on the anterior lower legs as a result of frequent rubbing) ultrastructural study demonstrated changes in the cutaneous nerves (DOYLE et al 1979).

BAKER, B. L. and WHITAKER, W. L.
Growth Inhibition in the Skin Following Direct Application of Adrenal Cortical Preparations. Anatomical Record 102:333, 1948.
BAKER, B. L. and MONTES, L. F.
Histochemical Changes in the Skin Following Local Application of Cortisol of Prednisolone. Anatomical Record 139:133, 1961.
DOYLE, J. A.
Prurigo Nodularis: A Reappraisal of the Clinical and Histologic Features Journal of Cutaneous Pathology 6:392, 1979.

A

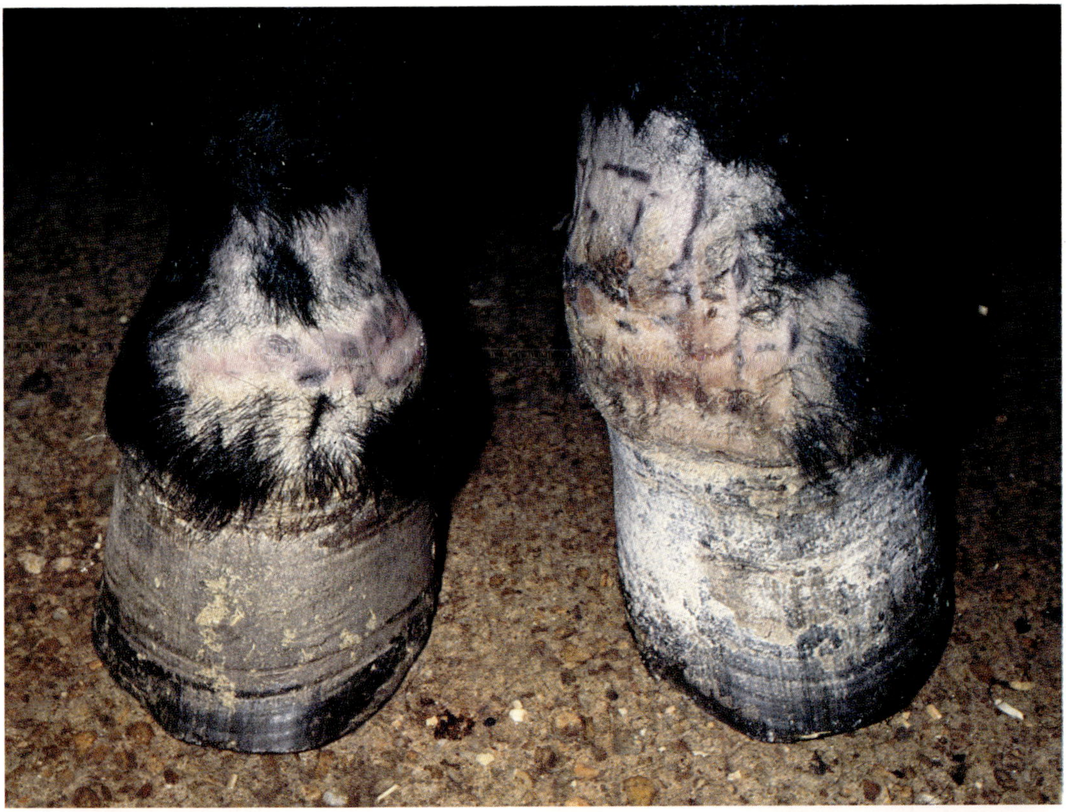

B

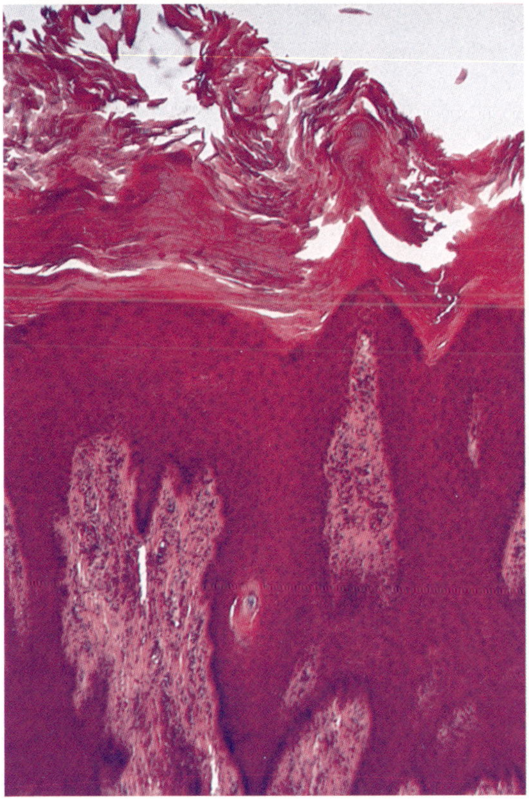

C

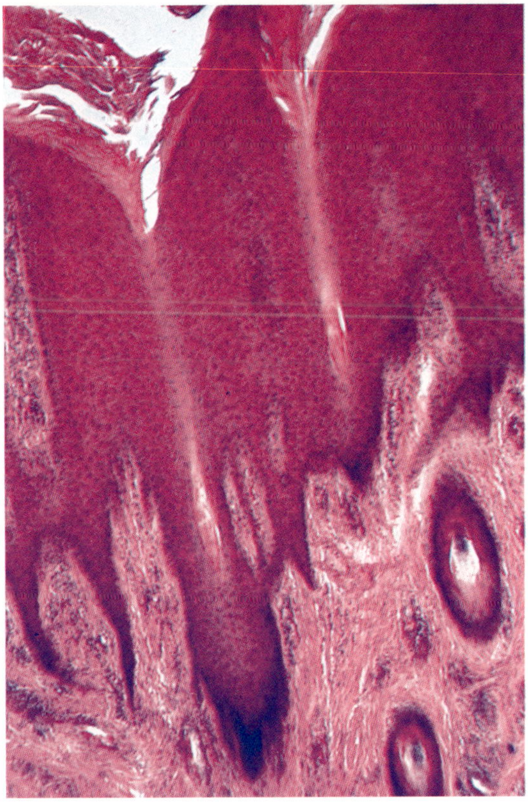

Chemical Burn

A 5-year-old bay Thoroughbred gelding was admitted for treatment of severe chemical burns of the fetlocks of the front legs that had resulted from the overzealous use of topical counterirritant medication.

Clinically, the affected skin consisted of an area with sharply demarcated and partially circinate borders covering the posterior surface of the fetlock joint (Fig. A). The upper part of the process had a bleeding surface with a few islands of granulating tissue. The lower part was mostly displaying granulating tissue in various stages of maturation as shown in a close-up view in Fig. B.

Radiologically, the metacarpophalangeal joints displayed thickening of the joint capsule and osteophyte formation around the joint margins. No reduction of joint space or clear evidence of osteochondrosis was apparent; however, flexion of the joint and range of motion were inhibited by loss of elasticity of the soft tissues as well as by pain from the burned areas.

Treatment consisted of superficial debridement of loosened sloughs and wound toilet, followed by continuous medication under nonadhering, sterile dressing strips (e.g., petrolatum gauze or Telfa pads) under absorbent cotton and gauze bandages until healing by epithelialization was complete (Fig. C). If neglected, wound fatigue further delays healing with even greater scarring the result. The choice of medications for such use is determined by the objectives of treatment: 1) Control of surface infection, 2) enzymatic debridement of necrotic tissue, 3) suppression of inflammation, and 4) control of exuberant granulation without inhibition of healing by epithelialization from the wound margins and from any surviving islands of epidermis within the wound. The use of strong antiseptics and astringents accomplishes some of these objectives, but tends to retard regrowth of epithelium. A tough, dry scab on the open wound may be practical in some cases, but can also contribute to wound fatigue. Therefore, when justified by economics and other local circumstances, the treatment of such wounds is best managed under bandage. One example of a reliable medication is a broad spectrum antibiotic in combination with a fungicide and a corticosteroid (Physicians' Desk Reference, 1980, 1661). Another combines extract of papaya (papain) with Balsam Peru. An important function the bandage serves is to prevent self-mutilation. If the patient persists in removing the bandage, the use of a neck cradle, cross-tie or bibbed halter can be tried. Most simply, the bandage can be painted with a saturated solution of picric acid to discourage removal.

The owner should be cautioned against further use of strong liniments and blisterings that contain concentrated iodine, phenol, salts of heavy metals (Hg, Pb, etc.), certain volatile oils, croton oil, cantharides, and other agents that may be corrosive when in direct contact with the skin, especially when reapplied at daily intervals or when applied under occlusion.

A

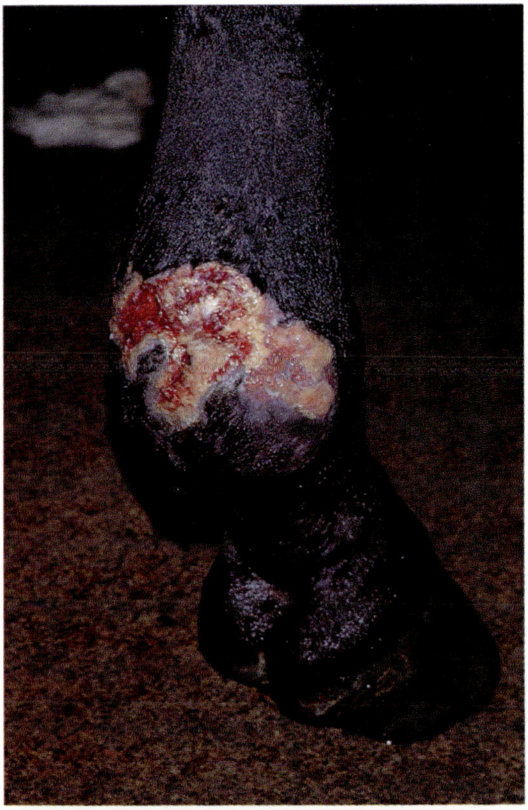

C

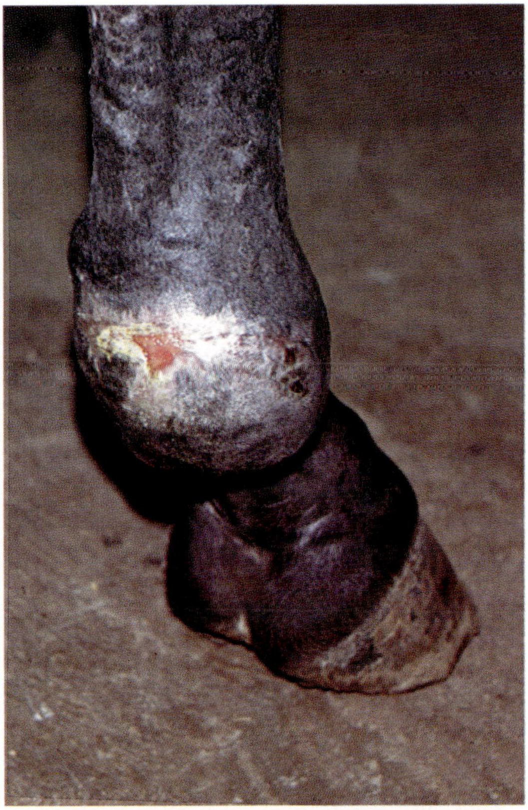

B

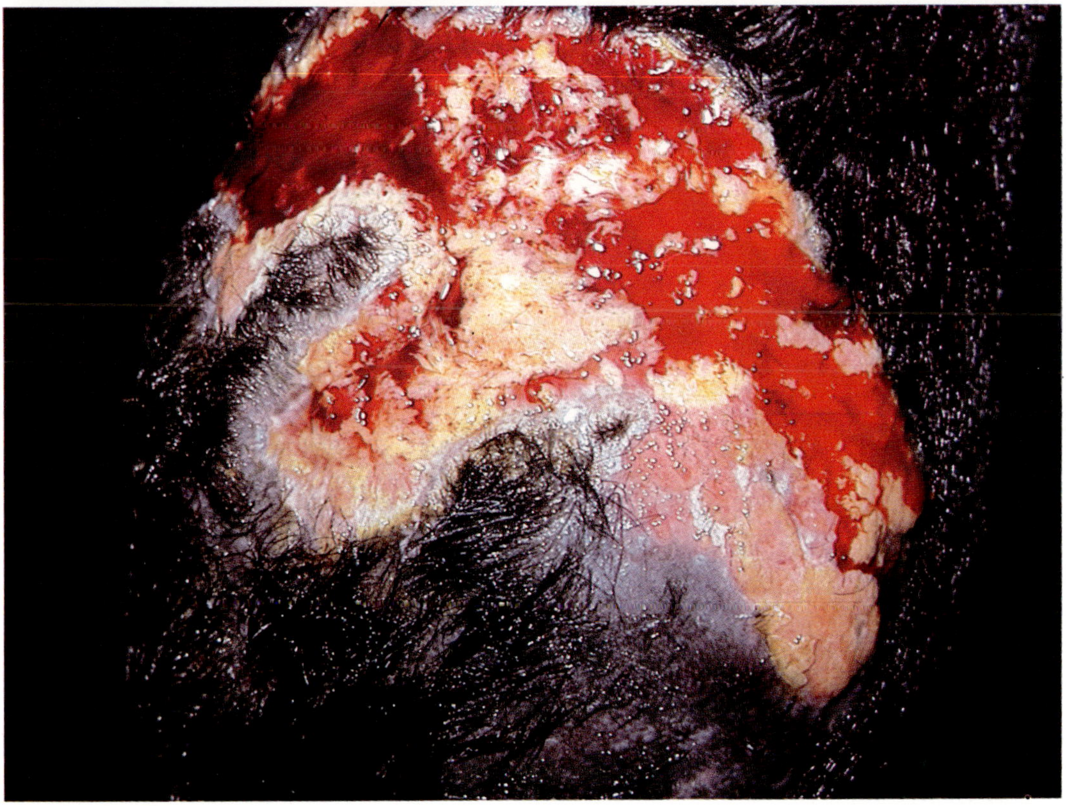

Hypertrophic Scar

A 5-year-old grey Mixed Breed gelding suffered abortive healing of an old rope burn on the right hind pastern that led to a large scar.

Clinically, a crescent shaped hypertrophic scar in the flexor surface of the pastern extended through 180° of its circumference on the posterior aspect. The surface of the lesion was generally scaly with a few excoriations covered by crusts and presented also some smooth areas. Although there was no definite multilobulation, a number of shallow perpendicular grooves could be noticed upon close inspection (Fig. A).

Histopathologically, the epidermis was markedly hyperkeratotic and extremely acanthotic. The acanthosis was of such magnitude as to approach in some places the degree, although not the irregularity, needed to call it pseudoepitheliomatous hyperplasia (Fig. B). The rete pegs displayed budding proliferation downwards into the dermis. Numerous dilated capillaries with prominent endothelium and connective tissue cells were seen throughout the dermis (Fig. C). Between the capillaries, the collagen was arranged in intertwining and anastomosing bands (Fig. C and D).

Treatment was wide surgical excision with second intention healing fostered by meticulous postoperative management of the wound under bandage. Exuberant granulation was controlled in part by use of a hydrocortisone-antibiotic ointment. Complete healing ensued and recurrence was not observed. It may be argued that this tumor could be called a keloid rather than a hypertrophic scar. Clinically, the surface of a keloid is more smooth and glossy, and the tumor contrasts more sharply with the surrounding normal skin than in this patient's lesion. Furthermore, a keloid usually presents irregular borders. Microscopically, these two conditions are very difficult, if not impossible, to distinguish from each other (LEVER 1975). As a matter of fact, MANCINI and QUAIFE (1962) in their careful study suggested the term »hypertrophic healing« to embrace all forms of abnormal wound healing in which the duration and the degree of fibroplastic response may vary considerably leading to these tumors. The same investigators also observed that keloids and hypertrophic scars begin with the formation of perivascular nodules. These nodules were considered the histological units of these growths. Therapeutically, the lack of recurrence following excision supports the diagnosis of hypertrophic scar rather than keloid. Because of their almost invariable recurrence after removal, keloids have been called the nemesis of cutaneous surgery.

CONWAY, H. B.
Tumors of the Skin. p. 53. Charles C. Thomas, Springfield, Illinois 1956
LEVER, W. F.
Histopathology of the Skin. p. 576. J. B. LIPPINCOTT and Co. Philadelphia, 1975.
MANCINI, R. E. and QUAIFE, J. V.
Histogenesis of Experimentally Produced Keloids. Journal of Investigative Dermatology 38:143, 1962.

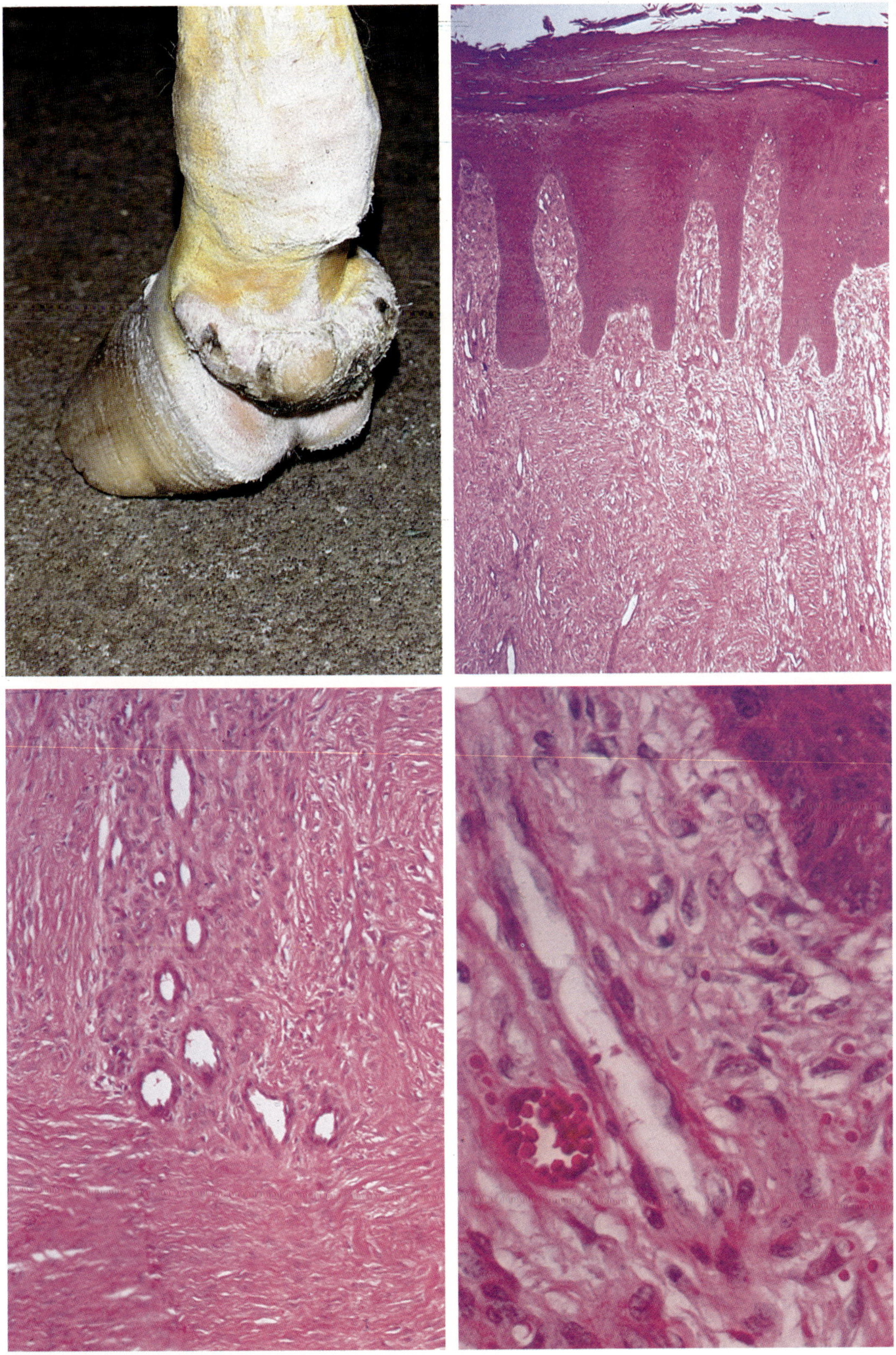
A B C D

Bacterial Infections

Eight interesting patients affected in different manners by bacterial infections are presented.

While some of the lesions are superficial, others are rather deep. The need for precise microbiological studies, specific antimicrobial therapy and sometimes surgical treatment should be considered.

The possibility of bacteremia followed by systemic dissemination and a fatal outcome must always be kept in mind.

Fistulae and Sinuses

A 10-year old Tennessee Walking Horse gelding was presented with a 4-month history of bilateral draining fistulae of the withers. The fistulae had been noticed over the past 4 weeks following rupture of an area of swelling.

Clinically, there were ulcerated areas covered by crusts, blood and exudate. A copious purulent discharge issued spontaneously from the ulcers (Figs. A and B).

A 3-year old Chestnut gelding was presented for treatment of a phlegmonous swelling of the ventral neck which traced upward to the right jugular furrow (Fig. D).

Clinically, a slightly fluctuant swelling was surrounded and superimposed by a firm, edematous plaque that occupied most of the ventral cervical region down to the pectoral muscles.

Treatment. Fistulae and sinuses are frequent manifestations at the skin surface of underlying pathology. Although the terms are often used interchangeably, there is a nuance in the meanings that makes "fistula" more appropriate for reference to an abnormal passage or communication between two internal organs or from one internal organ to the body surface; thus, fistula of the withers in reference to a tract leading from the site of the supraspinous bursa. Other examples would be: salivary fistula, conchal fistula, dentral fistula, rectovaginal fistula, and enteric fistula. In the context of this discussion, "sinus" is an abnormal channel or fistula permitting the escape of pus, hence the somewhat confusing use of the expressions, sinus of the withers and conchal sinus. More appropriate is the use in costal sinus, which is purulent tract extending outward from a rib.

In the second case presented here, a perivascular abscess had resulted from the accidental escape of an irritating I.V. solution outside the jugular vein.

The accumulated pus was drained via surgical incisions kept open with a collapsible latex Penrose tube (Fig. D'). Although created by planned surgical incision, this could be referred to as a sinus of the jugular furrow or, simply, a perivascular sinus.

In the first case, the abscess of the supraspinous bursa that had drained spontaneously at the outset was subsequently explored and drained more effectively by incisions kept open for a time by indwelling drains (Fig. C).

In either case, successful treatment depends upon removal of necrotic tissue, sterilization of the pyogenic membrane, and provision of adequate ventral drainage. Reckoning on the body's ability to slough and discharge soft necrotic tissue (as opposed to bone and cartilage), it may not be an overstatement to say that ventral drainage is the most important single factor in the surgical management of such problems (see Cases 15 and 16).

A

B

C

D

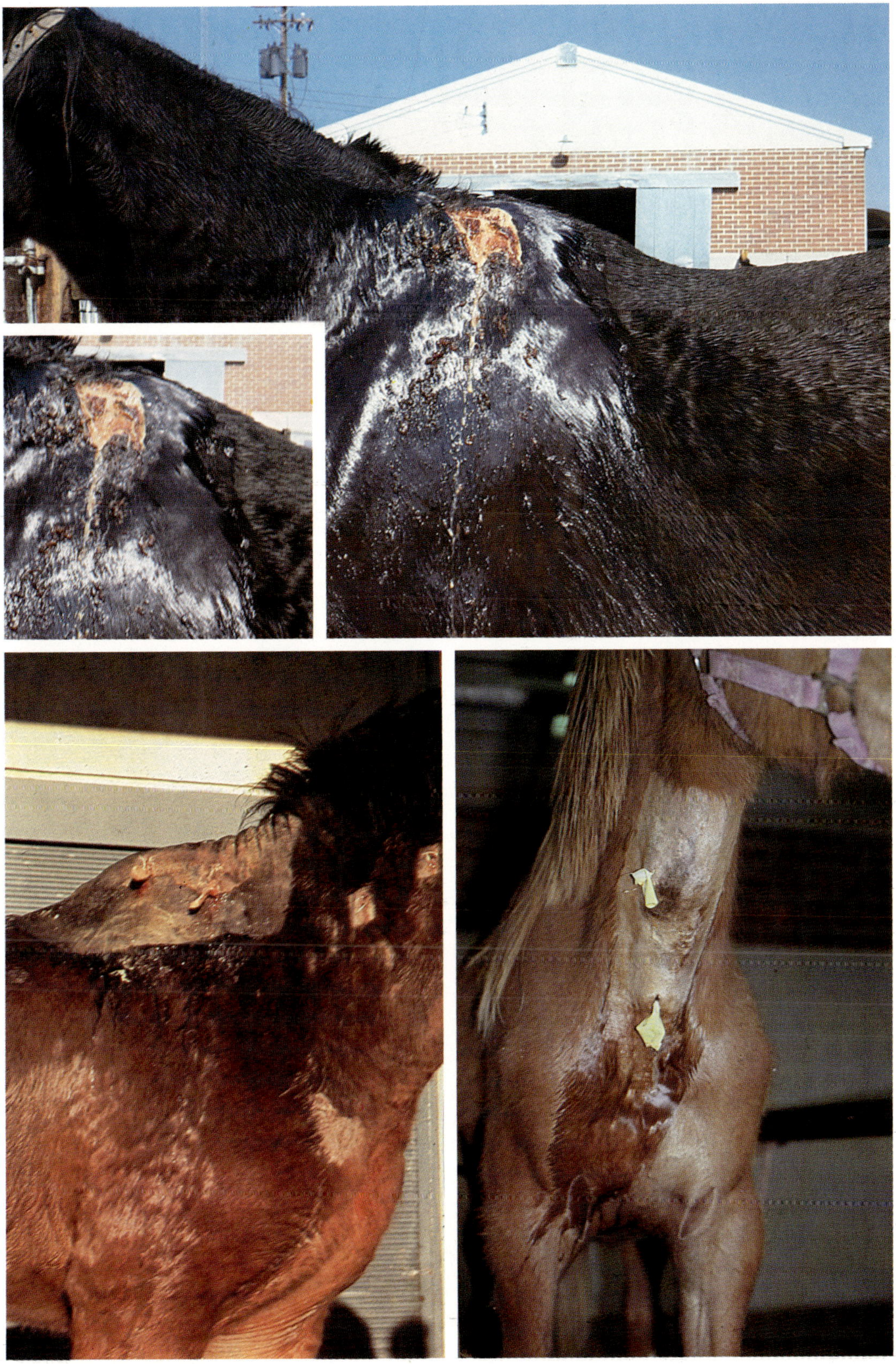

Fistula

A 9-year-old female Quarter Horse was presented for evaluation and management of an ulcerated area on the withers, the unhealed remainder of an extensive surgical incision for drainage of an abscess of the supraspinous bursa operated several weeks earlier.

Clinically, there was a triangularly shaped ulcer on the right side of the withers. The edges were sharply demarcated and nonindurated. The ulcer itself had a homogeneous fairly smooth red surface because it was completely filled with healthy looking granulation tissue.

Histopathologically, a 6 mm punch biopsy was performed on one edge of the lesion and included both the granulating area and the epidermis surrounding the ulcer. Fig. B shows the surface of a nonepithelialized site covered by thin exudate underneath which there were islands of epithelial cells. There were also several remnants of sweat ducts in the midst of healthy-looking collagen bundles. Fig. C shows the surface of an area almost completely epithelialized. The thin exudate was also present but the epidermis, although including a cleft was more developed than in Fig. B. The opening of a hair follicle is partially depicted on the left side of the field.

Treatment consisted of 1) gentle daily cleansing with povidone-iodine surgical scrub; 2) application of 1% silver sulfadiazine cream twice/daily; 3) maintenance of the patient in a stall and prevention of trauma; 4) ascorbic acid 2.2 mg/Kg daily. (ERRINGTON, 1942)

Epithelialization was complete in 2 months.

The rate of healing of ulcers at the site of old fistulas is a reliable indication of the successful management of the deeper pathology. If the ulcer periodically discharges pus and fails to heal, reexploration for faulty drainage or residual necrotic tissue is indicated.

ERRINGTON, B. J.
Ascorbic Acid in Certain Body Fluids of Horses. American Journal of Veterinary Research 3:242, 1942.
VAUGHAN, J. T.
Surgery of the Bursae, Equine Medicine and Surgery, 2nd Edition, p. 828-839. American Veterinary Publications, Wheaton, Ill., 1972.

A

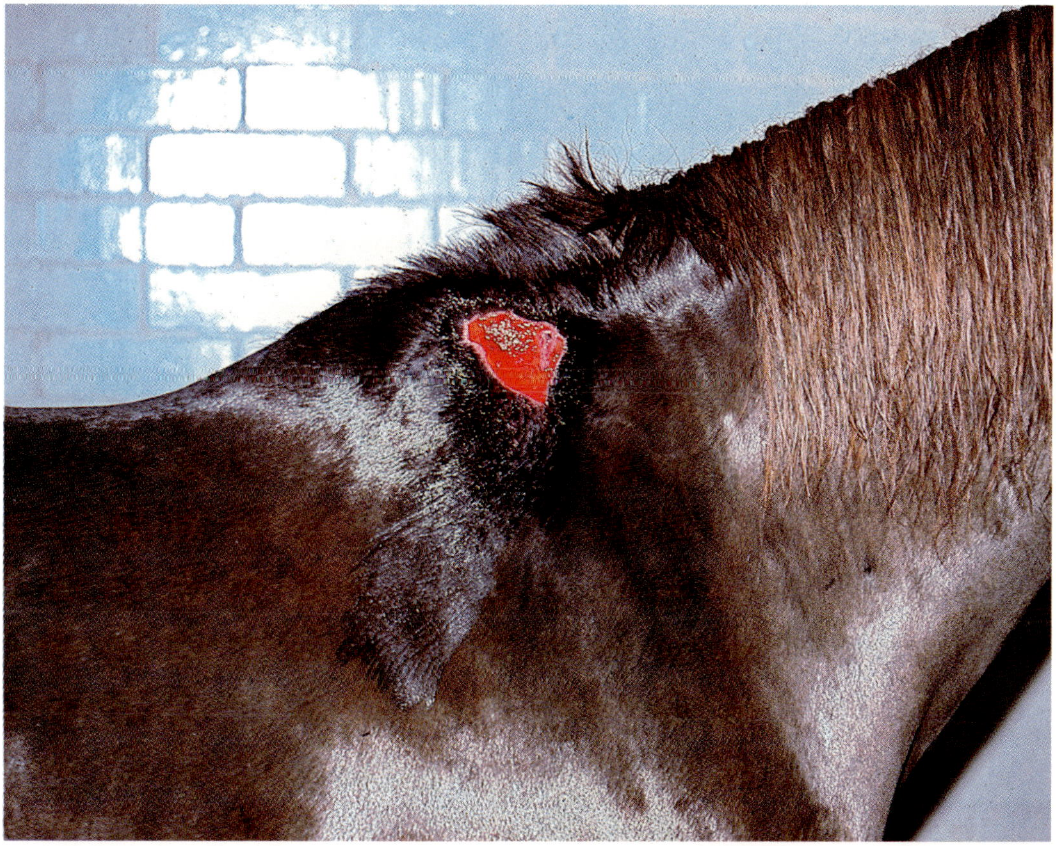

B

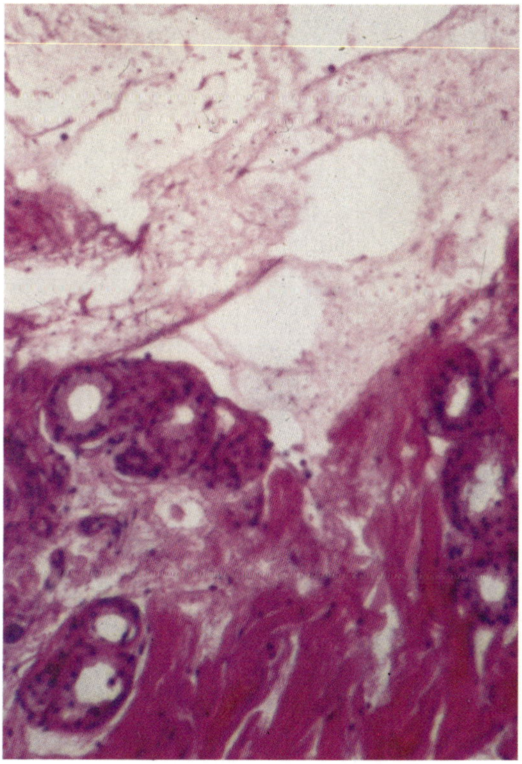

C

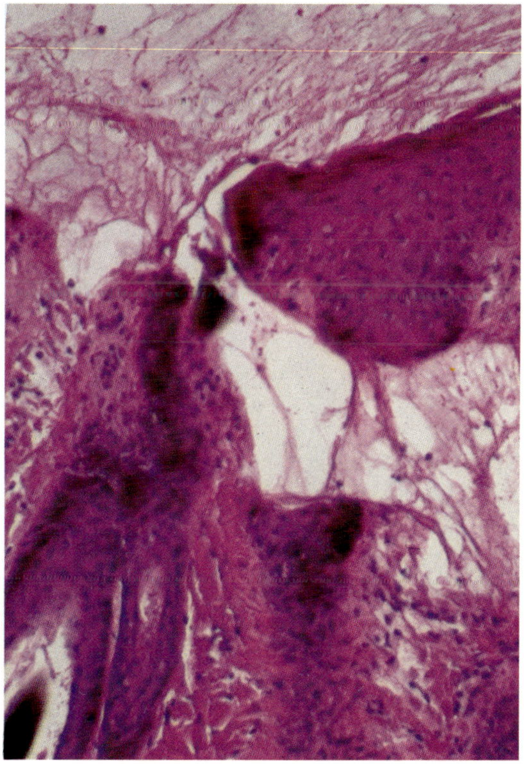

Pelvic Abscess and Sinuses

A 3-year old Chestnut Tennessee Walking Horse mare was referred for the complaint of a pelvic infection that had resulted from a complication of a per cutaneous ventral coccygeal myotomy (tailset operation).

Clinically, the mare was presented with a purulent sinus in the dorsal perineal region just under the base of the tail (Fig. A). This communicated with a pelvic abscess that had dissected forward in the pelvic fascia to a point beyond the pubic brim that was out of reach to palpation per rectum.

Treatment first consisted of stabilization of the mare's general condition by a vigorous regimen of systemic antibiotic therapy. At this time, the mare was prepared for surgery in dorsal recumbency under general anesthesia, and the caudal abdomen was explored to determine the location and extent of the abscess. The most convenient access for drainage was found to be through the right inguinal canal. A counterincision was made alongside the right mammary gland over the superficial inguinal ring, and retroperitoneal access to the lesion was created by blunt dissection through the inguinal fascia (extension of the pelvic fascia) until the abscess cavity could be identified by test puncture. Following the pathway of the puncture with blunt scissor dissection, the abscess was evacuated and a drain installed. The abscess cavity was packed with iodoform gauze dressing for the first few days. The gauze packing and the flexible plastic drain were retained with skin sutures (Fig. B). The plastic drain also communicated with the perineal sinus to permit through-and-through irrigation. This was subsequently replaced with a Penrose (latex) drain which was used until suppuration abated (Fig. C). Removal of the drain was followed by prompt healing of the tract and no further complications ensued.

WALKER, D.F. and VAUGHAN, J.T.
Bovine and Equine Urogenital Surgery. Lea & Febiger, Philadelphia, 1980.

A

B

C

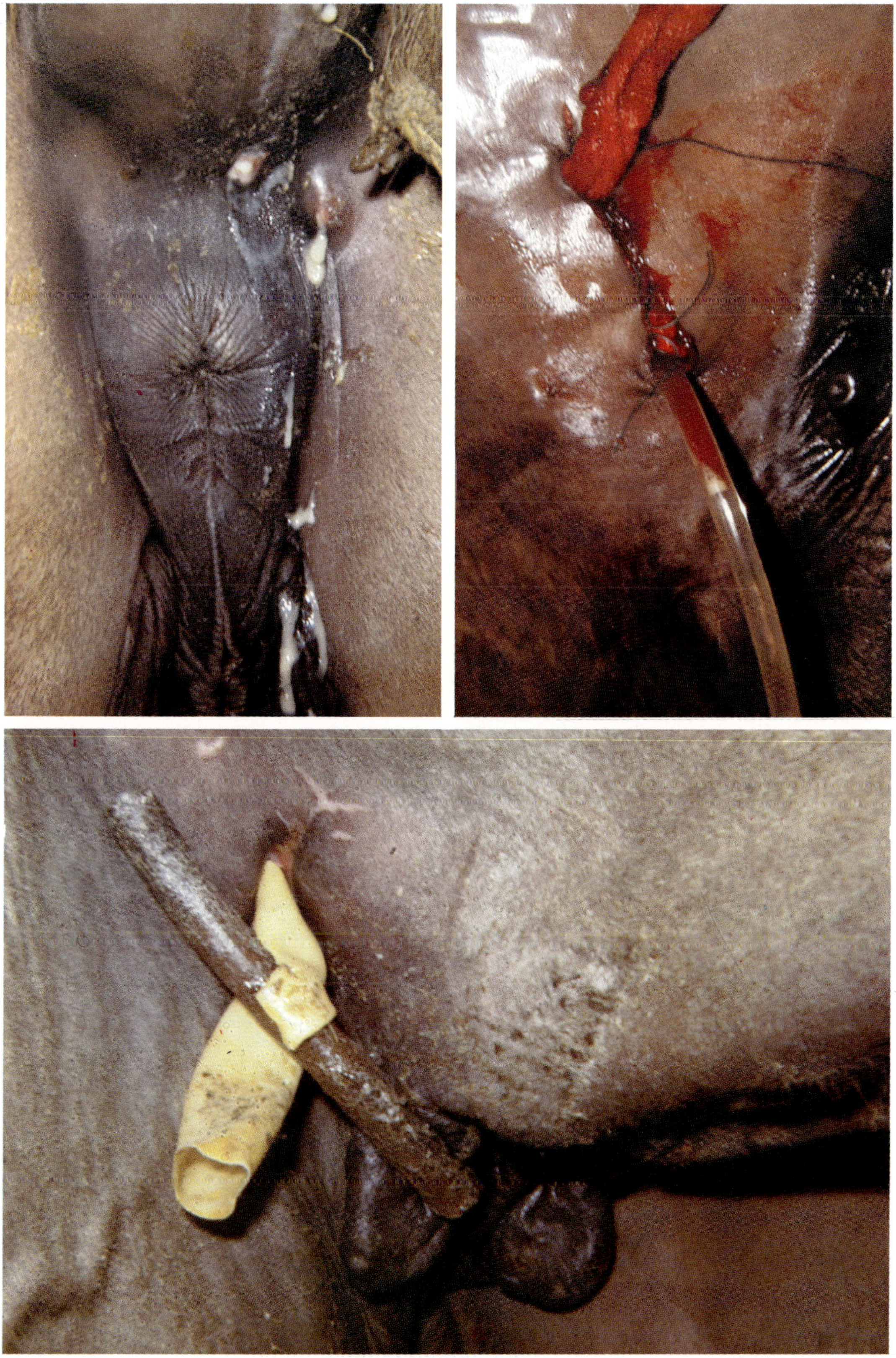

Pyoderma

A 3-year-old Pasofino gelding required dermatological care for a dermatosis of 6 weeks duration.

Clinically, there was an inflamed area over the right hip with its center covered by a large crust whose color ranged from yellow to red to brown-black. A purulent exudate was being spontaneously released in some parts of the lesion. The lower posterior edge of the affected area was hard, dry, and depigmented (Fig. A).

Histopathologically, the stratum corneum showed large deposits composed of fibrin, leukocytes and keratinized cells. There was also hyperkeratosis both outside the hair follicles and at the follicular openings. Moderate acanthosis characterized the stratum spinosum. Some focal spongiosis was noted in the deeper stratum spinosum. The papillary dermis was filled by polymorphonuclear leukocytes and erythrocytes (Figs. B and C). Sections stained with the Brown and Brenn technique showed many gram positive cocci in the stratum corneum and few cocci in the stratum spinosum and upper dermis.

Bacteriologically, cultures were performed with samples (exudate and crusts) obtained from several different areas of the involved skin. *Staphylococcus aureus* and *Streptococcus equi* were isolated.

Hematologically, marked leukocytosis with neutrophilia were noticed.

Treatment. According to the results of antibiotic sensitivity studies, cephalothin sodium was administered intramuscularly 20 ml (2 gm) every 12 hours for 7 consecutive days. Topical treatment consisted of thorough washing with povidone-iodine skin cleanser, followed by topical application of 0.2% nitrofurazone in a water miscible base once daily. The clinical response was rapid and the patient could be discharged after 1 month in the hospital.

Microscopically, the early sequence of events in cutaneous pyoderma cannot be easily detected in natural infections (like in this patient) because biopsies are taken when the process is already fully developed. In view of this, it is interesting to look at the findings in JORDAN's model (JORDAN et al 1974) whereby *Streptococcus zooepidemicus* was inoculated to observe carefully the development of experimentally induced pyoderma in guinea pigs. BRYANS (1972) has discussed extensively the importance of *Streptococcus zoopidemicus* as an infectious agent in the horse.

BRYANS, J.T.
Streptococcal Diseases in Equine Medicine and Surgery. p. 79. Edited by E.J. CATTCOT and J.F. SMITHCORS. American Veterinary Publications, Wheaton, Illinois, 1972.
JORDAN, W.E.
The Experimental Inductions of Superficial Cutaneous Infections in Guinea Pig. Journal of Investigative Dermatology 55:149, 1970.
JORDAN, W., MONTES, L.F. and PITTILLO, R.F.
Microscopic Features of Pustule Formation in Experimental Impetigo of Guinea Pig. Journal of Cutaneous Pathology 1:54, 1974.

A

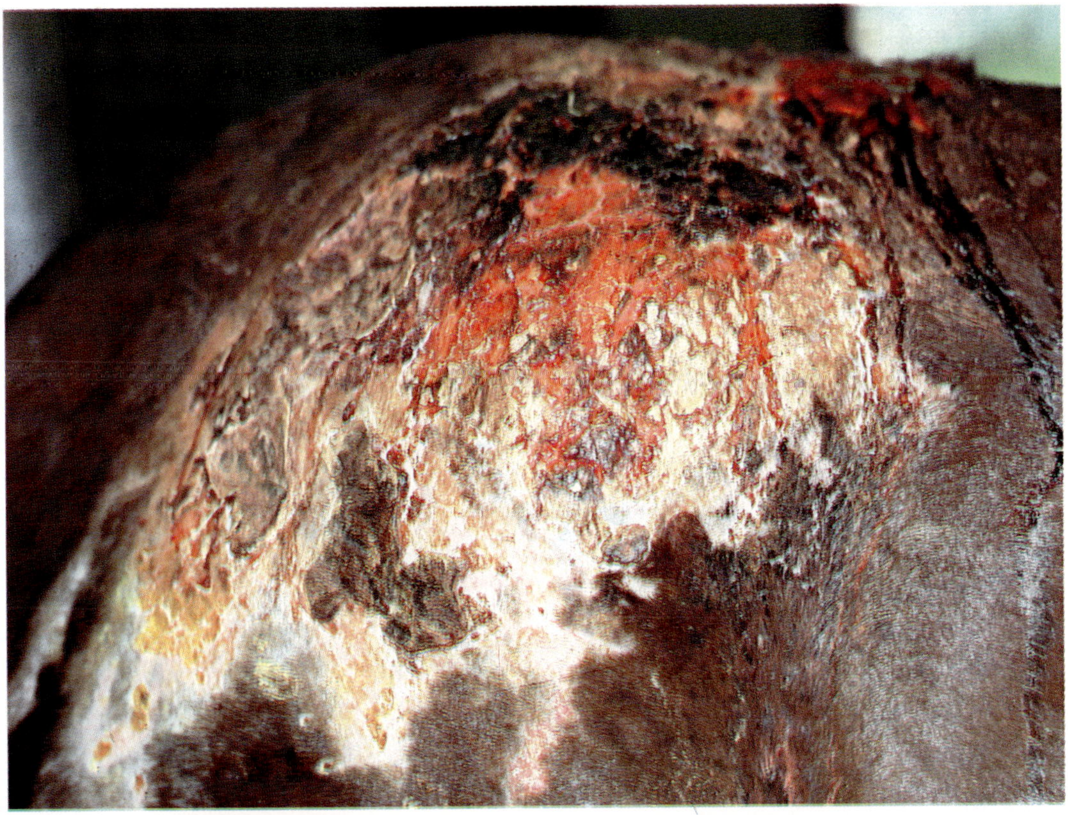

B

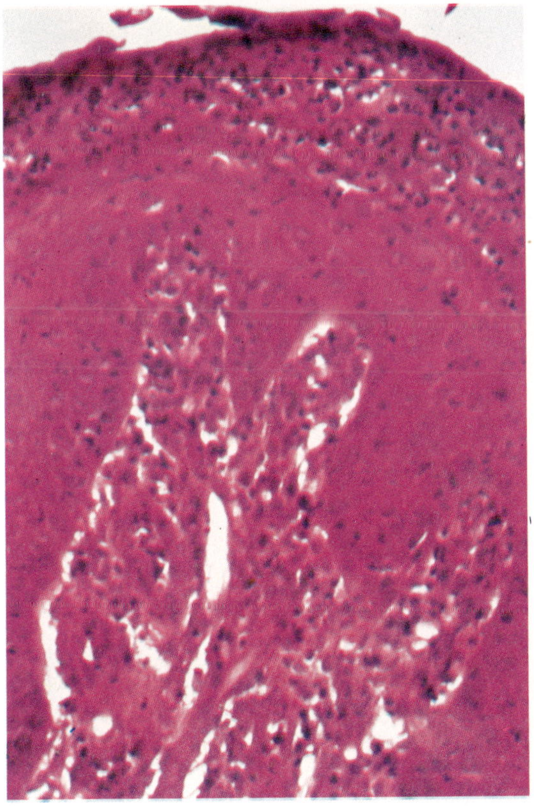

C

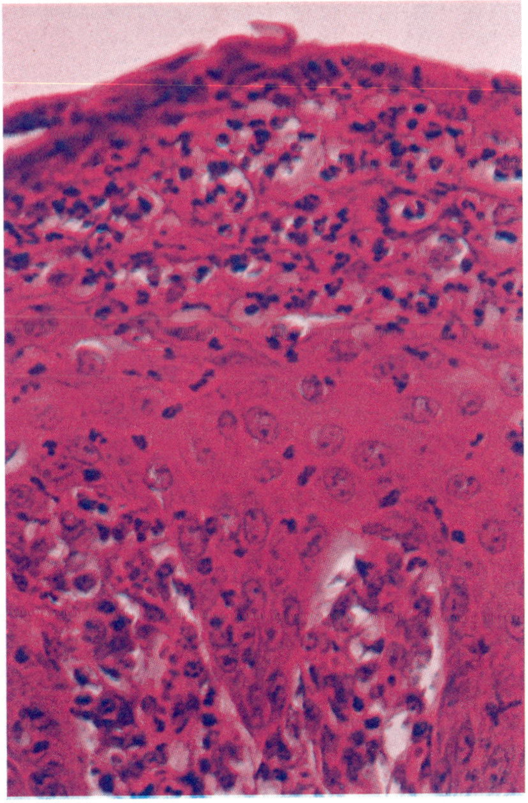

Burn

A 4-year-old Thoroughbred mare was seriously burned during a stable fire and referred to the Large Animal Clinic for intensive care.

Clinically, there was a very extensive, 2nd to 3rd degree burn. The affected areas, involving approximately 50% of the body surface, were fiery red and oozing serum. Close inspection revealed in some places malodorous greenish yellow scabs and profuse suppuration. In the midst of the burned areas there were some healthy epithelial islands that had been spared. The mare was extremely irritable due to the intense pain and pruritus. Upon arrival to the clinic, 20 days after the accident, it became apparent that the process had already become complicated by a superimposed infection (Fig. A).

Bacteriologically, cultures obtained through gentle swabs of the red oozing areas and also planting the crusts directly on culture media yielded *Pseudomonas aeruginosa* in large numbers.

Treatment consisted of 1) wet dressings using aluminum acetate 1:40 solution (Burow's solution) for one hour twice daily, 1% silver sulfadiazine cream applied gently over the entire affected areas B.I.D. (Fig. B), 2: sedation, 3) pinch grafts on selected sites, 4) supportive therapy. After 3 months of continued therapy the improvement was dramatic (Fig. C). All treatment was discontinued after approximately 650 days. The mare was retired for breeding and subsequently pronounced in foal to a Thoroughbred stallion.

Silver sulfadiazine is available in a 1% water miscible cream (SILVADENE) which spreads easily (FOX 1968). It has broad activity against Gram-positive and Gram-negative bacteria, *Candida albicans* and *Herpes simplex* virus.

Silver sulfadiazine was chosen in this patient in particular because of its great activity against *Pseudomonas aeruginosa* (FOX 1968, FOX et al 1969) and the fact that it has proven very effective and safe in severely and extensively burned humans (DICKINSON 1973). It must be kept in mind, however, that in patients with large burns significant amounts of silver sulfadiazine are absorbed, therefore close monitoring to prevent any of the reactions due to sulfonamides is necessary. In cases like this one, preparations containing hexachlorophene should be avoided because of the serious complications of systemic absorption of the compound.

DICKINSON, S.J.
Topical Therapy of Burns in Children with Silver Sulfadiazine. New York State Journal of Medicine 73:2045–2049, 1973.
FOX, Jr., C.L.
Silver Sulfadiazine. A New Topical Therapy for Pseudomonas in Burns. Archives of Surgery 96:184–188, 1968.
FOX, Jr., C.L., RAPPOLE, B.W., and STANDFORD, W.
Control of Pseudomonas Infection in Burns by Silver Sulfadiazine Surgery, Gynecology and Obstetrics 128:1021–1026, 1969.
(Grateful acknowledgement to Dr. J.M.Humburg, School of Veterinary Medicine, Auburn University, AL 36849.)

A

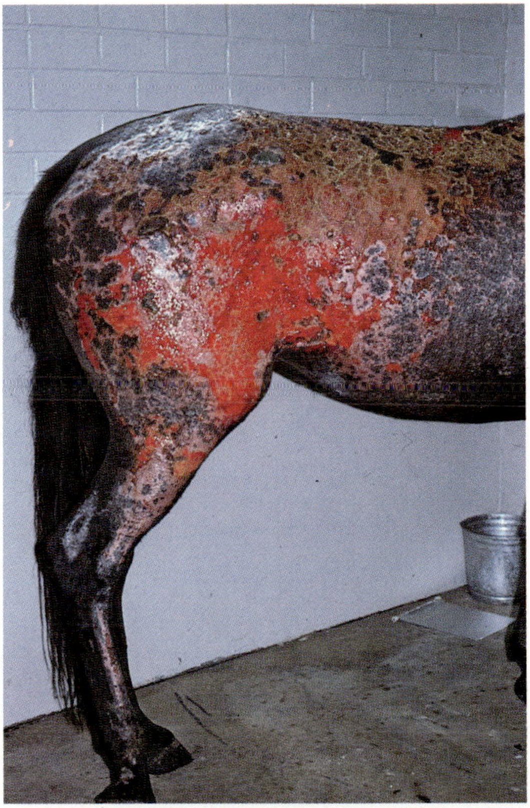

C

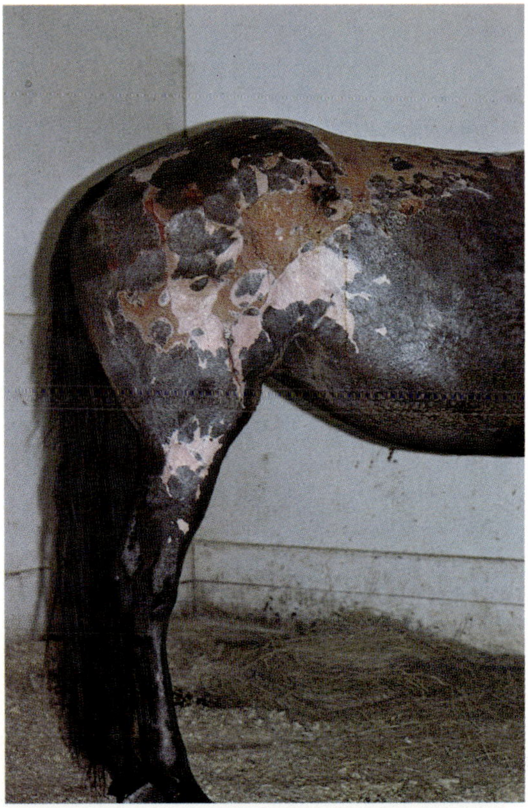

B

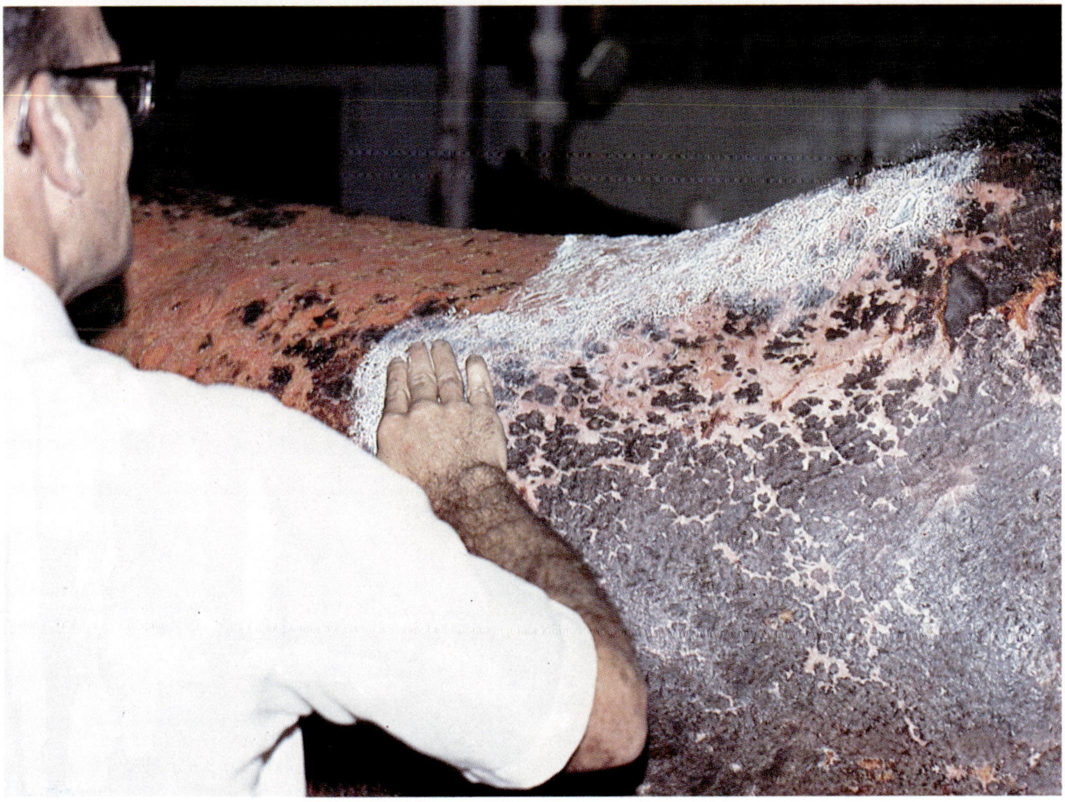

Healing Burn

A 6-year-old Thoroughbred mare necessitated evaluation and management of a chronic dermatitis that was a sequela of a third-degree burn which occurred during a barn fire 5 months earlier.

Clinically, there was involvement of the upper back and right hip by marked black hyperpigmentation with irregular edges (Fig. A). The center of the affected area was covered by adherent yellow to reddish crusts that appeared dry (Fig. B). Hairs were either absent or very thin and short.

Histopathologically, a biopsy specimen from the hyperpigmented zone revealed that the stratum corneum was hyperkeratotic and contained large amounts of small melanin granules. The stratum spinosum, although not strictly atrophic, lacked rete pegs and had a fairly uniform thickness throughout the specimen. An impressive accumulation of melanin was present in the basal cell layer and also in higher levels of the stratum spinosum. An increased number of fibroblasts was associated with young collagen arranged in thin, fairly parallel bundles and dilated dermal vessels were evident in the dermis. Melanin was found in the upper dermis both free and phagocytized by melanophages (Figs. C and D). Hair follicles were significantly reduced in number in many areas and completely absent in other areas.

Treatment consisted of 1% silver sulfadiazine cream once daily applied mostly on the central crusted area (BAXTER 1971). Epithelialization progressed steadily and complete coverage of the area by intact although thin epidermis took place about 2 months later.

The horse's owner was advised to expect a persistence of the pigmentary changes and of the alopecia. To what degree those alterations were permanent it was difficult to prognosticate, but in part, at least, a correlation of the clinical features with the histopathology suggest that much of the changes were going to persist. In this situation one can speak of permanent alopecia because the destruction of hair papillae was complete. The microscopic features are reminiscent of those found in some types of human scarring alopecia (PINKUS and MEHREGAN 1976). It should be remembered as PINKUS and MEHREGAN (1976) have pointed out that "a peculiar situation exists in epidermis that has regenerated after a burn or other denudation. The new epidermis usually carries a few melanocytes with it as it migrates over the wound surface. It is repopulated with melanocytes secondarily some weeks later (STARICCO 1961) by migration from hair follicles and from the wound border, and by local multiplication."

BAXTER, C.R.
Topical Use of 1% Silver Sulfadiazine. In Contemporary Burn Management. Edited by H.C. Polk, Jr. and H.H. Stone. p.217. Little Brown, Boston, 1971.
PINKUS, H. and MEHREGAN, A.H.
A Guide to Dermatohistopathology. p.271, p.416. Appleton Century Crofts. New York, 1976.
STARICCO, R.G.
Mechanism of Migration of the Melanocytes from the Hair Follicle into the Epidermis Following Dermoabrasion. Journal of Investigative Dermatology 36:99, 1961.

A B C D

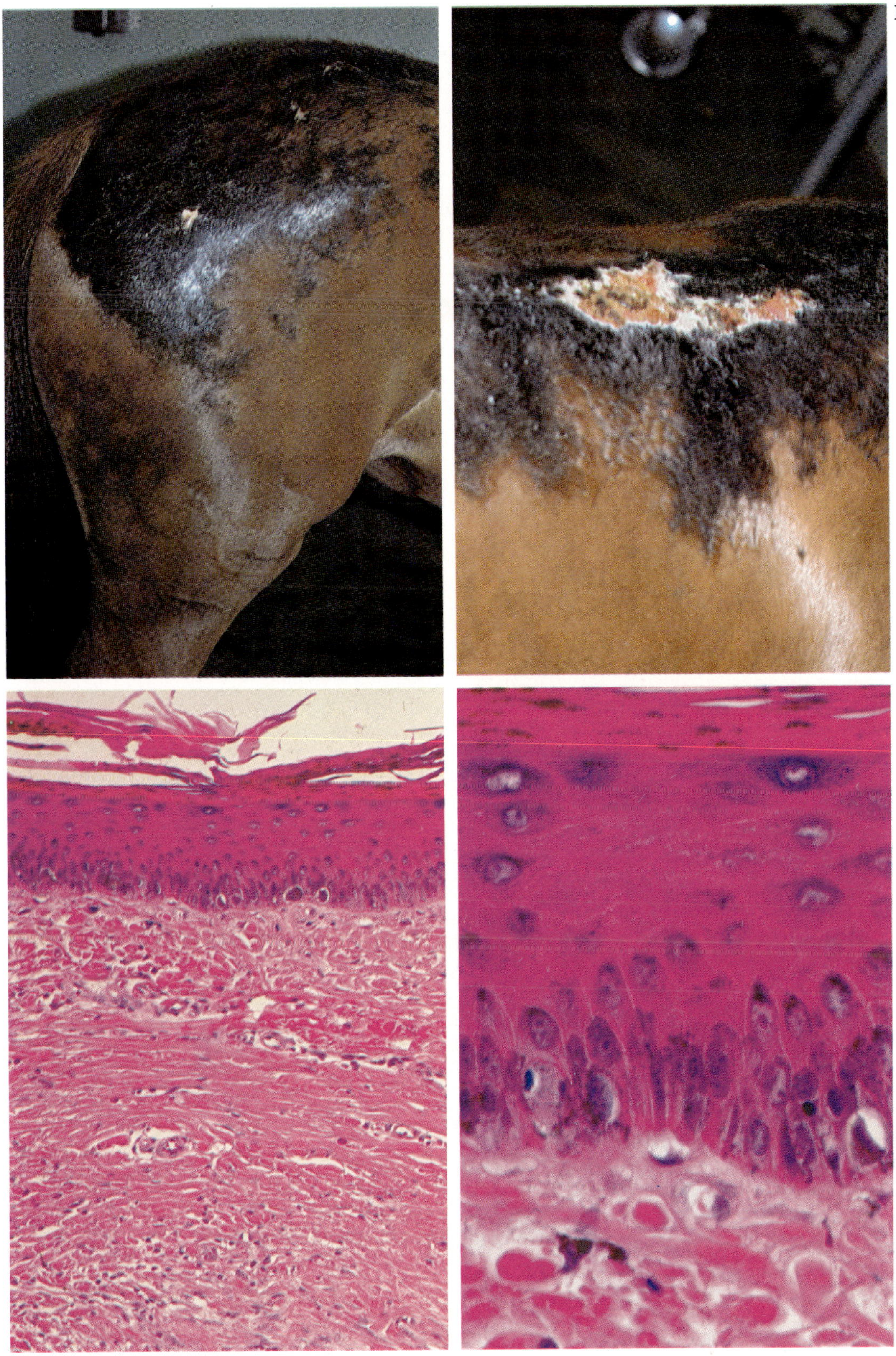

Ulcerative lymphangitis

A 10-year-old bay gelding was admitted for treatment of a chronic, inflammatory swelling of the right foreleg that was attended by cutaneous eruptions and cording of the lymphatic vessels, most conspicuous on the medial aspect of the leg. Edema of stasis extended to the foot.

Clinically, the area of the limb surrounding the chesnut showed bullae together with purplish spots of blood extravasated into the skin and dilated veins (Fig. A). Culture of exudate from an unopened pustule revealed *Corynebacterium pseudotuberculosis (OVIS)* showing *in vitro* sensitivity to chloramphenicol, erythromycin, gentamycin, and kanamycin.

Histopathologically, only a 4 mm punch biopsy was obtained from one of the areas near the bullae where clinically the changes were minimal and appeared to represent early stages of the condition. In the stratum spinosum, spongiosis was observed, cells showing "alteration cavitaire", and many neutrophils migrating into the stratum corneum with microabscess formation. The upper dermis showed dilated vessels and an inflammatory infiltrate composed of neutrophils and lymphocytes (Fig B).

Treatment consisted of daily wound toilet with povidone-iodine scrubs and spray, in addition to local drainage and swab of pustules and ulcers. The extensive abscessation of pectoral, ventral abdominal, and inguinal regions commonly associated with the disease (Knight, 1968) was not a feature of this case. Systemic treatment was by intramuscular injections of chloramphenicol 10 mg/kg T.I.D. for 7 days. Fly control and stable hygiene were important to the overall management of the patient. Healing was attended by gradual recession of edema and drying of the cutaneous lesions.

Ulcerative lymphangitis must be differentiated from cutaneous glanders (farcy) caused by *Malleomyces mallei* and epizootic lymphangitis caused by *Histoplasma (Cryptococcus) farciminosus,* both troublesome in the Near and Far East. A third possibility is the nonspecific lymphangitis (primarily of the hind legs) which is a feature of other diseases from which a variety of pyogenic organisms have been recovered (Jubb and Kennedy 1970), including the streptococci, staphylococci, clostridia, and *Shigella equirulis*. This was noted in Tufvesson (1952) who attributed predisposing influence to lowered resistance due to low protein rations, exhaustion, and concurrent disease, as well as to overcrowding and seasonal factors. More recently, Reid (1965) credited the high incidence of chest abscesses *(Corynebacterium pseudotuberculosis)* in California horses to transmission by arthropod vectors (genera Musca or Stomoxys) also carrying the infective larvae of Habronema spp., suggesting an interrelationship between ulcerative lymphangitis and cutaneous habronemiasis (Reid 1965).

The use of antibiotics is usually futile and may predispose to exacerbations of pyemia resulting in fatal spread to lungs and kidneys in contrast to an ordinarily low mortality rate with conservative, local therapy (Knight 1968). The infection is relatively refractory to antibiotics because it is due to a facultative, intracellular parasite, rendered still more inaccessible to systemic therapy by the isolating effect of abscess wall encapsulation (Hagan & Bruner 1981). The use of autogenous bacterins is alluded to by Knight (1978) and Blood & Henderson (1974).

BLOOD, D.C. and HENDERSON, J.A.
Veterinary Medicine, Fourth Edition, p. 304. The Williams & Wilkins Company, Baltimore, 1974.
GILLESPIE, J.H. and TIMONEY, J.F.
Hagan and Bruner's Infectious Diseases of Domestic Animals, Seventh Edition, p. 233. Comstock Pub. Assoc., Cornell University Press, New York 1981.
JUBB, K.V.F. and KENNEDY, P.C.
Pathology of Domestic Animals, Second Edition, V. 1, p. 141. Academic Press, New York and London, 1970.
KNIGHT, H.D.
Journal of the American Veterinary Medical Association, V. 155, 446, 1969.
KNIGHT, H.D.
Cornell Veterinarian, V. 68, 220, 1978.
REID, C.H.
Veterinary Medicine/Small Animal Clinician, March, p. 233, 1965.
TUFVESSON, G.
Nordisk Veterinärmedicin, 4, 529–729–817, 1952.

A

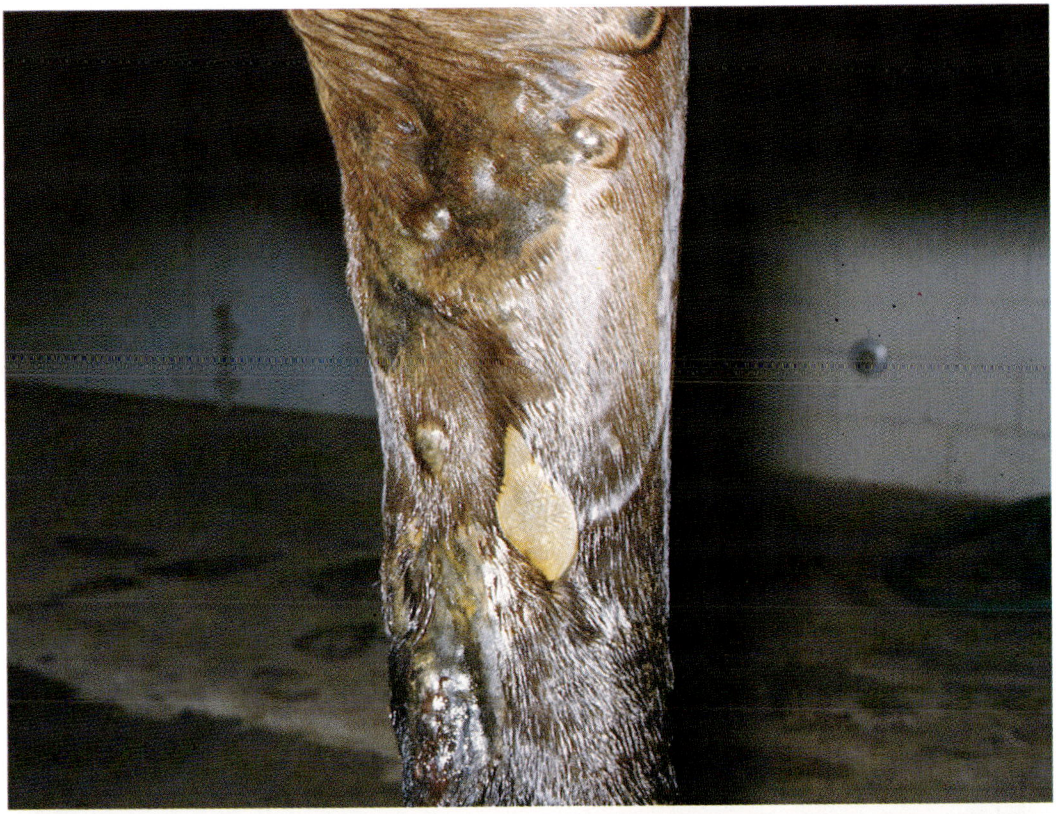

B

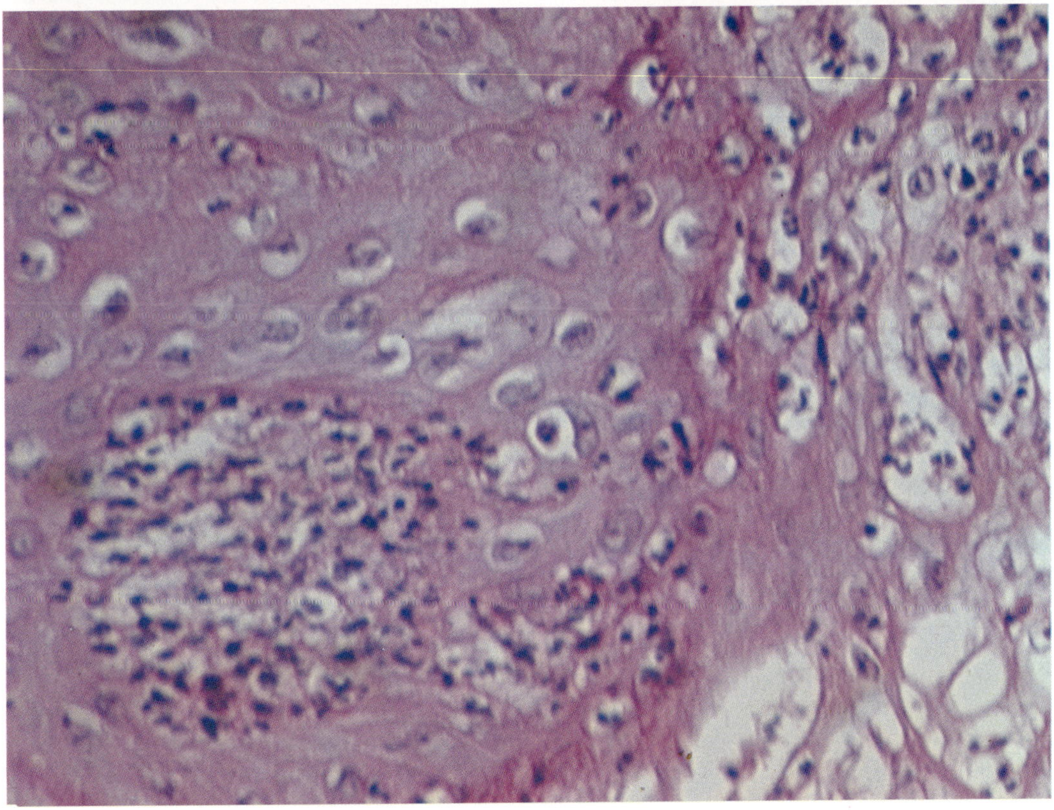

Unguilysis

(Canker)

A 13-year-old Tennessee Walking Horse required hospitalization during the late part of a rainy winter season because of a severe destructive process which had gradually developed over a 6-month period and involved all 4 feet.

Clinically, a severe moist, malodorous, invasive pododermatosis of the frogs and sulci was striking. Upon scraping and curettage of the hoofs, soft scales mixed with amorphous yellowish brown material could be obtained. In Fig. A the bluish green color of the hoofs was the result of impregnation with copper sulfate that had been applied as a home remedy prior to admission to the hospital.

Histopathologically, loose masses of keratinized cells were enclosing masses of neutrophils, mononuclear cells and erythrocytes. In many areas these cells were concentrated in large numbers forming microabscesses. PAS stained sections failed to show fungal cells. Brown and Brenn stained sections demonstrated many Gram-positive and some Gram-negative bacteria.

Treatment consisted of the following: 1) topical 10% benzoyl peroxide acetone gel applied once daily under a sterile dressing followed after a time by B.I.P. when daily changes of bandage were no longer required; 2) gradual excision of the infected layers of keratinized cells using a scalpel, until the level of healthy epithelium was reached; 3) intramuscular penicillin and streptomycin; 4) prolonged maintenance of the horse under hygienic stable conditions. After 12 consecutive weeks under this program, there was marked improvement (Fig. B). The patient was discharged but instructions were given to the owner to continue the use of benzoyl peroxide at home once daily without occlusion.

Canker is not a cause of lameness as frequently now as it was in the past (FESSLER 1972). It should not be dismissed, however, as a mild disorder because once microorganisms invade the multilayered keratinized tissues they are difficult to eradicate. Although the bacteria play an important role, canker is the result of other factors such as moisture, trauma, poor hygiene, and occlusion from the common practice in saddle horses of shoeing over pads. Ultrastructural studies of canker are needed to elucidate the precise location of the microorganisms in the affected hoof. If, by electron microscopy, it becomes apparent that bacteria and/or fungi penetrate the keratinized cells as in erythrasma (MONTES et al 1965) or in candidiasis (WILBORN and MONTES 1980), then a more primary role for the microorganisms will have to be considered. If this becomes the case, some systemic antimicrobial treatment will have to be developed.

FESSLER, J.F.
Surgery of the Foot and Hoof. Equine Medicine and Surgery. Edited by E.J. Cattcot and J.F. Smithcors. p. 810 American Veterinary Publications, Wheaton, Illinois, 1972.

MONTES, L.D., McBRIDE, M.E., JOHNSON, W.P., OWENS, D.W. and KNOX, J.M.
Ultrastructural Study of the Host-Bacterium Relationship in Erythrasma 90:1489, 1965.

WILBORN, W.H. and MONTES, L.F.
Scanning Electron Microscopy of Oral Lesions in Chronic Mucocutaneous Candidiasis. Journal of the American Medical Association 244:2294, 1980.

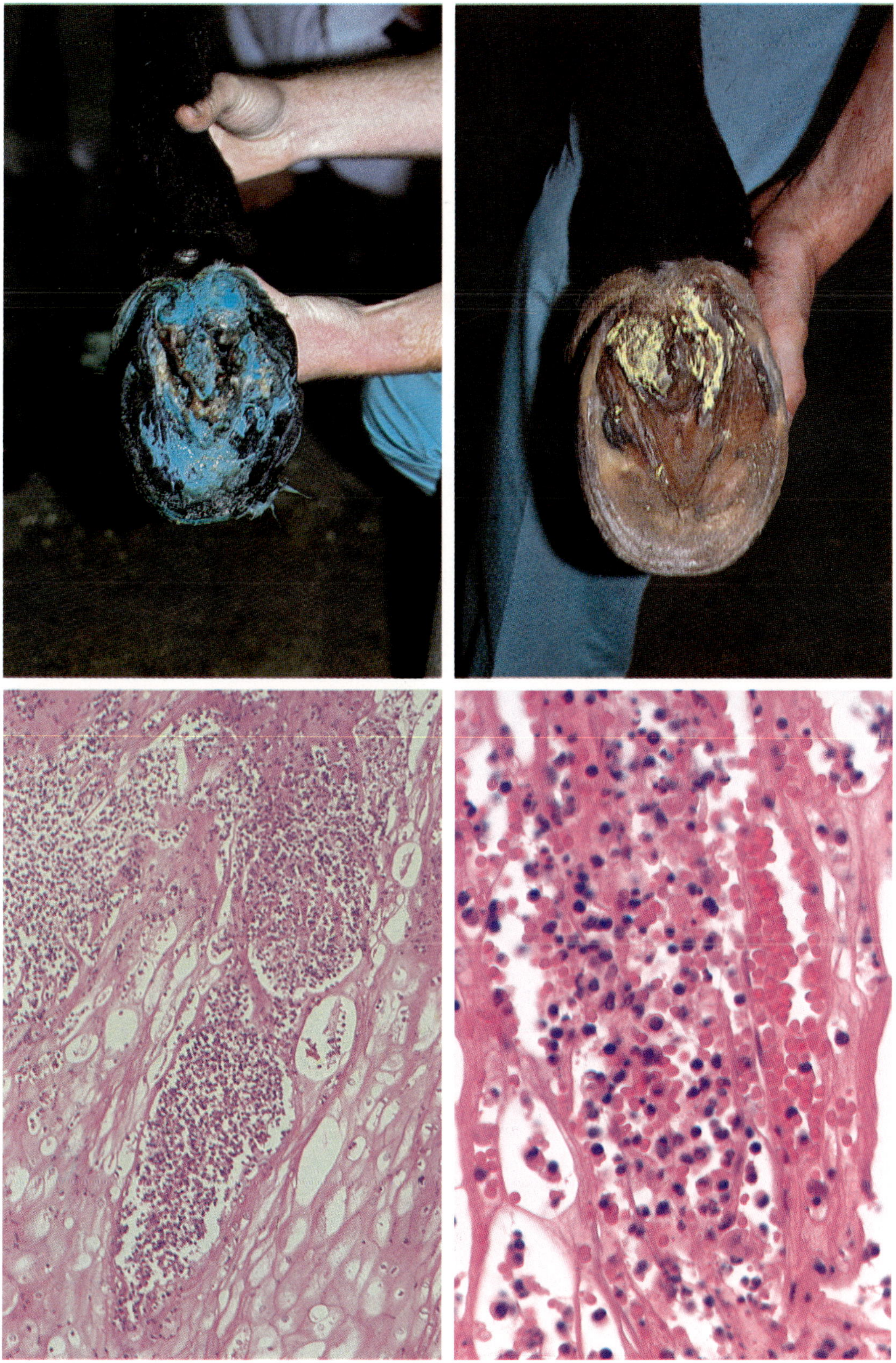
A
B
C
D

Fungal and Related Infections

Fungi differ from bacteria because of the higher complexity of their cellular structure (they possess true nuclei, mitochondria, and endoplasmic reticulum).

Fungal infections are usually more chronic than bacterial infections. Mycological diagnosis must precede the institution of specific therapy. Patients described in this chapter were handled keeping this in mind.

Microorganisms like *Dermatophilus SP* and *Nocardia SP* because of their large size have classically been grouped with the fungi, although they should be regarded as bacteria.

Dermatophilosis

A 3-year-old Thoroughbred mare was admitted because of chronic intractable diarrhea of several weeks duration that led to a very poor physical condition with marked weight loss and extreme debilitation. During the course of the internment and while the patient was in an air conditioned stall, a generalized rash, partilarly severe over the croup was noticed requiring dermatological evaluation and treatment.

Clinically, the involved areas of the croup and also to a lesser extent the back and the loin showed prominent scabs whitish or grey in color of variable size and thickness, firmly adherent to the underlying skin (Figs. A, B, C). Upon removal of the scabs using a wooden tongue blade, the skin underneath the scabs displayed intensely red, abraded areas with an oozing, bloody appearance (Figs. A and B).

Microbiologically, scabs taken from several different places were ground in a mortar with sterile saline solution to make up a suspension with which smears were prepared. The smears were stained with Giemsa for 45 minutes. Microscopic examination demonstrated coccoid cells as well as branching filaments, 1.0–1.5 microns wide. These organisms were attached to the scales or free between them. The filaments when studied carefully under oil immersion, revealed septation and fragmentation into cuboidal packets of coccoid cells (Fig. D).

Cultures performed as recommended by KAPLAN and JOHNSTON (1966) yielded colonies of *Dermatophilus congolensis*. The isolates were Gram positive, nonacid-fast, catalase positive and hydrolyzed urea and casein.

Treatment consisted of removal of the crusts and loose hair by gentle currying and brushing, followed by thorough cleansing with povidone-iodine surgical soap. After rinsing, the affected areas were sprayed with povidone-iodine surgical antiseptic and allowed to dry. Daily treatment for 2 weeks resulted in complete clearing.

Dermatophilosis, also known as streptothricosis, is caused by *Dermatophilus congolensis*, an actinomycete first described by VAN SACEGHEM in cattle in the Belgian Congo (LLOYD and SELLERS 1976). KAPLAN and JOHNSTON (1966) consider this infection an exudative dermatitis followed by the formation of scabs. Although it was earlier regarded as an exotic disease it is now apparent that the distribution is world wide.

As clearing of the infection takes place, the previously infected sites may show alopecia but this is only temporary because *Dermatophilus congolensis* infects the keratinized layers of the epidermis and hairs without reaching the dermis (LLOYD and SELLERS 1976). VANBREUSEGHEM et al (1976) observed high sensitivity of this organism to erythromycin, an antibiotic which has not been widely used but may well become an important agent in the management of dermatophilosis.

KAPLAN, W. and JOHNSTON, W. J.
Equine Dermatophilosis (Cutaneous Streptothricosis) in Georgia. Journal American Veterinary Medical Association 149:1162, 1966.
LLOYD, D. H. and SELLERS, K. C.
Dermatophilus Infection in Animals and Man. Academic Press, New York 1976.
VANBREUSEGHEM, R., TAKASHIO, M., EL NAGEH, MM, PRESLER, D., SELLY, M. and VAN WETTERE, P.
Some Experimental Research on Dermatophilus Congolensis in Dermatophilus Infection in Animals and Man. Edited by D. H. LLoyd and K. C. Sellers, p. 202. Academic Press, New York 1976.

PLATE 22

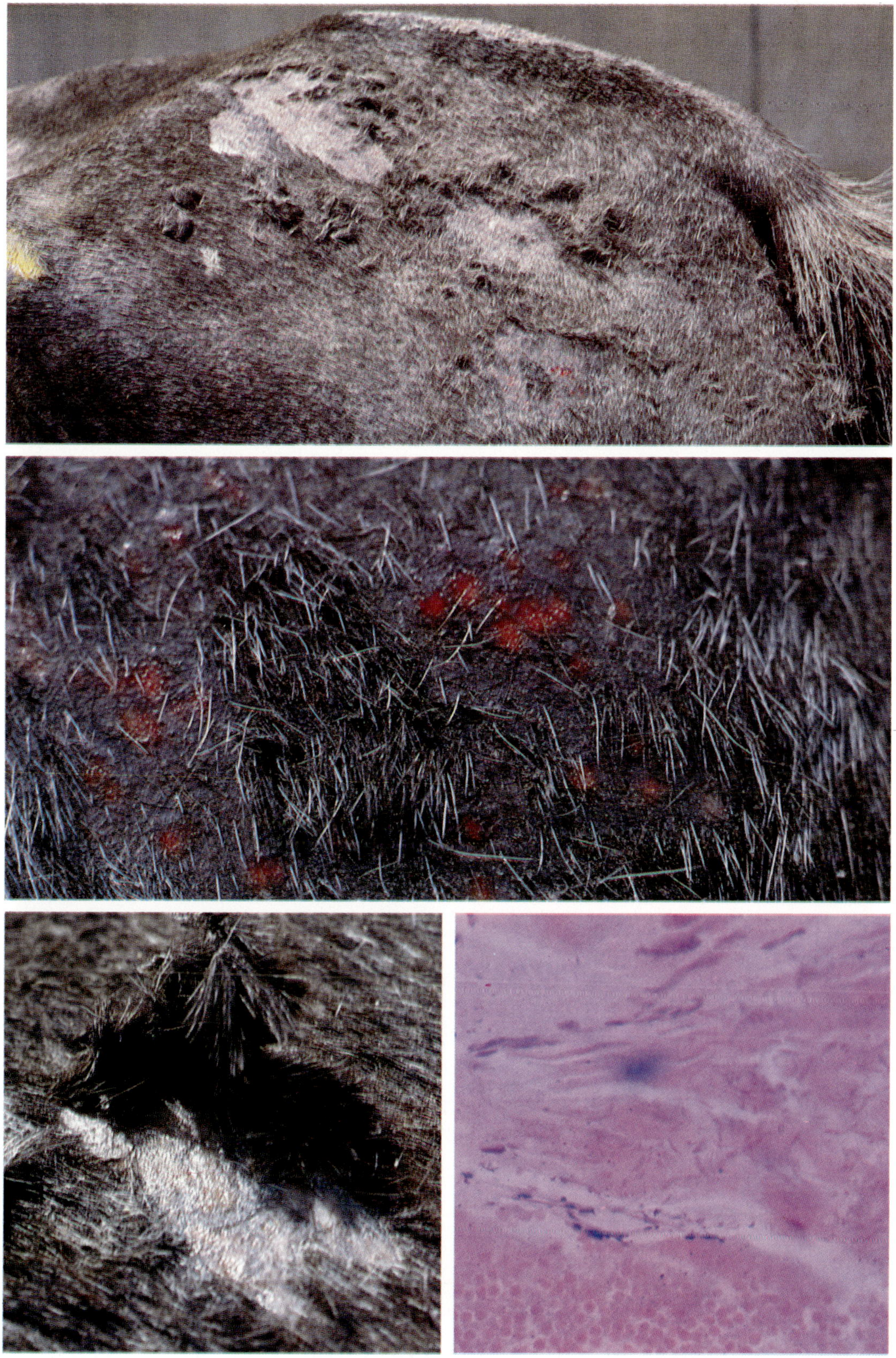

A B C D

Candidiasis

A 2-week-old Thoroughbred filly foal delivered by an agalactic mare was fed ENTERAL formula and developed nosocomial diarrhea with fever and leukocytosis. Following treatment with oral chloramphenicol for seven days a perianal rash developed.

Clinically, there was a symmetrical acute irritation in areas covered by the stools. The involved areas were the undersurface of the tail and the buttocks, which displayed erythema, mild exudate and minor superficial erosions (Fig. A).

Mycologically, smears prepared with exudate from the involved areas and stained with Gram and periodic acid-Schiff (PAS) showed yeast cells in the form of blastospores and pseudohyphae. Swabs obtained from the same areas were planted in Sabouraud's dextrose agar and in Sabouraud's dextrose agar with cycloheximide and chloramphenicol. Cultures incubated at room temperature and at 37°C yielded large colonies of a yeast which was identified as *Candida albicans* after subculturing in special media. The same yeast was isolated in large numbers from the stools.

Treatment consisted of gentle daily cleansing with careful removal of the stools, application of white petrolatum and control of the diarrhea. One week later, the involved areas showed marked healing. Temporary residual pigmentation was the only visible change (Fig. B). This disappeared rapidly and one month later the skin looked normal.

Candidiasis is the most common yeast infection. Cultures in Sabouraud's dextrose agar yield whitish creamy colonies of *Candida albicans* composed of pseudohyphae and blastospores that react strongly to periodic acid-Schiff staining (Fig. C). In special media, such as corn meal agar, *C. albicans* develops the typical larger chlamydospores (Fig. D) which are not produced by other yeasts. This patient's problem could not be more similar to the human diaper rash that follows diarrhea induced by broad spectrum antibiotics (BOUND 1956) (MONTES et al 1971). *C. albicans* can produce cutaneous disease through two different mechanisms. One is direct invasion with digestion of keratin. The other is primary irritation as in contact dermatitis. Whether only one of these mechanisms or both played a role in this case remains to be demonstrated. Another factor in candidiasis is occlusion, in this case provided naturally by the horse's tail. Any of the anticandidal topical treatments would be useful in patients like this one.

BOUND, J. P.
Thrush Napkin Rashes. British Medical Journal 1:782–784, 1956
MONTES, L. F., PITTILLO, R. F., HUNT, D., NARKATES, A. J. and DILLON, H. C.
Microbial flora of infant's skin. Comparison of types of microorganisms between normal skin and diaper dermatitis. Archives of Dermatology. 1971:103:640–648
PITTILLO, R. F., MOORE, W. J., PANZER, J. D. and MONTES, L. F.
Bacterial Flora of Infants Skin: Comparison Between Diaper-Occluded and Unoccluded Areas. International Journal of Dermatology 12:245–249, 1973.

A B C D

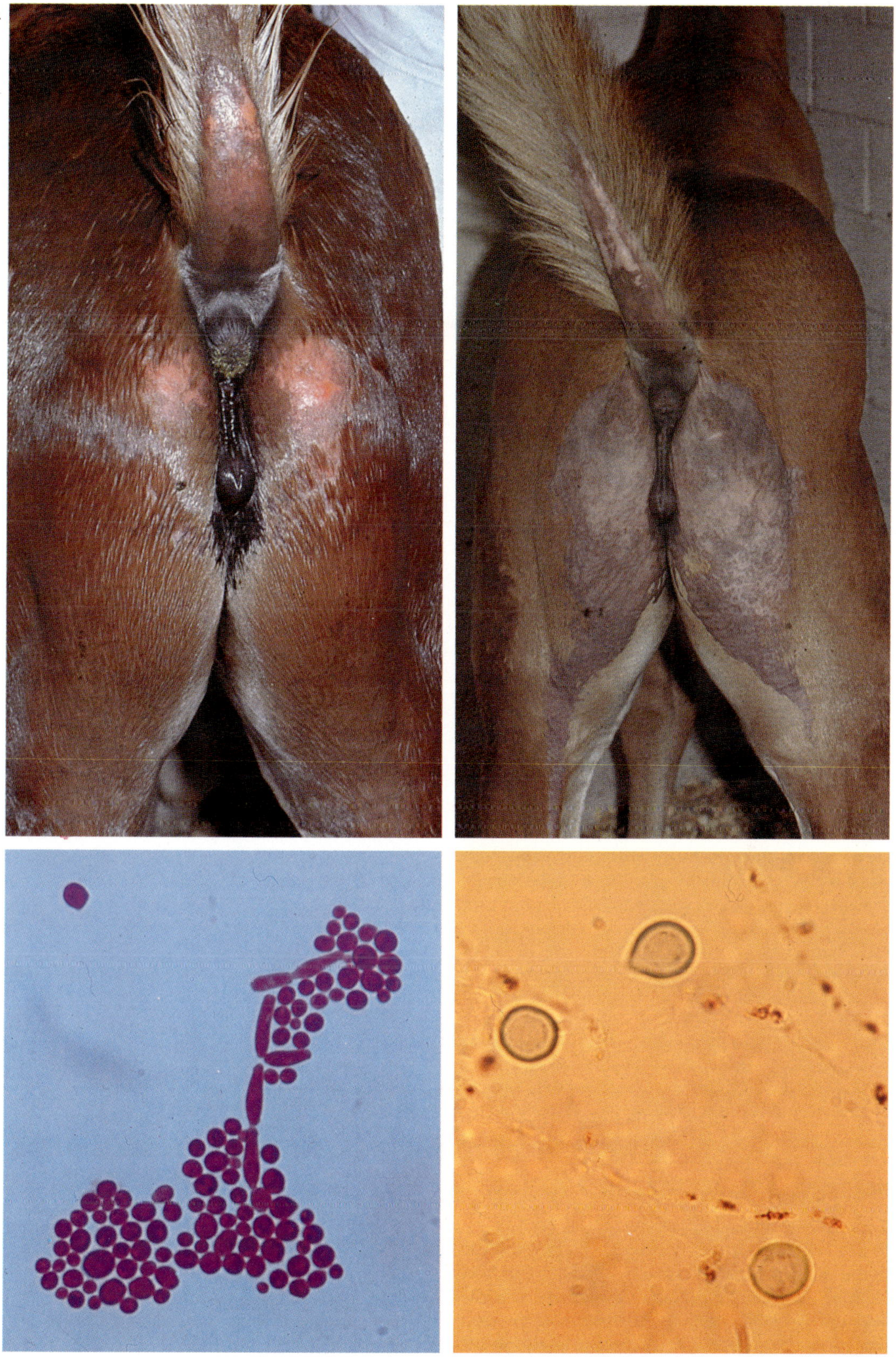

Dermatophytosis

(Tinea)

A 4-year-old Thoroughbred mare presented a rash of approximately 8 weeks duration which had developed during the latter part of the summer.

Clinically, there were multiple round circinate scaly patches ranging in diameter from 1 to 5 centimeters. The lesions had a slightly raised hyperpigmented border and a depressed scaly center. They were more numerous and prominent over the brisket and legs. In some areas they showed a tendency to become grouped (Figs. A and B).

Histopathologically, the stratum corneum was moderately hyperkeratotic. The stratum spinosum showed focal areas of minimal spongiosis. There was a very mild subacute inflammatory infiltrate in the upper and mid-dermis. PAS stained sections showed positively stained hyphae and arthrospores in the stratum corneum outside the hair follicles. The follicles themselves did not show fungal cells.

Mycologically, potassium hydroxide (KOH) preparations of scales removed by scraping the affected areas revealed many septate hyphae as well as arthrospores. Scales were treated with several drops of a 30% solution of potassium hydroxide on a glass slide for thirty minutes. In addition, other scales were directly planted in Sabouraud's dextrose agar and in Sabouraud's dextrose agar containing chloramphenicol and cycloheximide and incubated at room temperature. Colonies developed rapidly and were initially identified as *Microsporum gypseum* by the appearance of a light brown powdery surface with radiating furrows. The observation of numerous ellipsoid macroconidiae with 4 to 6 septations confirmed the identity of the fungus (Conant et al 1971). These typical cells of *M. gypseum* could be further evaluated by transmission electron microscopy. A thick cell wall and numerous intracellular organelles were apparent (Figs C and D).

Treatment was carried out by topical application of 1% clotrimazole solution on the affected areas twice daily (SPIEKERMANN and YOUNG 1976). In addition, a shampoo containing salicylic acid and benzalkonium chloride was used to wash the horse every other day. Clearing of the infection occurred rapidly and after four weeks on this program there was no evidence of skin lesions.

Topical treatment was preferred over systemic griseofulvin because the infection was not very severe. It should be remembered that griseofulvin is not free of side effects and of resistance by fungi (HILDICK-SMITH et al 1964).

CONANT, N.F., SMITH, D.T., BAKER, R.D. and CALLAWAY, J.L.
Manual of Clinical Mycology. W.B. Saunders Company, Philadelphia 1971.
HILDICK-SMITH, G., BLANK, H. and SARKANY, I. Fungus Diseases and Their Treatment. P. 436 Little Brown and Company, Boston 1964.
SPIEKERMANN, P.H. and YOUNG, M.D.
Clinical Evaluation of Clotrimazole Archives of Dermatology 112:350, 1976.

A B C D

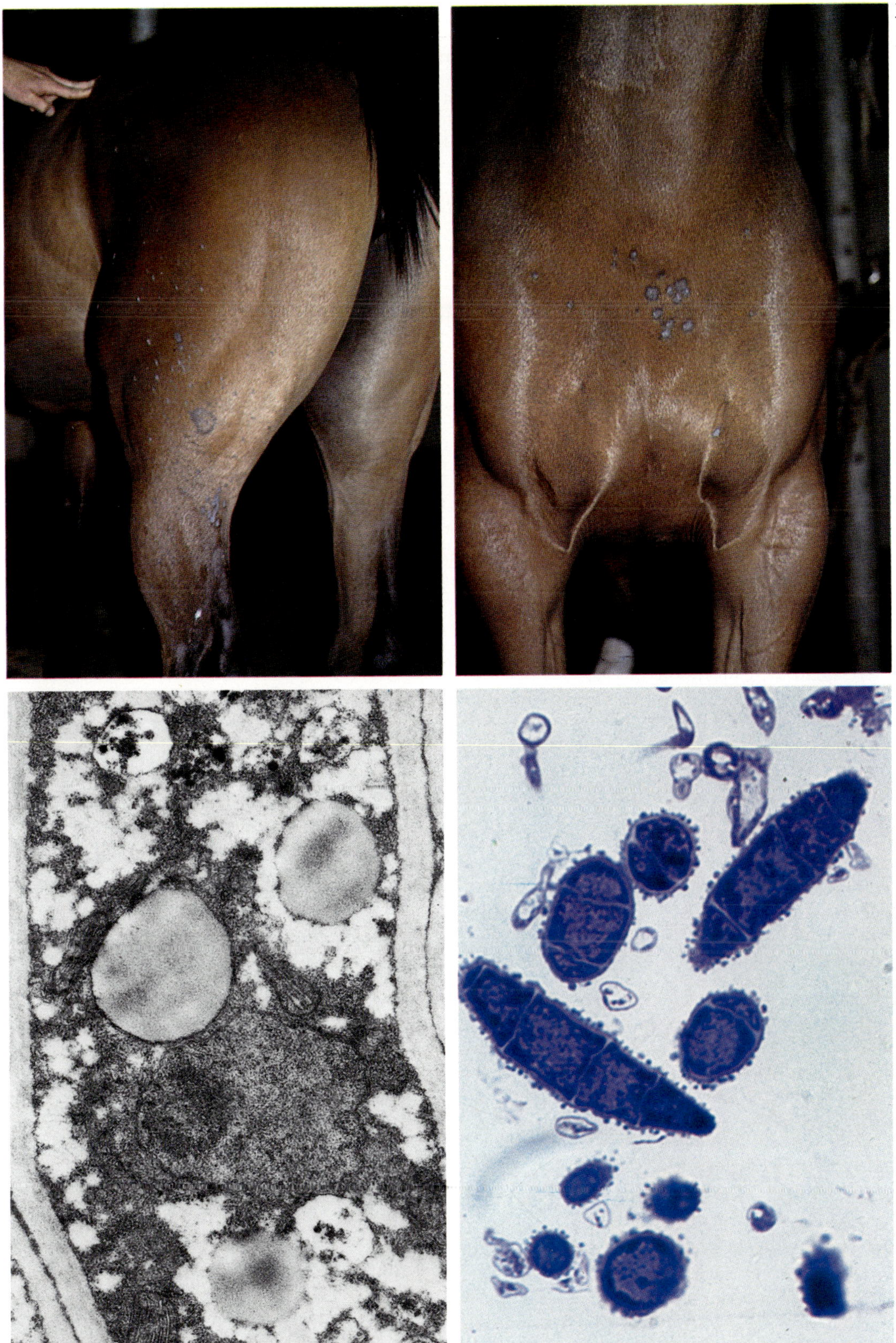

Sporotrichosis

A 9-year-old male Quarter Horse was referred because of multiple lesions that had developed on the left hind leg over a 2-month period.

Clinically, many intradermal nodules were found over the inner aspect of the leg. In general the smaller were covered by intact epidermis. The larger nodules were partially eroded or covered by a dark bloody crust. Most of the nodules were surrounded by edematous skin. The entire affected leg was also edematous (Fig. A).

Histopathologically, one of the nodules with intact epidermis was removed through an excisional biopsy. Half of the specimen, following fixation and embedding, was serially sectioned and stained with hematoxylin and eosin and PAS-hematoxylin. The epidermis showed pseudo-epitheliomatous hyperplasia while the dermis was filled with a granulomatous reaction. The features shown in Figs. B and C are very similar to those described by LURIE (1971). There were giant cells of the foreign body type in the center of a granuloma surrounded by lymphocytes, plasma cells and histiocytes. It was interesting to notice several clear zones surrounded by darkly stained bodies within the cytoplasm of the giant cells (Fig. C). Electron microscopic examination would be required to determine if such bodies were cells of *Sporothrix schenckii*. A few asteroid bodies were detected.

Mycologically, the other half of the biopsy specimen was homogenized and the material used for smears and cultures. Smears stained with Gram and PAS demonstrated cigar-shaped organisms although in small numbers. Cultures planted in Sabouraud's dextrose agar alone and in Sabouraud's dextrose agar with added chloramphenicol and cycloheximide grew typical colonies of *Sporothrix schenckii*.

Treatment was carried out with iodide therapy. A loading dose of 50 gm in 20% aqueous solution (250 ml) I.V. was followed by daily administration of 30 gm organic iodide on feed until iodism appeared. Thereafter, the dosage was reduced until appetite and body temperature returned to normal, and was maintained at that level until the lesions regressed (about 30 days). Rough hair coat, dandruff and mattering of the eyes were other signs of iodism. Sporotrichosis may respond to other forms of treatment such as sulfonamides, stilbamidine, griseofulvin (DAVIS and WORTHINGTON 1964) and amphotericin B. On the other hand it may undergo spontaneous cure (LURIE 1971). Nevertheless, to leave a patient untreated may be risky because one never knows whether the infection is limited to the skin or if it is also systemic. A precautionary note is that the use of iodides may be contraindicated in pregnancy.

DAVIS, H.H. and WORTHINGTON, W.E.
Equine Sporotrichosis. Journal American Veterinary Medical Association 145:692, 1964.
FISHBURN, F. and KELLEY, D.C.
Sporotrichosis in a Horse. Journal American Veterinary Medical Association 151:45, 1967.
LURIE, H.I.
Sporotrichosis Human Infection with Fungi, Actinomycetes and Algae. Edited by R. D. Baker, p. 614 Springer Verlag. Berlin 1971.

A

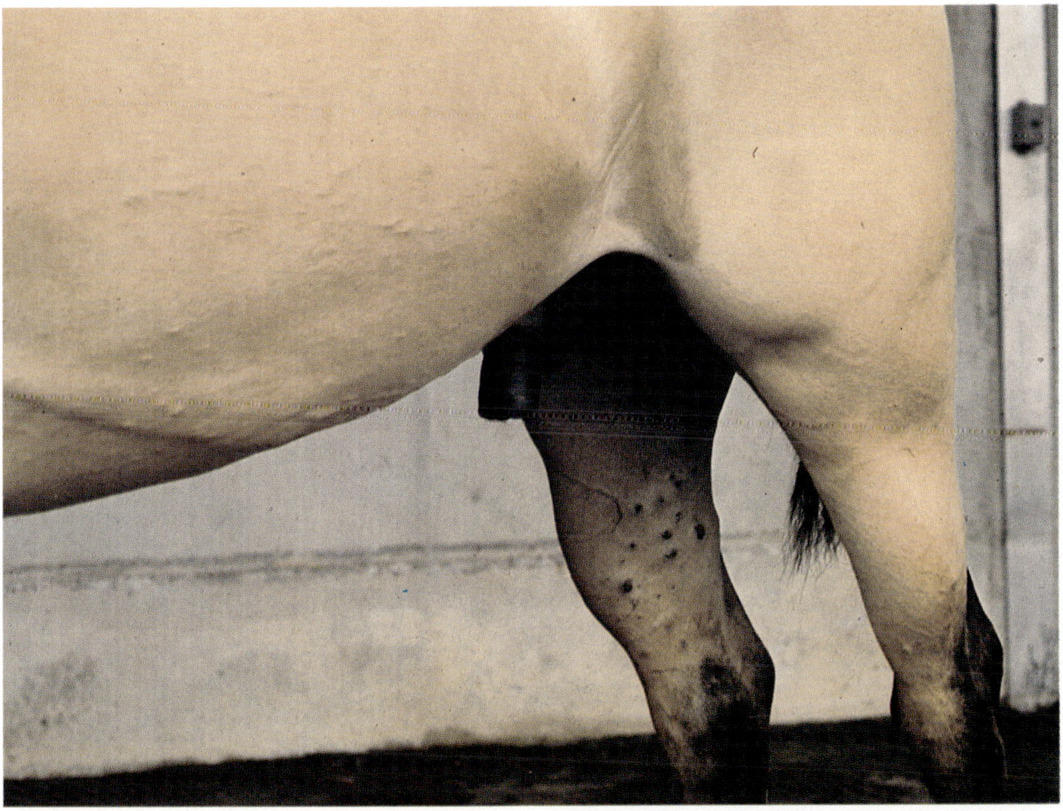

B

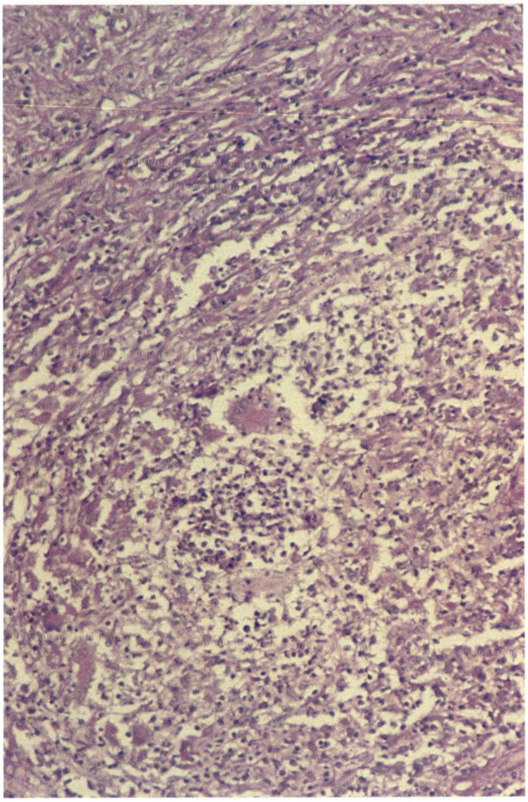

C

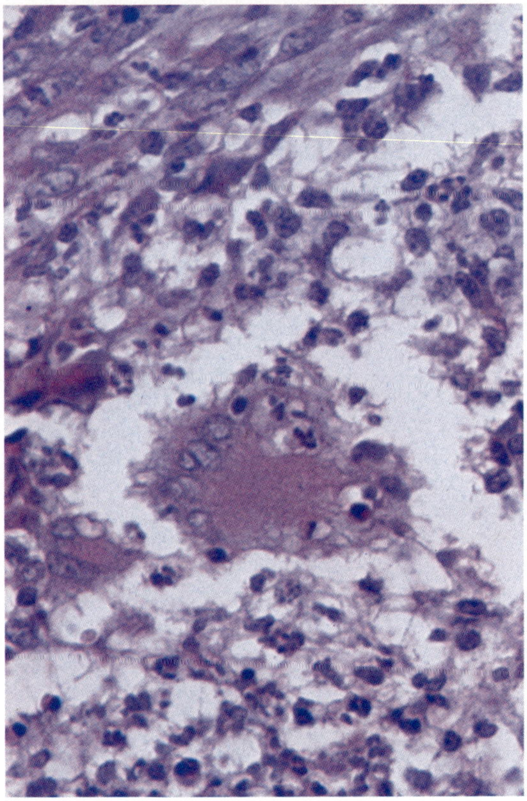

Nocardiosis

A 15-year-old Mule required evaluation and management of multiple ulcerated lesions which had developed gradually over a period of six months.

Clinically, there were several draining ulcers with an irregular border over the neck, left side of withers and girth. The ulcers were partially covered by a serous exudate and by yellowish crusts the removal of which induced superficial bleeding (Fig. A).

Histopathologically, the epidermis and upper dermis were completely destroyed and replaced superficially by an admixture of polymormophonuclear leukocytes and fibrin. The epidermis surrounding the ulcers displayed pseudoepitheliomatous hyperplasia. The deeper dermis showed "grains" which stained positively with the McCallum-Goodpasture technique. There were also well-stained, Gram-positive, isolated organisms throughout the deeper dermis in the midst of newly formed vessels and a subacute inflammatory infiltrate (Fig. B).

Mycologically, smears were performed using the deeper portions of exudate obtained through surgical incision. Gram stains showed Gram-positive branching filaments about 1 mm in diameter which broke into bacillary forms. Cultures (GEORG et al 1961) were planted in Sabouraud's dextrose agar without antibiotics and using Petri dishes instead of slants. Incubation at room temperature yielded *Nocardia asteroides*.

Treatment consisted of initially wide and deep surgical drainage that was repeated 5 weeks later. Systemic treatment was carried out using sodium iodide I.V., first for 13 days and organic iodide P.O. (see Case 25). When the diagnosis of nocardiosis was confirmed, the treatment was changed to I.V. triple sulfas 500 mg/day for 7 days. After one week rest, the triple sulfas were repeated at the same dose for 10 more days. The patient responded very well but remained confined to the stall for 2 months. At the time of discharge, there were still small areas of alopecia but the lesion was otherwise almost healed (Fig. C).

CONNAR et al (1951) and CONANT et al (1971) have long emphasized that sulfonamides are very effective in the treatment of nocardiosis and that treatment must be continued until the active infection is controlled. This was the approach followed with this patient.

CONANT, N.F. SMITH, D.T., BAKER, R.D. and CALLAWAY, J.L.
Manual of Clinical Mycology. P. 58. W.B. Saunders Co. Philadelphia 1971.

CONNAR, R.G., FERGUSON, T.B., SEALY, W.C. and CONANT, N.F.
Nocardiosis. Report of a Single Case with Recovery. Journal of Thoracic Surgery 22:424, 1951.

GEORG, L.K., AJELLO, L., McDURMONT, C. and HOSTY, T.S.
The Identification of *Nocardia asteroides* and *Nocardia brasiliensis*. American Review of Respiratory Diseases 48:337, 1961.

A

B

C

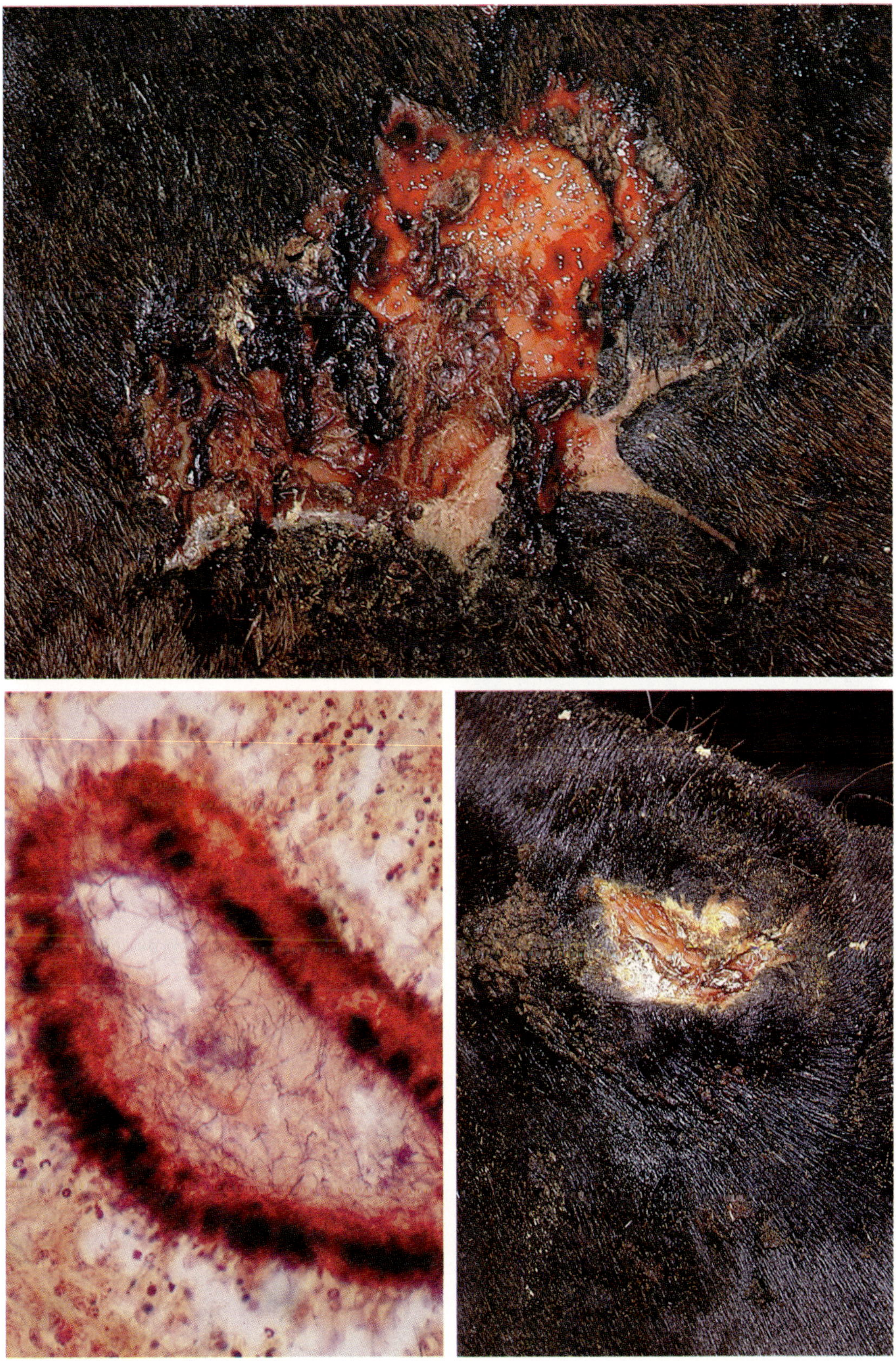

Phycomycosis

(Leeches)

A 19-year old Chestnut Thoroughbred mare was admitted for treatment of a chronic intractable granuloma referred to as leeches, or more specifically, Florida Leeches.

Clinically, a large (10×15 cm) indolent ulcer distorted the architecture of the lateral heel and extended from midway the pastern down onto the bearing surface of the foot (Fig. A). The fairly sharp though irregular border demarcating the lesion is misleading since leeches are characteristically of a phagedenic nature, undermining apparently normal skin and breaking out in an insidious, spreading process. A few satellite nodules outside the ulcer could be observed over the fetlock. The raw, granulomatous surface bled freely, especially at times when the mare would stamp the foot forcefully or chew at the lesion in agitation over what was interpreted to be intense pruritis. The loss of blood was sufficient to warrant identification of compatible donors. To further complicate matters, the mare was in advanced pregnancy.

Mycologically, cultures were planted in Sabouraud's dextrose agar without cycloheximide and chloramphenicol and incubated at 37 °C as recommended by BRIDGES and EMMONS, 1961. *Hyphomyces destruens* was isolated. Cycloheximide which is routinely employed as part of the culture media in the isolation of dermatophytes was avoided because it inhibits the growth of phycomycetes.

Histopathologically, the excised tissues contained yellowish branching masses of coagulation necrosis infiltrated by leukocytes and giant cells. Sections stained with PAS, Gridley and Gomori's silver methenamine showed wide branching hyphae (Fig. E).

Treatment consisted of local wound therapy under bandage and of systemic medication for an assortment of constitutional disorders, including purpura hemorrhagica, bacterial lymphangitis, herpesviral myelitis, and abortion due to rhinopneumonitis, and adrenocortical fatigue. The only unrelated problem was the equine herpesvirus infection presumptively due to an immunity break.

Sequential regimens of systemic antibiotic therapy, consisting of penicillin, gentamicin, cephalothin, and chloramphenicol were used to control bacterial infection. Phenylbutazone I.V. and P.O. and meclofenamic acid P.O. were used to suppress local inflammation and lameness. Adrenocorticosteroids and fresh whole blood transfusions were used in conjunction with antibiotics, antihistamines, and supportive medication to treat the purpura hemorrhagica. Adrenocorticotrophic hormone was used to treat the adrenal fatigue.

Local wound management included both electrofulguration and cryosurgery in addition to topical agents incorporating caustics, antiseptics, astringents, fungicidals (amphotericin), antibiotics, and stimulating embrocations. Cryosurgery was most impressive. Performed under local anesthesia, the procedure was repeated 3 times--on the 21st, 48th, and 69th hospital days according to the double or triple freeze-thaw cycle using a liquid nitrogen spray and an imbedded thermocouple to measure subsurface temperatures from minus 20° to 40°C. The wound was kept bandaged at all times. It was not until after the third cryosurgery had sloughed that the granulating tissue bed ceased to yield the caseous cores so typical of phycomycosis and seen in the cut surface of the biopsy specimen (Fig D).

Despite the stormy clinical course of complications, both local and systemic, the foot continued to respond to treatment (Fig. B) and was healing satisfactorily when discharged (Fig. C). It is perhaps noteworthy that the mare was transported to Kentucky for the final healing processes to occur before being returned to Florida. Four years later, the foot has healed completely (Figs F and G), bears weight, and conforms well in relationship to the fetlock and pastern (Figs. H and I). The mare is also breeding sound.

In Indonesia *Basidiobolus ranarum* was first isolated from a mare observed with this condition (VAN OVEREEM, 1925). The study by BRIDGES AND EMMONS (1961) including 23

A B C D E

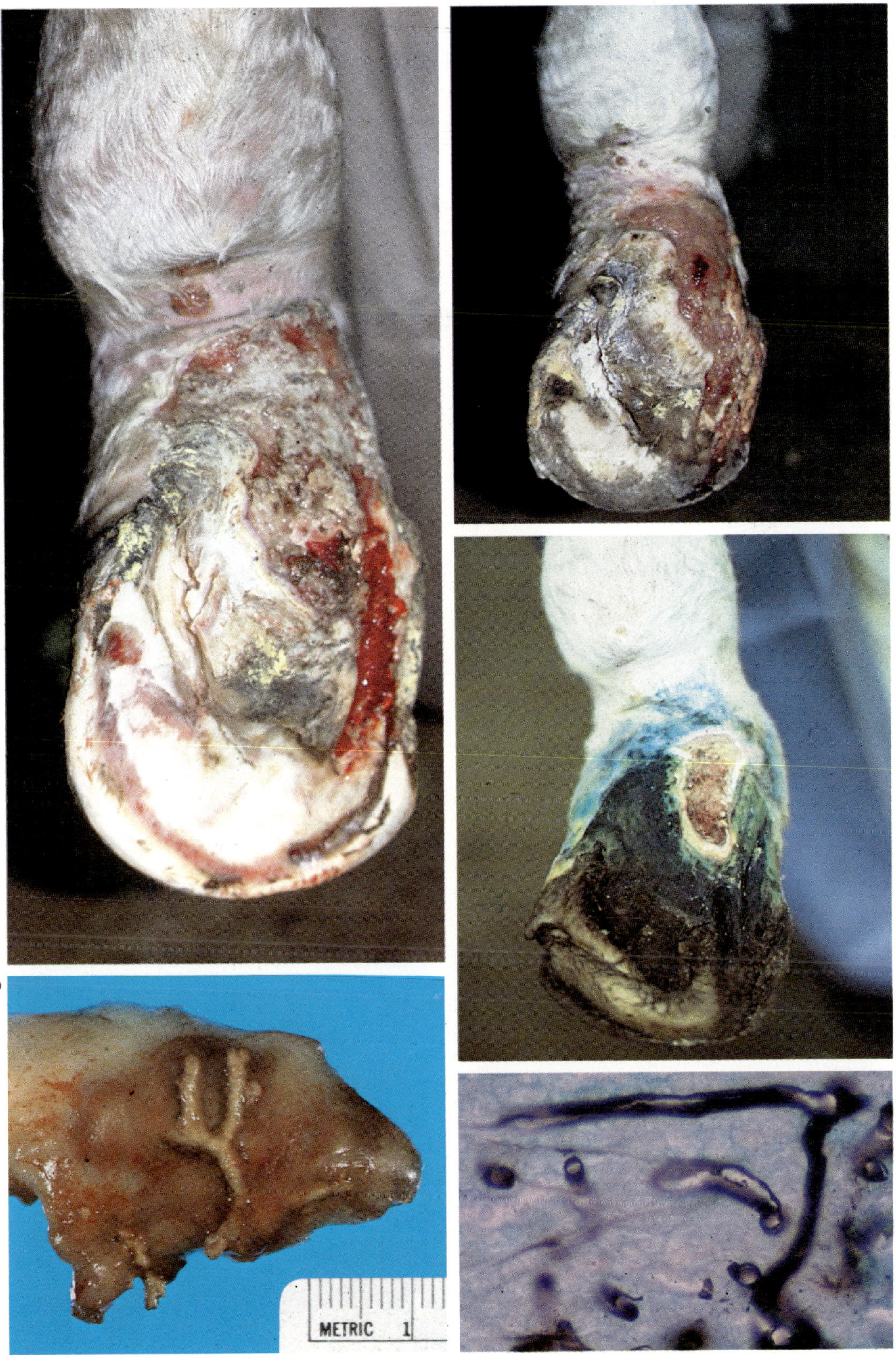

Phycomycosis

(Leeches)

A 19-year old Chestnut Thoroughbred mare was admitted for treatment of a chronic intractable granuloma referred to as leeches, or more specifically, Florida Leeches.

cases has contributed enormously to the understanding of phycomycosis in horses. The most common fungus isolated in this series was *Hyphomyces destruens*. It is noteworthy that the six patients described in detail by BRIDGES and EMMONS were mares like our patient. BRIDGES et al (1962) in another study reported *Entomophotora coronata* as another etiologic agent of phycomycosis in horses.

BRIDGES, C.H. and EMMONS, C.W.
A Phycomycosis of Horses Caused by *Hyphomyces destruens*. Journal of the American Veterinary Medical Association 138:579, 1961.
BRIDGES, C.H., ROMANE, W.M. and EMMONS, C.W.
Phycomycosis of Horses Caused by *Entomophotora coronata*. Journal of the American Veterinary Medical Association 140:672, 1962.
VAN OVEREEM, C.
Beiträge zur Pilzflora von Niederlandisch Indien. Bulletin Jardin Bot 7:423, 1925. (Grateful acknowledgement to Dr. Jay M. Humburg and Dr. Linda Dopson for assistance with this case.)

F

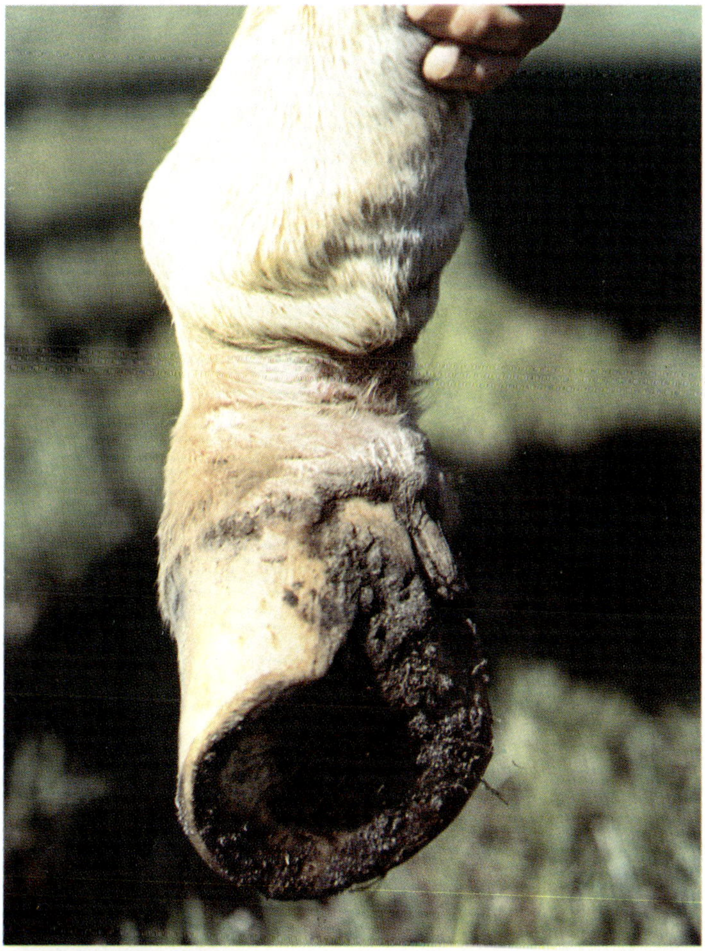

G

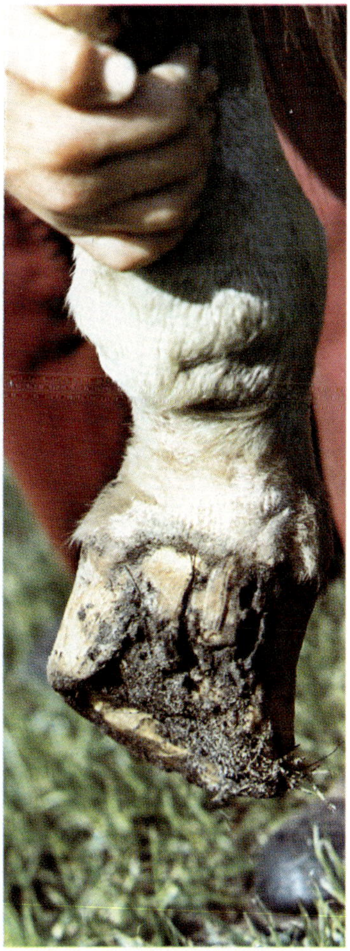

H

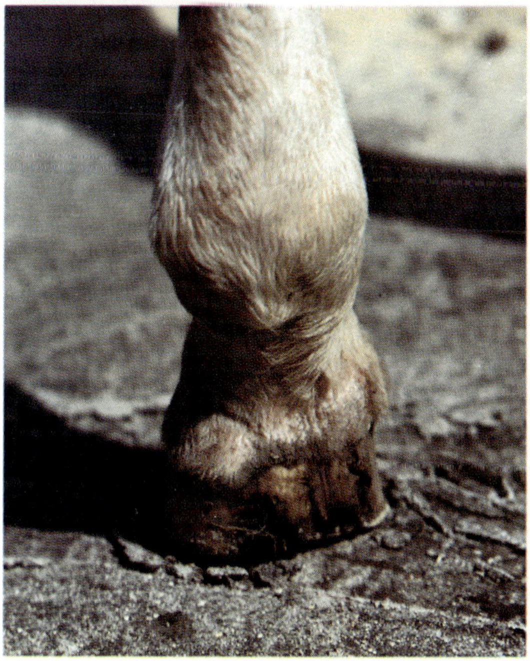

I

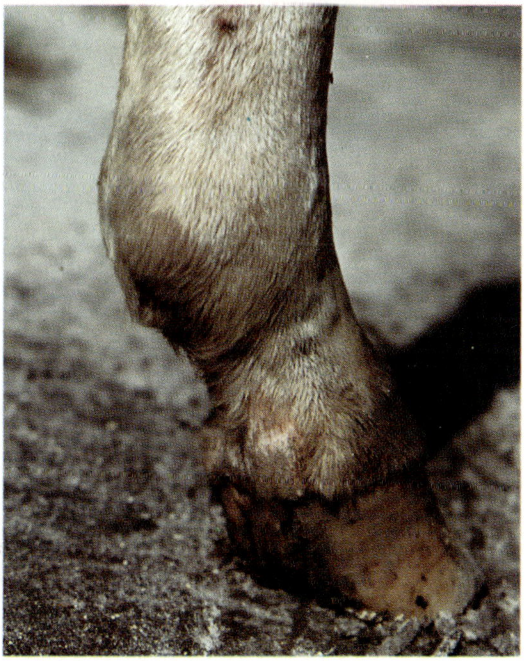

Viral Infections

Patients in this chapter are examples of viral infections of the epidermis where the keratinocytes become heavily invaded by *Papovaviridae*.

These DNA viruses invade mainly the nuclei of the keratinocytes. In the management of patients like these one must remember the need for steady and often prolonged treatment.

Recurrence of the lesions and frequent transmission to other horses can only be prevented by complete eradication of the infection.

Warts

A 3-year-old female Quarter Horse was brought for consultation because of an unusually large number of warts which began to develop about one year earlier.

Clinically, there were multiple, yellowish and brownish, firm, hyperkeratotic papules. Some lesions were isolated but many were grouped and concentrated forming large plaques and tumors around the muzzle and ears (Figs A and B).

Histopathologically, serial sections of many biopsy specimens showed hyperkeratosis, acanthosis, papillomatosis and vacuolated cells filled with deeply basophilic bodies of different sizes. A chronic dermal inflammatory infiltrate was also observed (Figs C and D).

Treatment of warts in horses is somewhat optional because active acquired immunity to the wart virus is usually sufficient to effect a spontaneous cure by the third year of life. In this patient, topical 0.1% retinoic acid cream was applied B.I.D. as recommended by DE BERSAQUES (1975) for human warts. Rapid involution with complete clearing occurred after three months of continuous therapy.

In such locations as in this patient, warts may cause much discomfort when aggravated by mechanical irritation from eating and rubbing, as well as by biting flies and gnats which are attracted to the face and ears of the horse. Accumulations of warts in the ears may cause conchal deformities. Soreness may increase the difficulty of bridling or grooming the head. As typical as is the gross appearance of warts on the horse's muzzle, the ear lesions must be differentiated from sarcoids and from the hyperkeratotic plaques that so often follow in the wake of chronic dermatitis caused by the bloodfeeding Buffalo gnat, *Eusimulium pecuarum* (Family Simuliidae). This underscores the need for microscopic study.

In humans, all the clinical forms of warts are caused by a single *Papillomavirus,* a member of the Papovavirus family. Warts virus can be transmitted to volunteers by intradermal inoculation of filtrates from warts. The incubation period varies from 6 weeks to a year. Antibody against the human wart virus can be detected by immunodiffusion or immunoelectronmicroscopy. (FENNER and WHITE 1976). In warts the virus grows abundantly within the nucleus of epidermal cells, sometimes invading also the cytoplasm through the nuclear pores. The vacuolated cells are not the only ones infected (LAURENT et al 1975).

DE BERSAQUES, J. Journal of Cutaneous Pathology 2:160, 1975.
FENNER, F. and WHITE, D.O.
Medical Virology. Academic Press, New York 1976.
LAURENT, R., AGACHE, P. and COUME;Marquet, J.
Ultrastructure of Clear Cells in Human Viral Warts. Journal of Cutaneous Pathology 2:140, 1975.

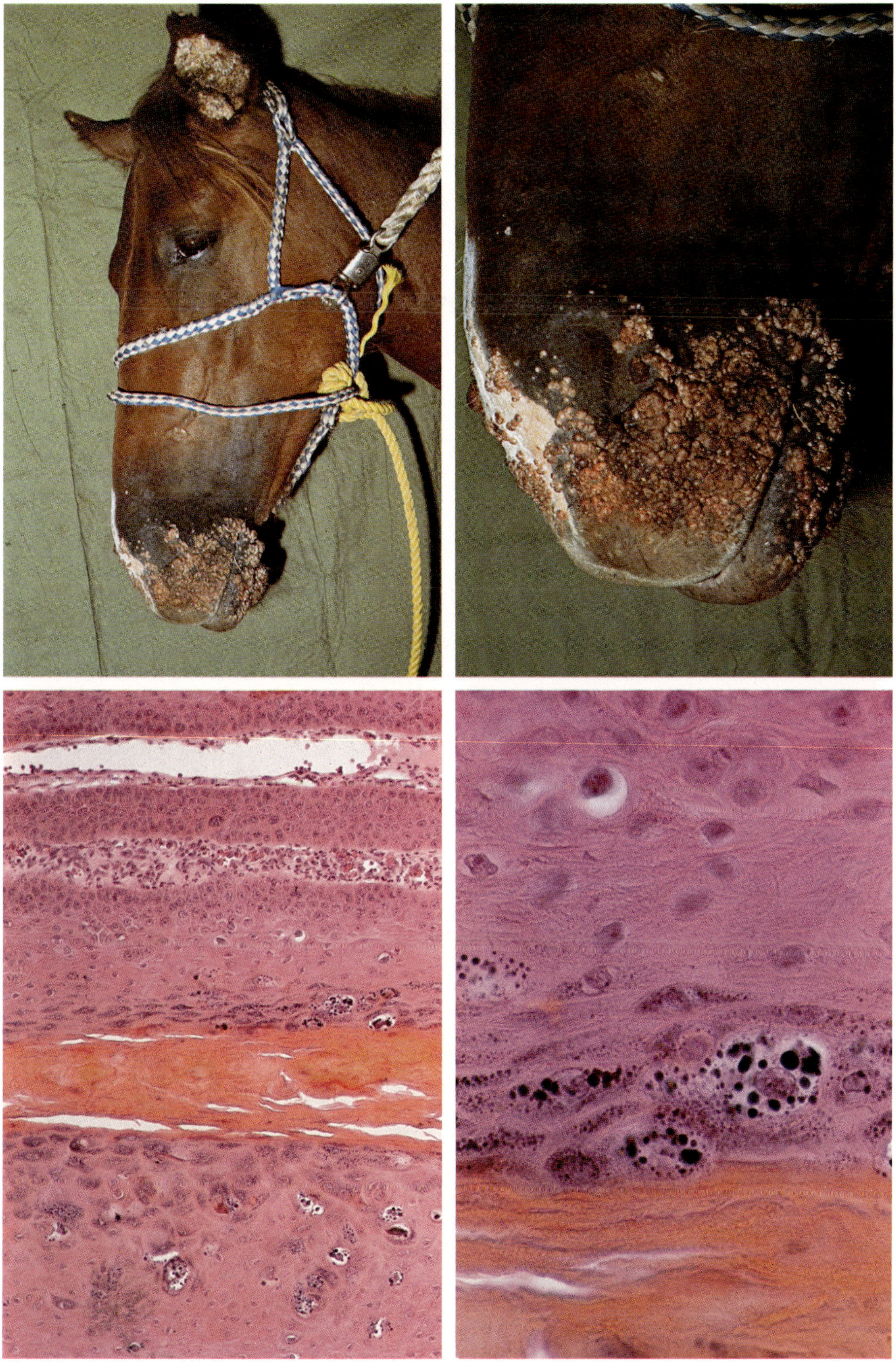

A B C D

Warts

A 2-year-old male Quarter Horse was referred for evaluation and treatment of warts on the left ear which had started to develop six months earlier.

Clinically, there were about ten acuminate whitish papillomatous lesions in the central area of the inner aspect of the left ear lobe. The size of the lesions was 3–5 mm in diameter at the base and 2–10 mm in height. The lesions were so close to each other that in several points their bases were confluent. Thus when observed from the distance the condition appeared at first as a single tumor. Close inspection, however, revealed the multiple nature of the warts. The uninvolved skin surrounding the warts showed loss of hair and was covered by scales. There was lack of induration, however (Fig. A).

Histopathologically, the stratum corneum was not only thickened (hyperkeratosis) but also displayed retention of nuclei (parakeratosis). The granular layer was very prominent not only because of its increased thickness but also because of the large vacuolated cells. There were various degrees of vacuolization: in some cells the vacuole occupied about half of the perinuclear zone in a crescent-like shape; in other cells the vacuole surrounded the entire nucleus. Keratohyalin granules were in some cells at the periphery of the vacuole and in other cells within the vacuoles (Fig. B). The superficial dermis contained a chronic inflammatory infiltrate.

Treatment was carried out by surgical removal according to the following steps: 1) washing of the ear with an hexachlorophene containing liquid cleanser; 2) topical antisepsis with 95% ethyl alcohol; 3) local anesthesia using 2 cm^3 of lidocaine; 4) excision employing curved scissors with removal of entire affected area plus a margin of three millimeters of the surrounding uninvolved skin; 5) electrofulguration of the bleeding points. The owner of the horse was instructed to apply neomycin cream 0.5% twice daily during the two weeks following the procedure.

It is advisable to recommend also, after complete healing has taken place, the institution of once/day applications of 0.1% retinoic acid cream. A normal metabolite of retinol (DE LUCA and SUTTIE 1969), this substance, when topically applied, induces an increase in epidermal mitotic activity, which in turn results in the production of less cohesiveness of horny cells enabling them to dehisce (KLIGMAN et al 1969, MONTES et al 1974).

DE LUCA, H.F. and SUTTIE, J.W.
The Fat Soluble Vitamins. The University Of Wisconsin Press Madison 1969.

KLIGMAN, A.M., FULTON, Jr., J.E. and PLEWING, G.
Topical Vitamin A Acid in Acne Vulgaris. Archives of Dermatology 99:469, 1969.

MONTES, L.F., HIRSCHOWITZ, B.I. and KRUMDIECK, C.M.
Acanthosis Nigricans and Hypovitaminosis A. Response to topical Vitamin A Acid. Journal of Cutaneous Pathology 1:88, 1974.

A

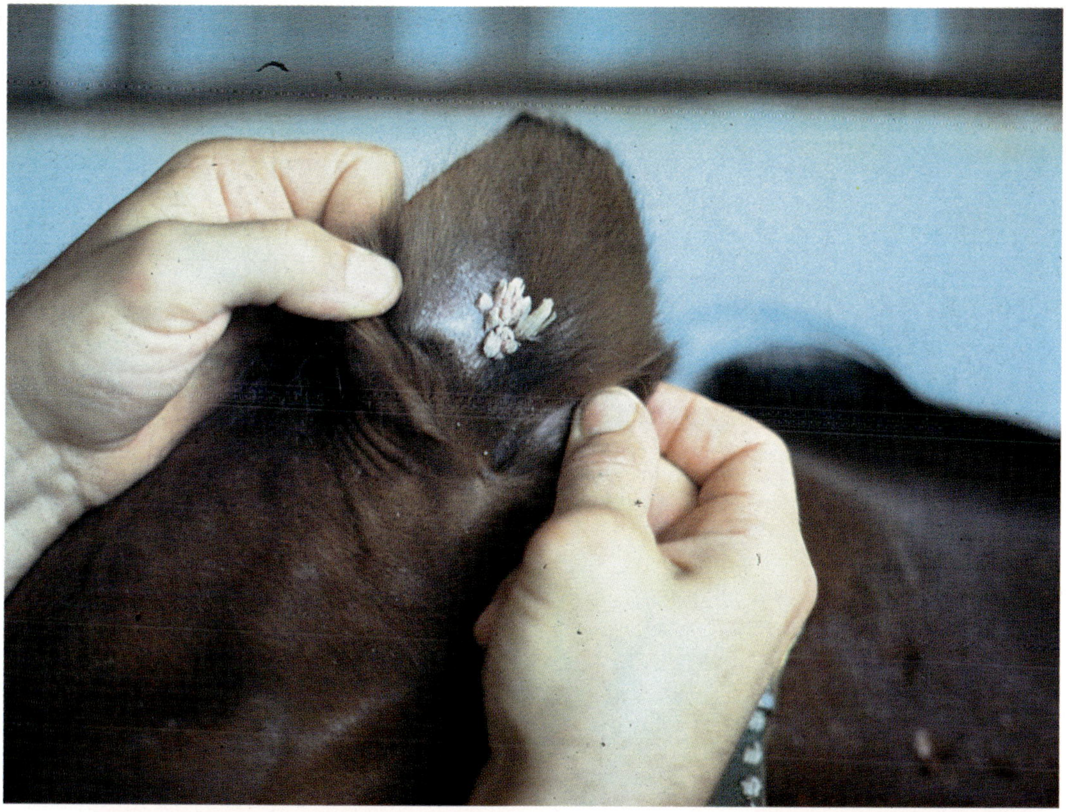

B

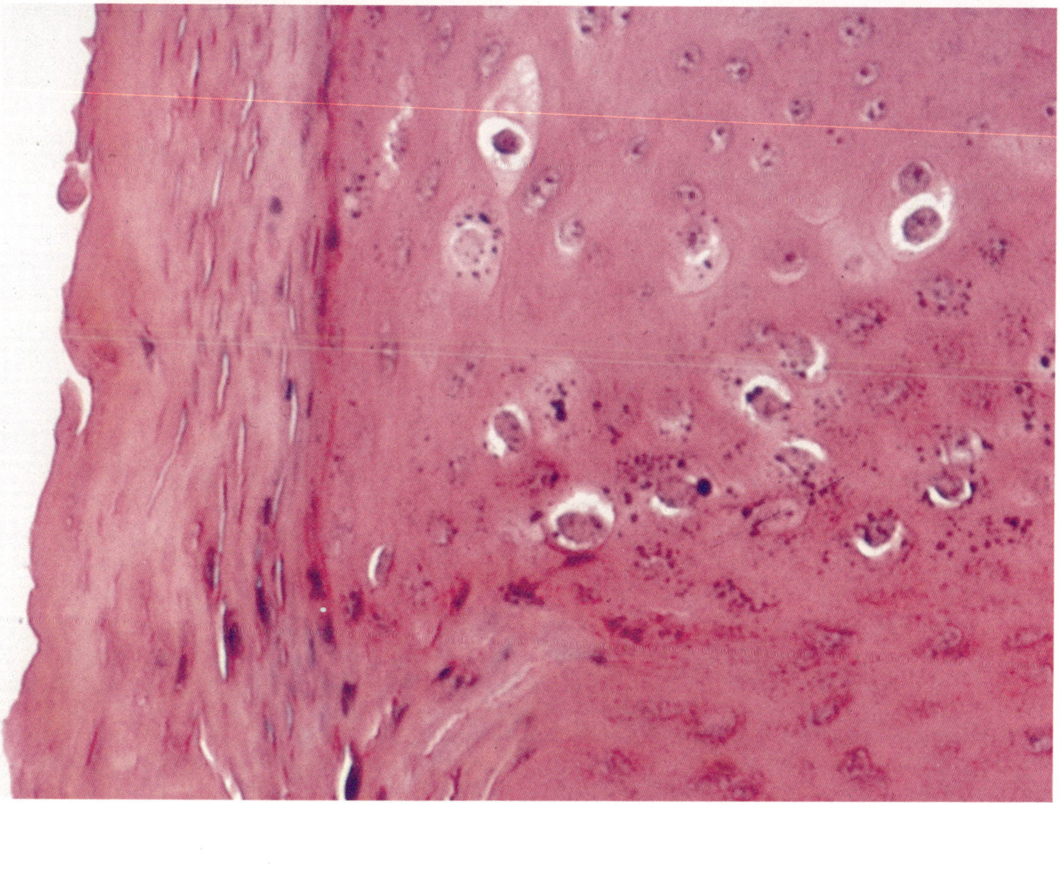

Warts

A 5-year-old male Tennessee Walking Horse required evaluation and treatment of multiple lesions on the muzzle of approximately one year duration which were gradually growing in size and number.

Clinically, there were about one hundred rounded lesions ranging from pinhead-sized papules to small tumors about 2 cm diameter (Fig. A). The lesions were hard in texture, and white to yellowish in color. Their surface was fairly smooth in the smaller lesions but rough in the larger ones, some of which were superficially eroded.

Histopathologically, there was marked hyperkeratosis, and pronounced ancanthosis. The characteristic vacuolization, together with increased accumulation of keratohyalin, were striking in cells of the granular layer (Fig. B and C). The superficial dermis revealed a subacute inflammatory infiltrate.

Treatment was carried out with very small amounts of 0.1% cycloheximide ointment, applied twice daily over a period of two months. The treatment resulted in mild desquamation and erythema over the area of application, but there was an almost immediate response. The warts gradually diminished in size and number and when the patient was examined again six months later there was no evidence of warts. Residual and temporary mild hyperpigmentation was the only visible change.

Cycloheximide ($C_{15}H_{23}NO_4$) is an antiviral, an antimitotic and an inhibitor of the synthesis of DNA and protein. This antibiotic has already been used systemically to treat human cryptococcosis. It was first isolated from the beers of *Streptomyces griseus.*

Despite its potency, the effects of cycloheximide on mammalian cells are reversible. Because of its strong action, however, this experimental drug – not yet available for clinical use – should be employed on very small areas and in minimal amounts and with extreme caution until a complete evaluation of its safety is accomplished (HERRMANN 1965, MONTES 1976).

In this patient, the topical chemotherapy was preferred over surgical treatment because of the very large number of lesions and the location. In this situation, it is practically impossible to achieve complete eradication of the infection by destructive methods alone which are usually followed by recurrence. Although the precise infective mechanisms in warts are not fully understood, transmission electron microscopy has provided an excellent view of the viral-host relationship in the keratinocytes (LUTZNER 1967).

HERRMANN, Jr. E.C.
Antiviral Substances. Annals of The New York Academy of Sciences 130:330, 1965.
LUTZNER, M.A.
Virus Diseases. In Ultrastructure of Normal and Abnormal Skin. Edited by A.S. Zelickson. Lea and Febiger. Philadelphia 1967.
MONTES, L.F.
Topical Cycloheximide in Psoriasis Journal of Cutaneous Pathology 3:1, 1976.

PLATE 30

A C

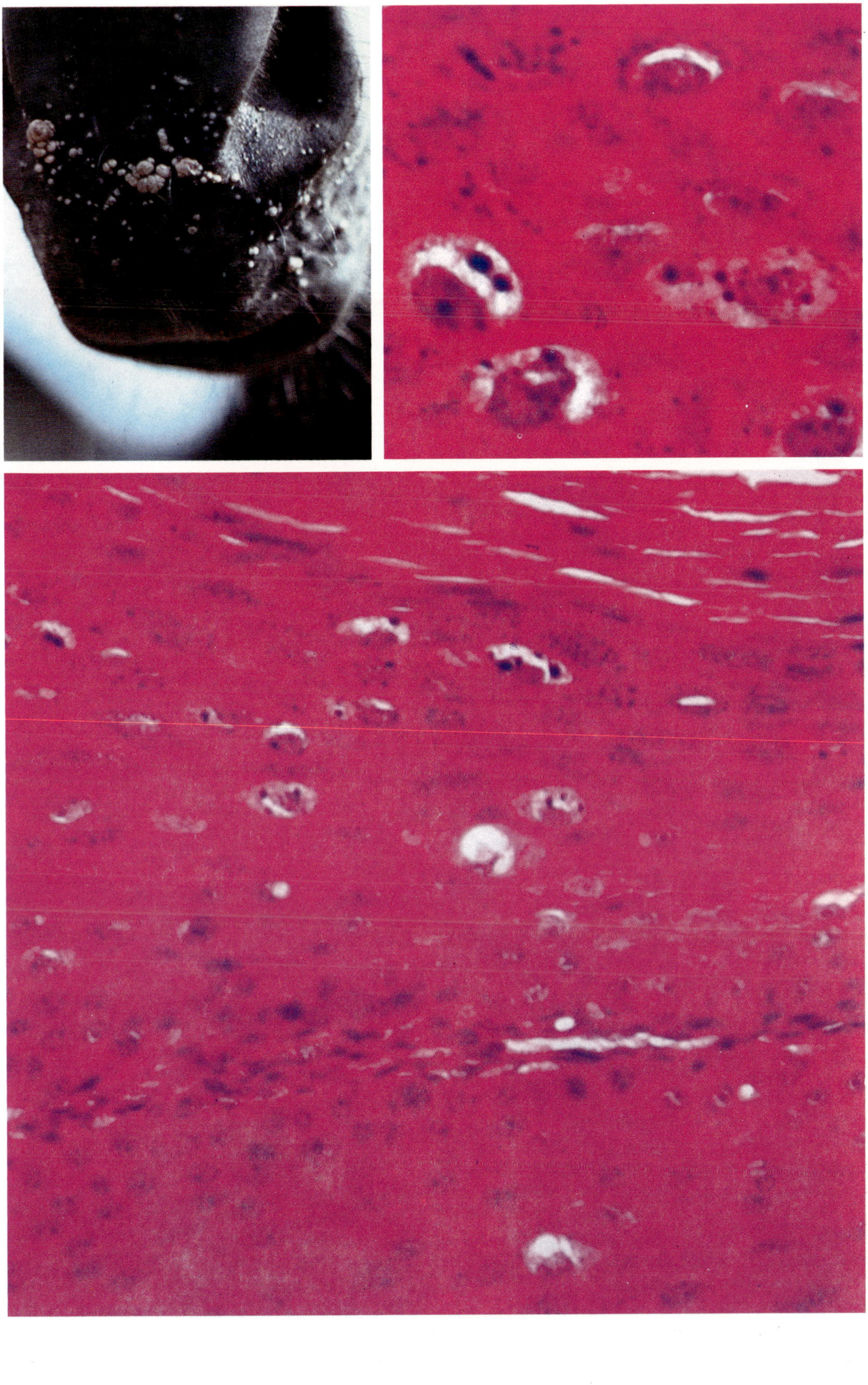

B

Condylomata Acuminata

(Venereal Warts)

A 5-year-old Thoroughbred chestnut mare was observed in a large breeding farm because of multiple gradually spreading lesions noticed for approximately one year over the vulva and the perianal areas.

Clinically, there were moist warts that stood out because of their whitish color which contrasted strikingly with the surrounding, normally pigmented, uninvolved skin. While many of the lesions were flat and not quite papillomatous, others were raised over the skin surface. A suggestion of Koebner phenomenon could be noticed upon close inspection (Fig. A).

Histopathologically, marked acanthosis, numerous mitoses, prominently vacuolated epidermal cells and a chronic dermal inflammatory infiltrate were seen (Fig. B) (LEVER 1975). Interestingly, melanin in the basal cell layer was not visible in the lesions, but was well apparent in the normal epidermis at the edges of the lesions. Thus the contrast between the affected and the nonaffected skin was also striking microscopically (Figs. C and D).

Treatment with repeated weekly topical applications of 20% podophyllin in 95% ethyl alcohol produced rapid involution and final cure. When using podophyllin in this fashion, the surrounding normal skin should be protected from irritation. It is then advisable to use a very small cotton applicator in order to dab the solution on the lesions only. Since some spreading of the podophyllin solution onto the normal skin is unavoidable, this can be minimized by applying petrolatum around the lesions just before the treatment. Although an accurate diagnosis had not been established, when first seen by the local veterinarian, the contagious nature of this condition was suspected. Hence the mare was kept isolated from the stallions, an important measure that most likely prevented dissemination of the infection in the farm.

Condylomata acuminata are caused by a virus believed to be the same one which produces common warts. Because these papovaviruses induce a true proliferative response, the papillomas can be regarded as one of the benign virus-induced tumors of the skin (STEIGLEDER 1978). However it should be kept in mind that malignant transformation of condyloma acuminatum into squamous cell carcinoma can occur (ROOK et al 1972), another important reason for complete eradication of this infection.

LEVER, W. F.
Histopathology of the Skin. J. B. Lippincott, Philadelphia, 1975.
ROOK, A. J., EBLING, F. J. G. and WILKINSON, D. J.
Textbook of Dermatology. Blackwell Scientific Publications, Oxford 1972.
STEIGLEDER, G. K.
Histology of Benign Virus Induced Tumors of the Skin. Journal of Cutaneous Pathology 5:45, 1978.

A B

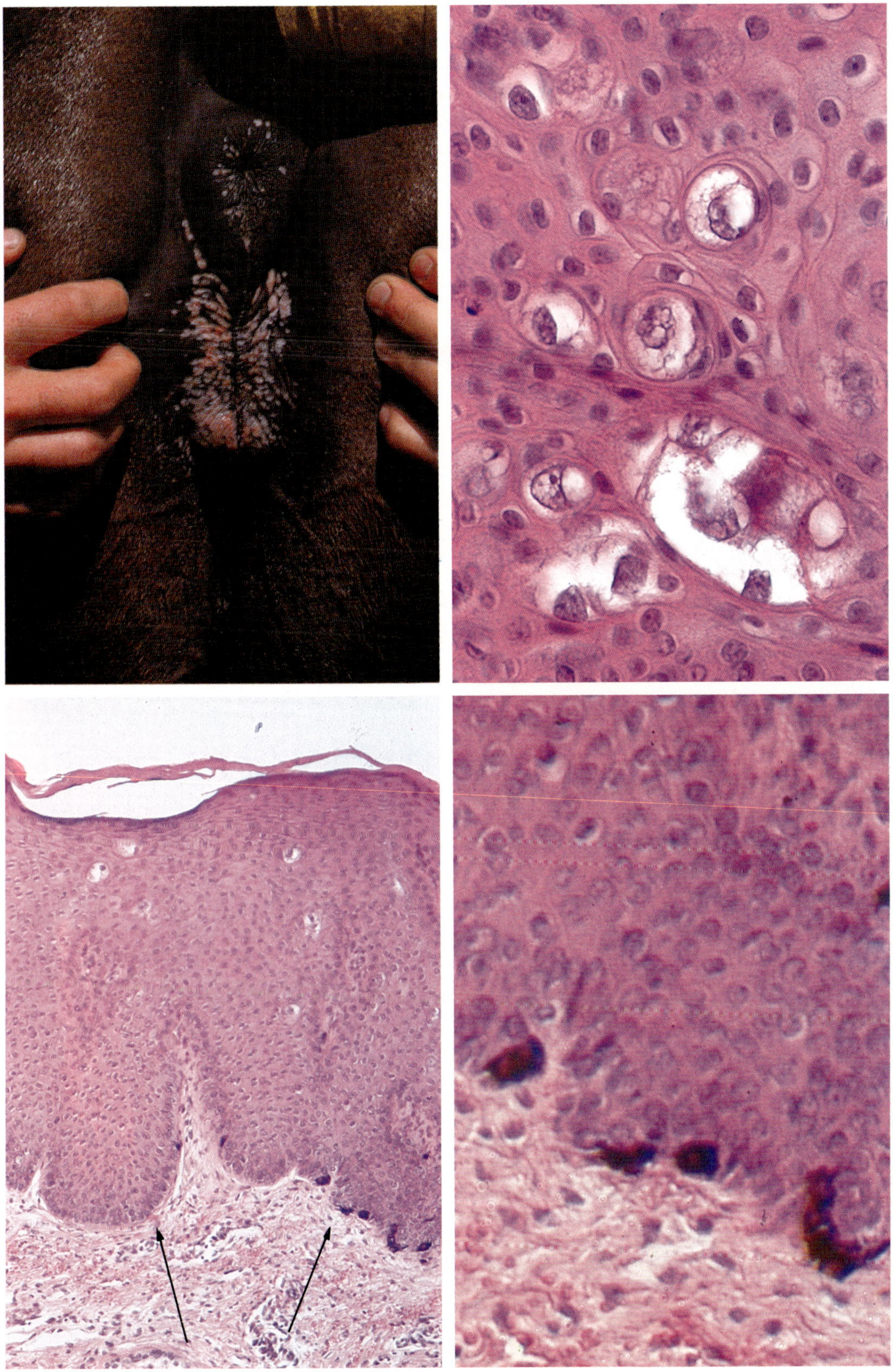

C D

Condylomata Acuminata

(Venereal Warts)

A 7-year-old male pony (gelding) was admitted to the Large Animal Clinic because of surgery for upward patellar fixation. Examination of the patient disclosed in addition a dermatological problem on the penis.

Clinically, there were many white moist warts spread over the surface of the shaft of the penis concentrated around the urethral orifice (Fig. A) and particularly confluent forming a solid plaque in parts of the balanopreputial sulcus. The surface of the lesions was in certain parts eroded, crusty or bloody. Some places in the vicinity of the warty growths were depigmented and scaly (Fig. B).

Histopathologically, the epidermis was hyperkeratotic and acanthotic. The most important finding was large clear cells throughout the stratum spinosum. These cells were more prominent near the stratum corneum and less prominent near the stratum basale. The nucleus of the clear cells was sometimes marginally displaced leaving a cytoplasm that was slightly basophilic and granular. A bandlike inflammatory infiltrate occupied the upper dermis and was mostly made up of lymphocytes and monocytes. While the basal cells showed little if any melanin, this was prominent in the basal cells of the uninvolved skin next to the lesion (Fig. C).

Treatment was carried out with topical application of 20% podophyllin ointment once daily during one month. The procedure was carefully performed using small cotton applicators and very small amounts of the medication. Only the affected skin was treated. When minimal irritation – a normal reaction to podophyllin – was noticed on a given site, treatment in that area was spared for one or two days. Regression of the lesions, estimated in about 80%, was accomplished after the first month of treatment. During a second month, the frequency of applications was reduced to one every other day. At the end of this second month complete disappearance of the lesions was noticed.

Podophyllin is a resin obtained from the roots of *Podophyllum peltatum* (Mandrake). It is a powder light brown to greenish yellow in color (OSOL and PRATT 1973) and has an antimitotic effect through interference of epithelial cells mitoses in metaphase (SULLIVAN and KING 1946). Podophyllin does not show the same effectiveness for common warts as it does for condylomata acuminata. The giant condyloma acuminata of Buschke-Lowenstein is an infrequent type which may develop in the anal or vulvar areas or in the prepuce with invasion of the corpora cavernosa of the urethra. Because of the resemblance of this type of lesion to squamous cell carcinoma, multiple biopsies from several different sites are sometimes necessary. For this tumor, surgical excision or cryosurgery are recommended.

MACHACEK, G. F. and WEAKLEY, D. R.
Giant Condylomata Acuminata of Buschke and Lowenstein. Archives of Dermatology 82:41, 1960.
OSOL, A. and PRATT, R.
The United States Dispensatory Lippincott Company, Philadelphia 1973.
SULLIVAN, M. and KING,
Effects of Podophyllin on Condylomata Acuminata and Verrucae Vulgares. Archives of Dermatology and Syphilology 56:30, 1947.

A

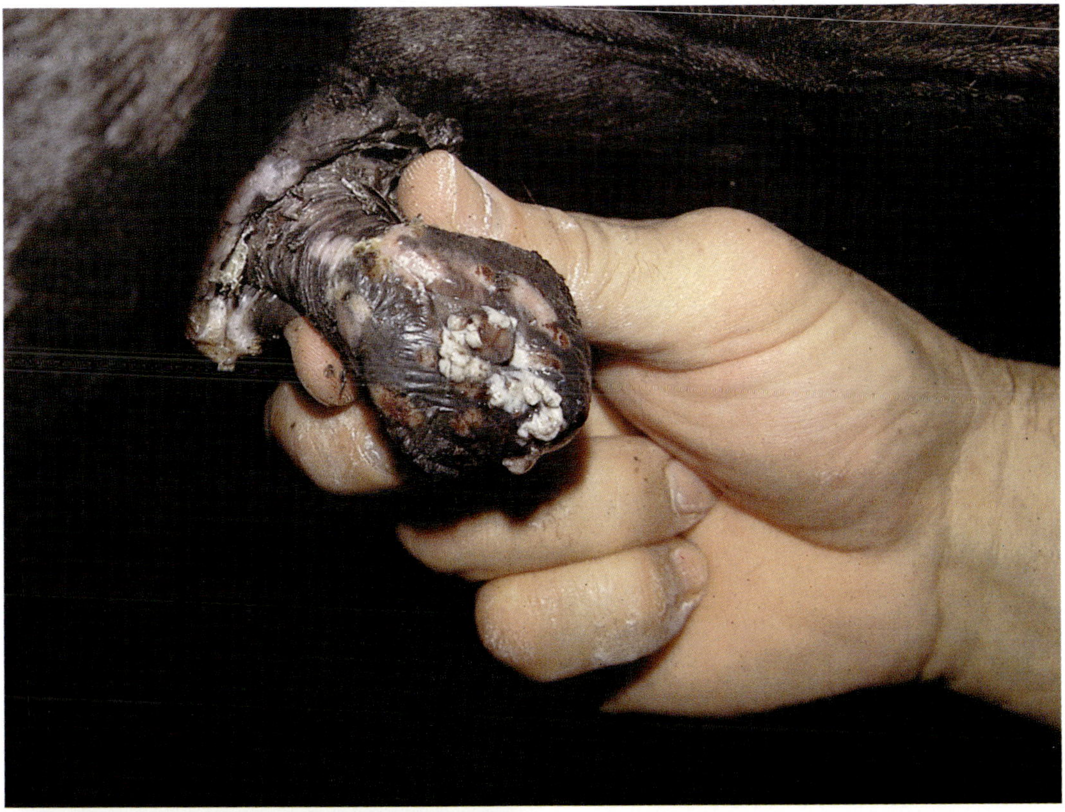

B

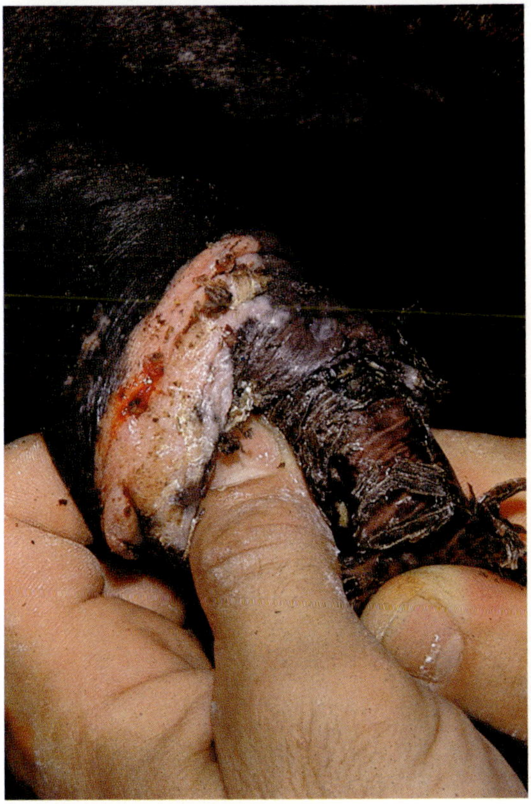

C

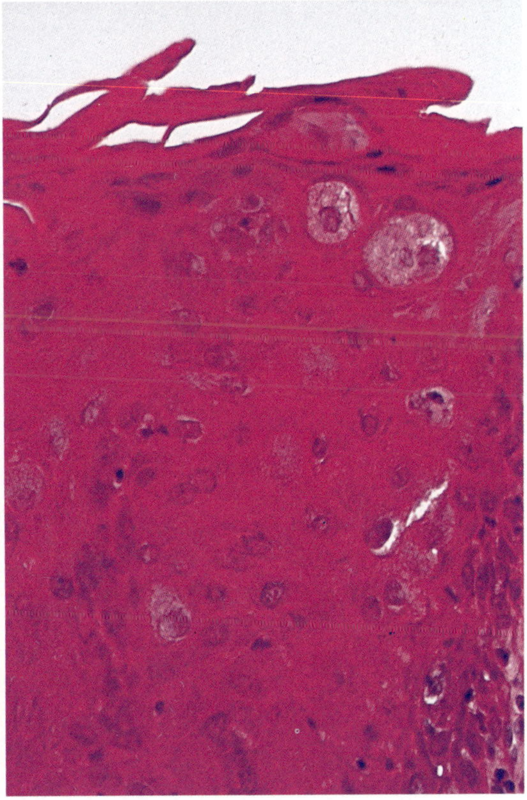

Parasitoses

The skin of the horse can be quite susceptible to infestation by parasites.

Notable examples are some members of the spirouidea family *(Habronema SP)* and some members of the onchocercidae family *(Onchocerca SP)*.

Cutaneous parasitoses can be accompanied by systemic infestation. Furthermore, if they reach a chronic stage and run a protracted course, serious impairment of important functions may occur.

DUNN, A. M.
VETERINARY HELMINTHOLOGY.
William Heinemann Medical Books Ltd. London 1978.

Habronemiasis

A 9 year old male Appaloosa was presented with severe "summer sores" of long duration, typified by exacerbation in the summer months.

Clinically, there were chronic indolent granulomas of the penis and prepuce with ulcerated red areas demarcated by edges of depigmented skin. Pressure on the lesions yielded caseous granules resembling, if not identical to, the Bollinger's granules seen in botryomycosis. The process showed also some predilection for the preputial ring (Figs. A and B). Incomplete retraction of the penis was the result of mechanical interference with the normal telescoping action of the preputial laminae caused by the space-occupying granuloma and chronic scar formation.

Histopathologically, there was a superficial crust in the ulcerated areas. The periphery of the ulcers displayed focal parakeratosis, marked acanthosis and intact epidermodermal junction. Dilated capillaries and an impressive number of eosinophils were seen throughout the dermis (Fig. C). A striking feature was also large lobulated granules made-up of eosinophils, nuclear remnants and nematode larvae. The larvae were few in number but impressive in size, measuring up to 60 microns in diameter and up to 15 mm in length. They were often undergoing septation and surrounded by a clear halo (Fig. D).

Treatment consisted of 1) the organophosphate, trichlorfon, by slow-drip intravenous administration, 22 mg/kg body weight diluted in 2 l of sterile physiological saline solution, for the active parasitism (BOYD and BULLARD 1968) and 2) revisionary surgery to excise the chronic scar formation. The incision was reconstructed under dermal mattress sutures. Nitrofurazone 0.2% dressing with trichlorphon incorporated for repellant as well as parasiticidal activity was used topically on a daily basis along with wound toilet. Sutures were removed in 10 days.

The seasonal prevalence of these "summer sores" is associated with the presence of flies which are intermediate hosts. Thus the control of flies in any stable or farm is of paramount importance for prophylaxis, particularly in those geographic areas where habronemiasis is endemic.

The clear zone surrounding the larvae indicates that some sort of lytic action may be exerted by the nematode on the tissue of the host. It is highly reminiscent of the phenomenon observed in cases of human candidiasis (MONTES and WILBORN 1968).

BOYD, C. L. and BULLARD, T. L.
Organophosphate Treatment of Cutaneous Habronemiasis in Horses. Journal American Veterinary Medical Association 153:324-, 1968.
DRUDGE, J. H.
Metazoal Diseases in Equine Medicine and Surgery. Pages 174–175. American Veterinary Publications Wheaton, Illinois 1972.
MONTES, L. F. and WILBORN, W. H.
Ultrastructural Features of Host-Parasite Relationship in Oral Candidiasis. Journal of Bacteriology 96:1349–1356, 1968.

A B

C D

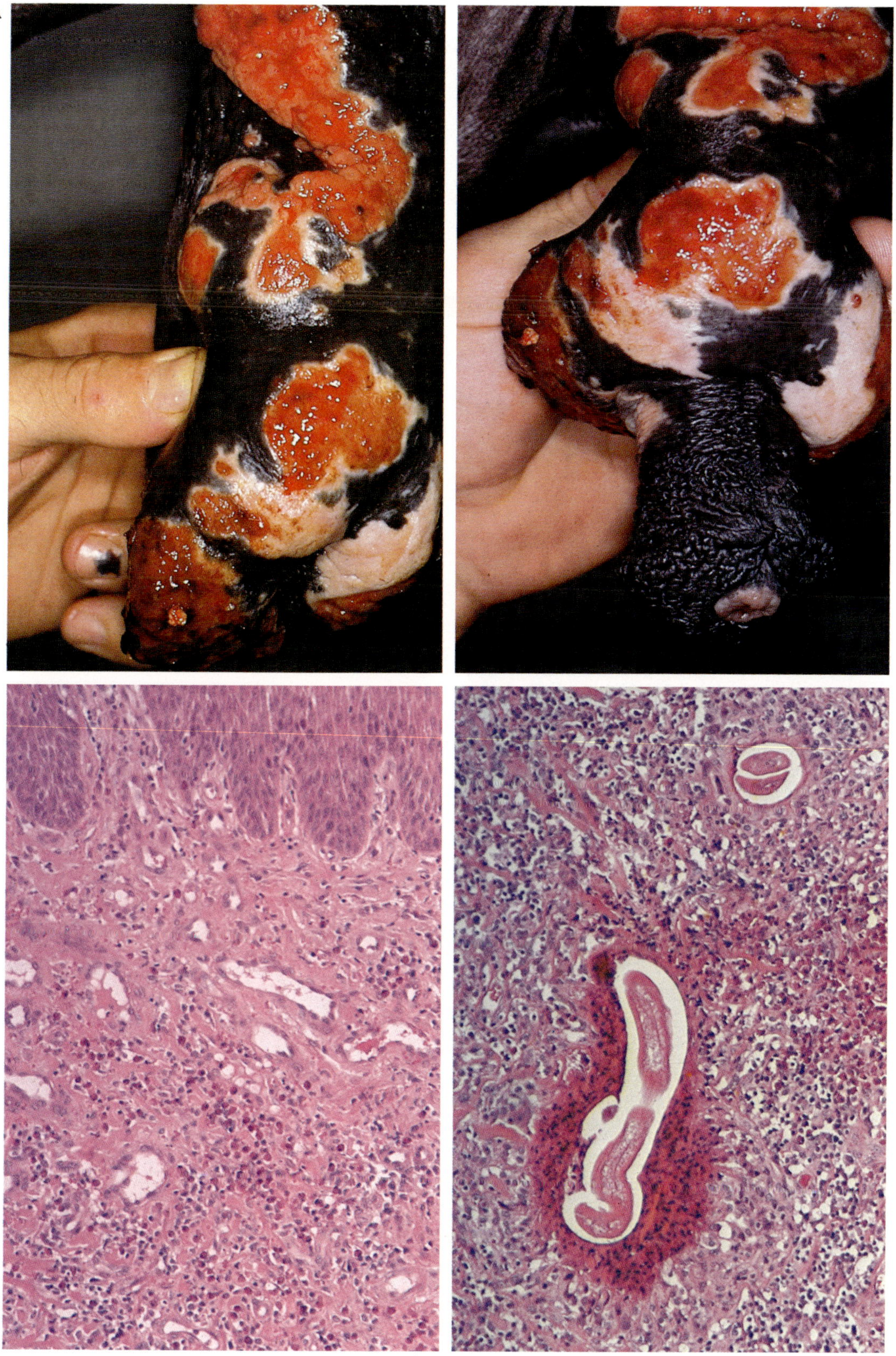

Habronemiasis

A 5-year-old Arabian stallion required treatment for a chronic "summer sore" under the lower jaw. The lesion had persisted for 8 weeks despite treatment by the owner and was complicated by aggravation of the halter.

Clinically, the lesion was an oval ulcer over the ventral border of the left ramus of the mandible, well demarcated by a fairly sharp elevated edge and displaying a moist but clean granulating surface, mostly with a red color but also including some yellow areas (Fig. A). In contrast to the exuberant characteristics of many parasitic granulomas, the ulcer had a flattened contour.

Histopathologically, there was a thin eosinophilic crust covering a superficial layer of edema, extravasated blood cells and dilated capillaries (Fig. B). Deeper into the dermis, vascular proliferation and an impressive degree of tissue eosinophilia were the striking features. The eosinophils were also prominent within the dermal capillaries (Fig. C). Careful study of serial sections revealed a very small number of nematode larvae.

Treatment consisted of a single intravenous dose of trichlorfon, 22 mg/kg, diluted in 2 l sterile physiological saline solution and given by slow drip as a precaution against organophosphate toxicity. Topical therapy with a trichlorfon-nitrofurozone paste was continued on a daily basis as the ulcer regressed in size and the surface underwent epithelialization. The rope halter, considered to be the source of the irritation, was replaced with a leather halter that avoided contact with the wound.

The topical preparation of trichlorfon as recommended by McMULLAN (1972) used in this horse was as follows:

Trichlorfon powder	4.5 gm
Nitrofurazone dressing	4–8 oz
DMSO qs ad	thick paste

The excellent results obtained in this case can be explained in part because of the relatively prompt treatment instituted before the ulcer became deeper and larger. It emphasizes the importance of an early and accurate diagnosis. The ulcer was also free of secondary bacterial infection. As an interesting sidelight, chronic chest abscesses in the horse have been attributed to a complication from secondary infection by *Corynebacterium tuberculosis* liberated by infected *Habronema* larvae (REID 1965). A preparation used earlier to prevent contamination by flies included topical phenol combined with tar in glycerine as a vehicle (UNDERWOOD 1936).

McMULLAN, W.C.
Equine Dermatology 4–7. College of Veterinary Medicine, Texas A and M University, 1976.
REID, C.H.
Habronemiasis and Corynebacterium "Chest" Abscess in California Horses. Veterinary Medicine Small Animal Clinic 60:233–242, 1965.
UNDERWOOD, J.R.
Habronemiasis Veterinary Bulletin. U. S. Army 16–28, 1936.

A

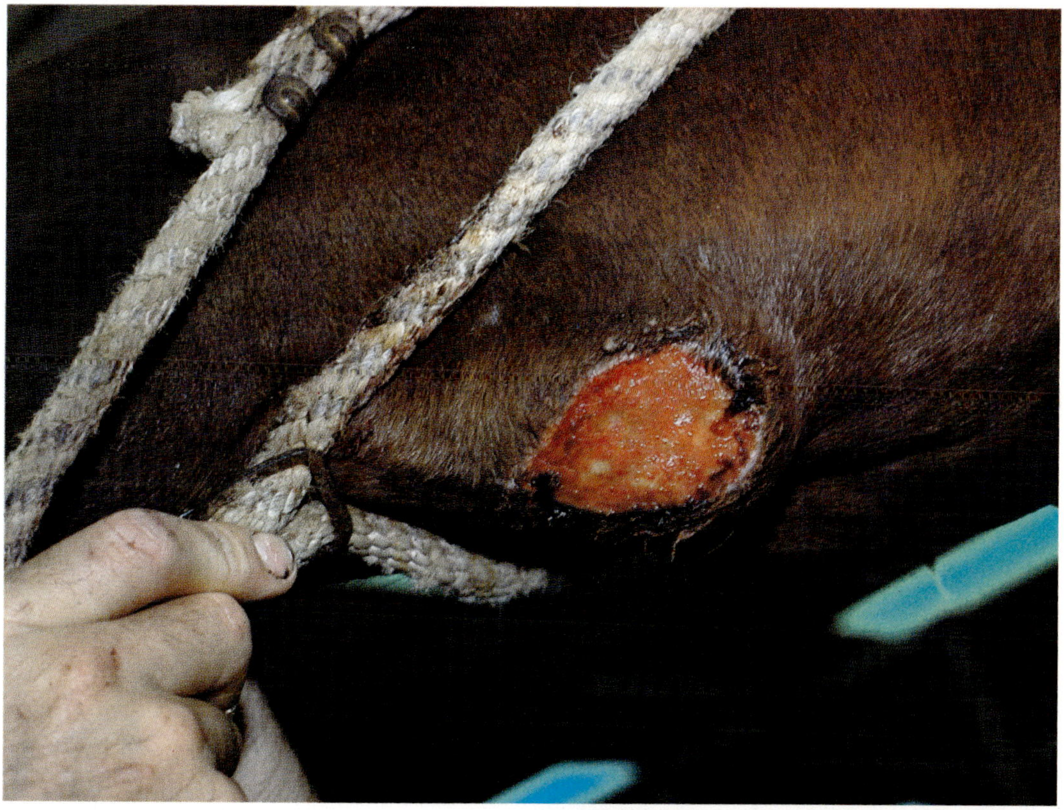

B

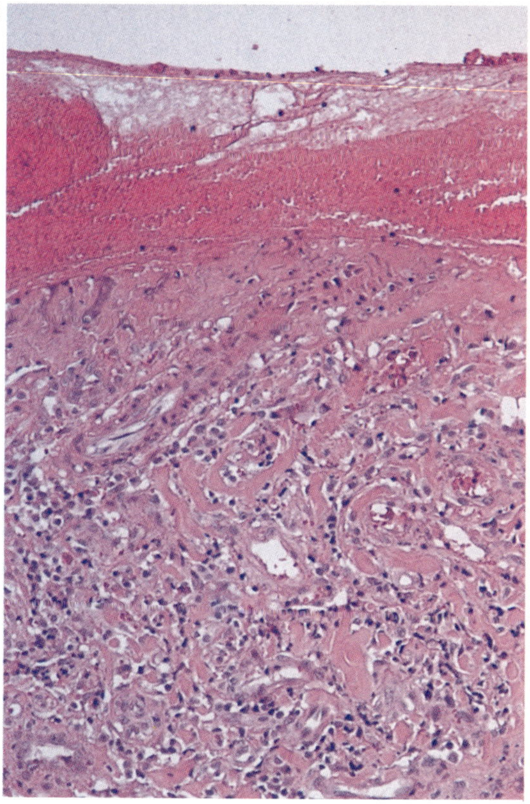

C

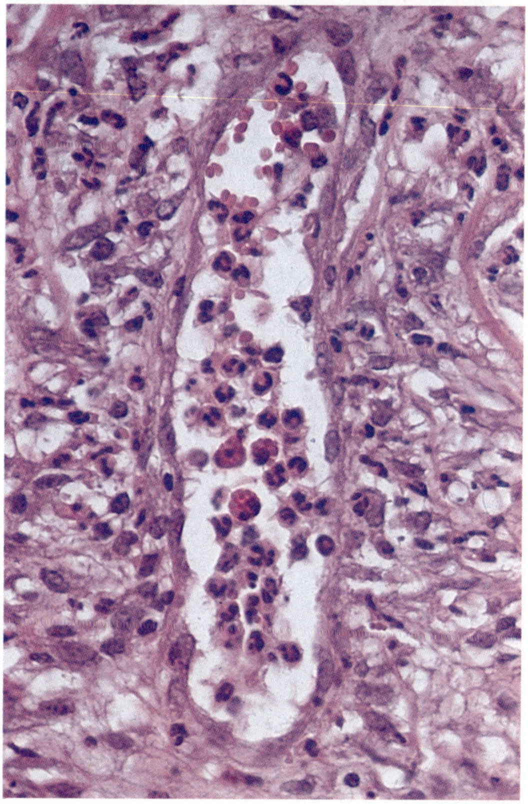

Habronemiasis

A 5-year-old chestnut mare was admitted for the complaint of a chronic, nonhealing sore on the dorsolateral surface of the hoofhead.

Clinically, a rounded ulcer about 10 cm in diameter was present on the external surface of the foot immediately above and in contact with the coronary edge of the hoof. The surface of the ulcer was partially covered by dark coagulated blood overlying the bed of granulating tissue (Figs. A and B).

Histopathologically, there was complete abscense of epidermis and papillary dermis. The main findings were eosinophils in massive numbers throughout the entire dermis. In some parts of the dermis there were concentrations of eosinophils in various stages of proliferation and degradation forming microabscesses that stood out because of their basophilia (Fig. C).

Treatment consisted of superficial excision under local anesthesia by planing the exuberant granulation tissue down to the contours of adjacent normal tissue, and subsequent medication with topical Trichlorfon in combination with a nitrofurazone-prednisolone cream for the parasiticidal effect as well as to control surface infection and excessive granulation. The use of a bandage serves to keep the medication in continuous contact with the wound, provides pressure to suppress granulation, and protects against reinjury and reinfestation during the healing period.

Alternative methods include the use of escharotics such as podophyllum, 25 to 50% in compound Tincture of Benzoin, and cryosurgery (MIGIOIA, 1978), employing a double freeze-thaw cycle method using liquid nitrogen.

An excellent description of the *Habronema* species has been presented by DUNN (1978). Two main species pathogenic to equines are: *Habronema microstoma* and *Habronema muscae*. They are small white worms resembling the ancylostomatids. The males may be up to 22 mm and the females up to 35 mm in length. The adults live in stomach wall and the eggs may hatch in the gut of the horse. *Hyperosia* and *Musca* are often attracted to cutaneous wounds in the summer. The fly larvae may emerge onto the damaged skin from the feeding fly. Then invasion of the already damaged tissue takes place and the classic "summer sore" develops.

DUNN, A. M.
Veterinary Helminthology. Butler and Tanner Ltd. Frome and London, 1978.
MIGIOIA, S.
Cryosurgical Treatment of Equine Cutaneous Habronemiasis Veterinary Medicine and Small Animal Clinician 73:1073, 1978.

A

B

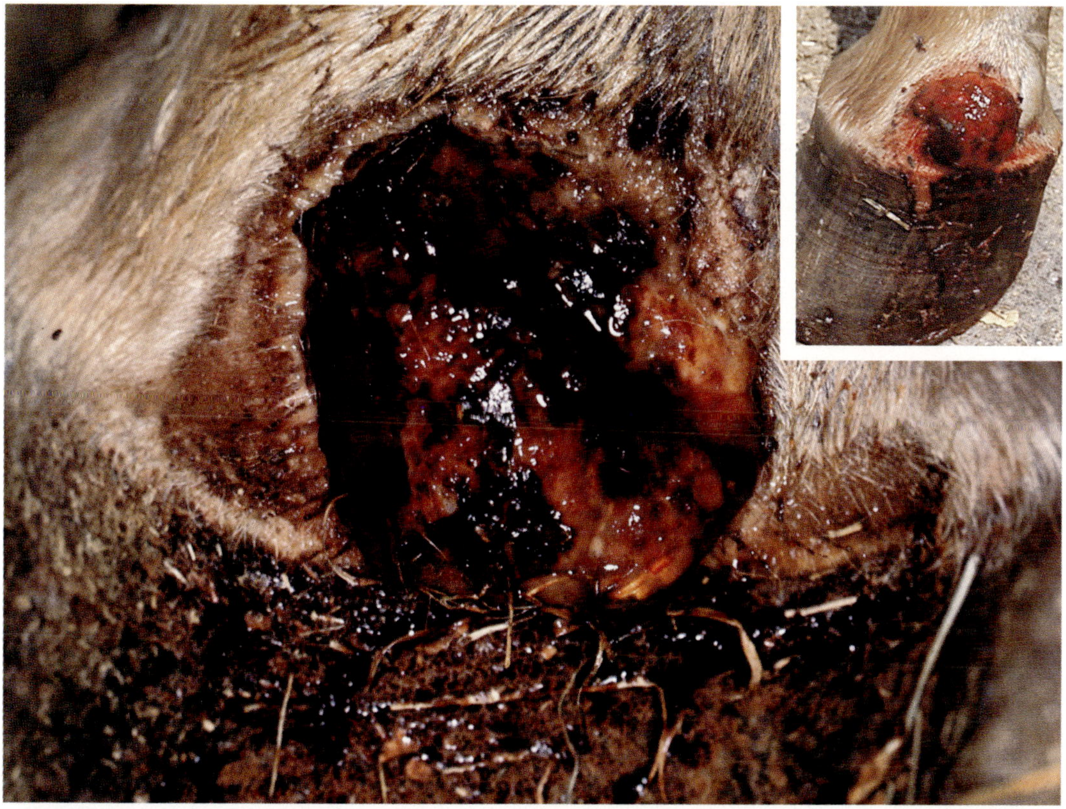

C

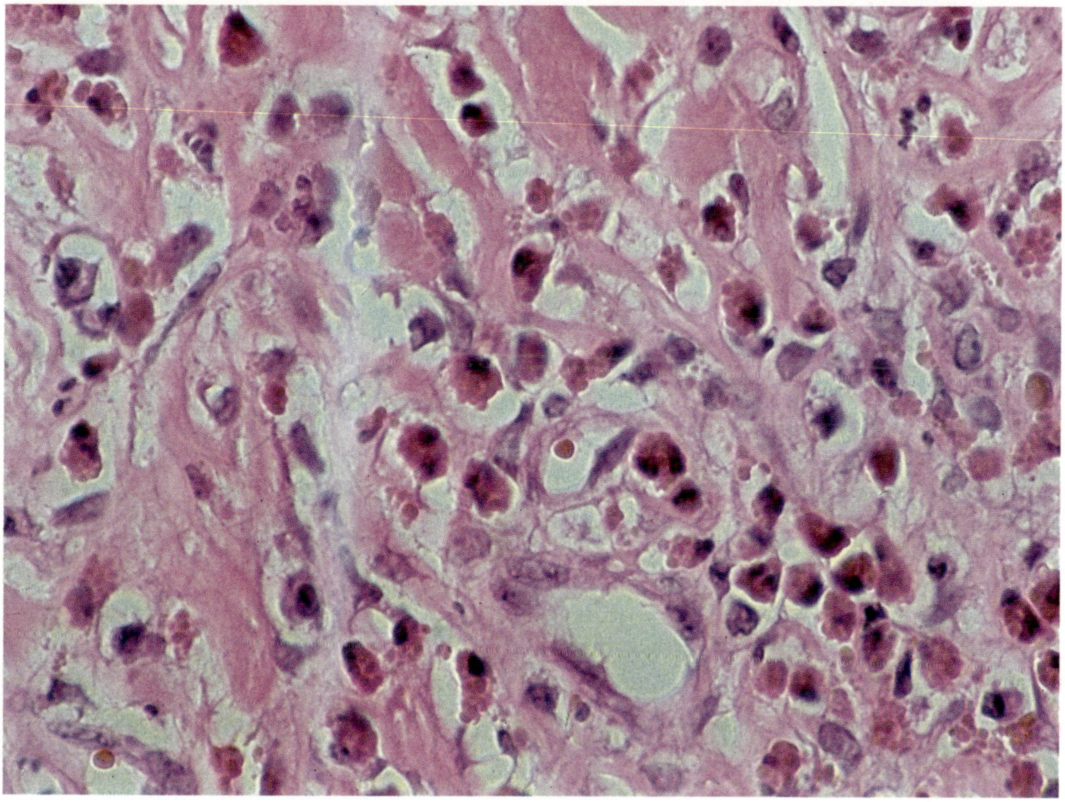

Habronemiasis

These two patients are presented to emphasize the importance of the differential diagnosis in cases of balanoposthitis.

The patient in Fig. A is a case of acute balanoposthitis.

The patient in Fig. B is a case of chronic posthitis due to habronemiasis in its inactive or quiescent stage.

Clinically, acute balanoposthitis (Fig. A) shows exudative erythema with a white yellowish discharge and marked acute preputial edema. Chronic habronemiasis (Fig. B) shows longstanding induration of the prepuce with depigmentation and indolent ulceration.

Mycologically, evaluation of the exudate in acute balanoposthitis by direct examination and cultures demonstrated *C. albicans* in large numbers (Montes, 1981).

Histopathologically, a 2 mm punch biopsy in chronic habronemiasis revealed the classic picture of massive dermal eosinophilia characteristic of this condition (Fig. C).

Treatment. Healing of the skin in these cases paralleled resolution of the deeper pathology. In the acute balanoposthitis, the skin was cleansed carefully with povidone-iodine surgical soap and covered with a nitrofurazone cream in a water miscible base, before being manually replaced in the prepuce and retained there by a nylon-mesh suspensory. This was repeated daily until edema and inflammation had subsided sufficiently so that retraction of the penis was spontaneous.

If manual replacement is deferred due to extreme swelling (phalloncus) and if hydrotherapy in the form of a pulsating spray is to be used to reduce edema, then it is preferable to use an oil-base protective ointment such as A and D ointment to prevent maceration and further excoriation of the irritated epidermis.

The chronic posthitis was complicated by deep scarring, the result of annual exacerbations of summer sores. It was necessary in this case to resect the scarred prepuce circumferentially (reefing operation) and reconstruct the normal edges of the wound under interrupted dermal mattress sutures of monofilament polypropylene. Healing thereafter was uneventful (Walker and Vaughan, 1980).

MONTES, L. F.
Candidal Balanitis. Current Dermatologic Management. Edited by S. Maddin. W. B. Saunders Co., Philadelphia, 1981.

WALKER, D. F. and VAUGHAN, J. T.
Bovine and Equine Urogenital Surgery Lea & Febiger, Philadelphia, 1980.

A

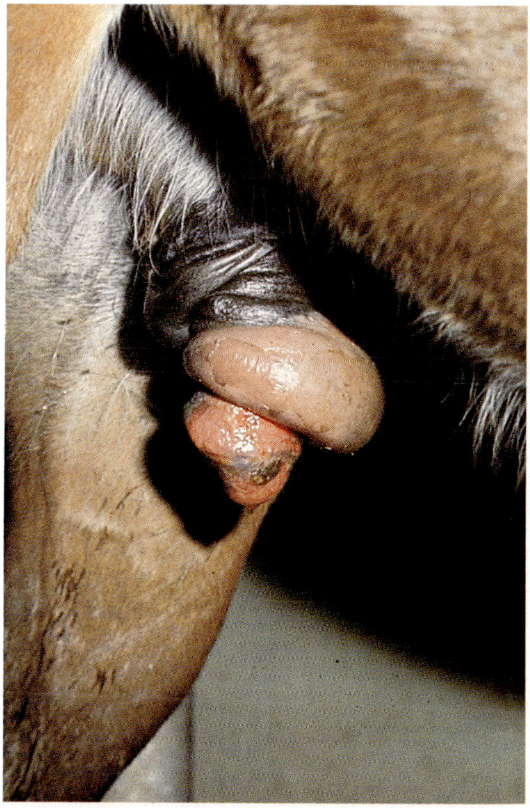

B

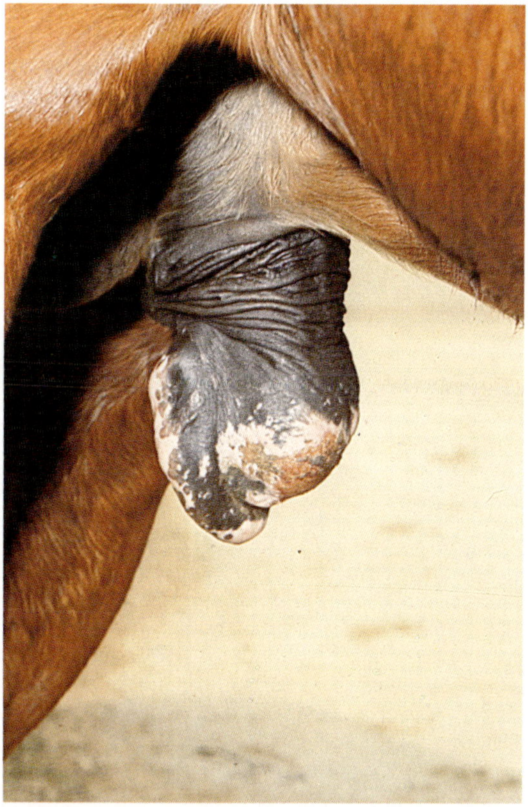

C

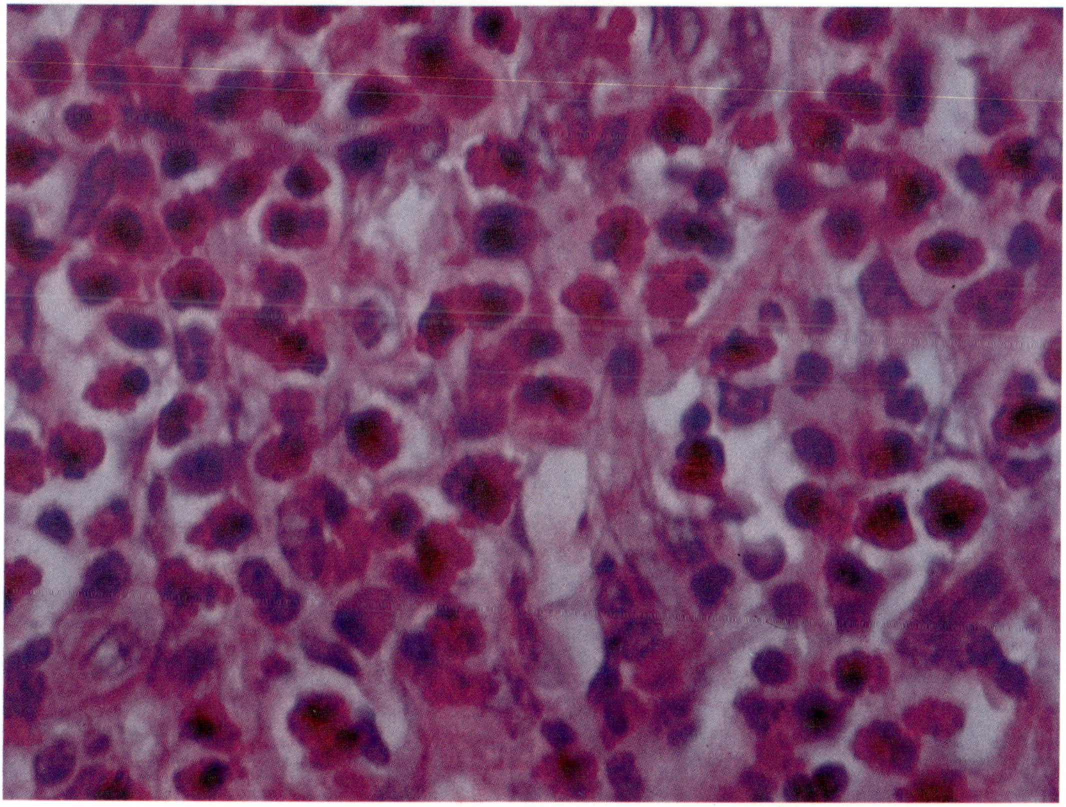

Onchocerciasis

A 3-year-old grey Quarter Horse mare needed treatment for a rash of 2 months duration which developed in late summer.

Clinically, the patient showed confluent scaly patches, excoriations, nodules and eczematous changes over the brisket, medial forelegs, withers, abdomen and head (Fig. A). There was also alopecia in many of the affected areas.

Histopathologically, the epidermis revealed slight hyperkeratosis, irregular acanthosis and small focal clefts at the epidermodermal junction. The papillary and subpapillary dermis was filled with microfilariae 5–10μ in diameter and 100–500μ in length. A mild chronic inflammatory reaction was also present in those areas of the dermis containing the parasites (Figs B and C).

Treatment was diethylcarbamazine citrate (D.E.C.) 6.6mg/kg given in the feed for 7 consecutive days in conjunction with 10mg (total dose) of dexamethasone q.d. for the first 3 days and 5mg q.d. thereafter for 4 days. After the first week, the steroid was discontinued and D.E.C. was continued through the 21st day. The response was rapid. The involved areas started to show regression of the cutaneous changes almost immediately. Temporary hyperpigmentation lasted for several weeks, although gradually faded. At the same time hair started to regrow, and, in approximately 3 months after completion of the treatment, the previously infested areas had reacquired their normal appearance.

The relative mildness of the inflammatory reaction observed in this patient seems to indicate that *Onchocerca cervicalis* did not elicit a very strong immunological response which may account for the chronicity of the infestation if left untreated. In previously unexposed guinea-pigs (STANNARD 1972), the intradermal injection of microfilariae resulted in very mild inflammatory response.

STANNARD and CELLO (1975) found microfilariae of *Onchocerca cervicalis* in skin samples of 48 of 100 slaughtered horses from the Western United States. The infection was more common in the older horses and seemed to occur with equal frequency in both sexes.

Like other investigators, RABALAIS and VOTAVA (1974) found that the skin of the umbilicus and periumbilical regions are the areas of greatest microfilarial density, thus biopsy specimens should be taken from those areas to insure diagnostic accuracy. Biopsy specimens from other areas had fewer microfilariae.

RABALAIS, F.C. and VOTAVA, C.L.
Cutaneous Distribution of Microfilariae of Onchocerca Cervicalis in Horses. American Journal of Veterinary Research 35:1369, 1974.
STANNARD, A.A.
Dermal Onchocerciasis: An Investigation of Naturally Occurring Onchocerca Cervicalis Infection in the Equine and Experimentally Induced Infection in the Guinea Pig. Dissertation. Univ. of California, Davis California, 1972.
STANNARD, A.A. and CELLO, R.M.
Onchocerca Cervicalis Infection in Horses from the Western United States. American Journal of Veterinary Research 36:1029, 1975.

A

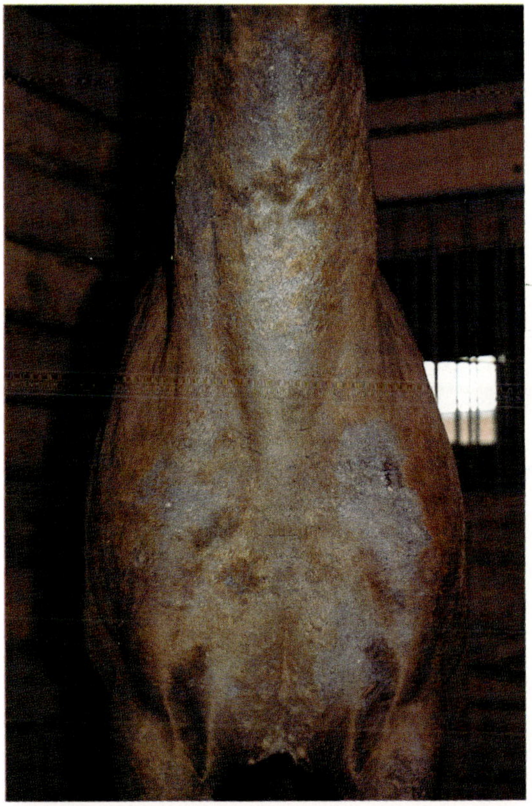

B

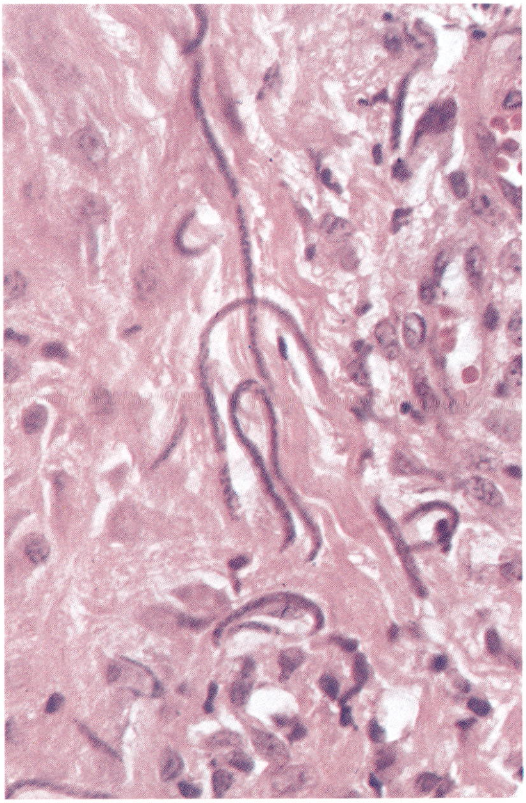

C

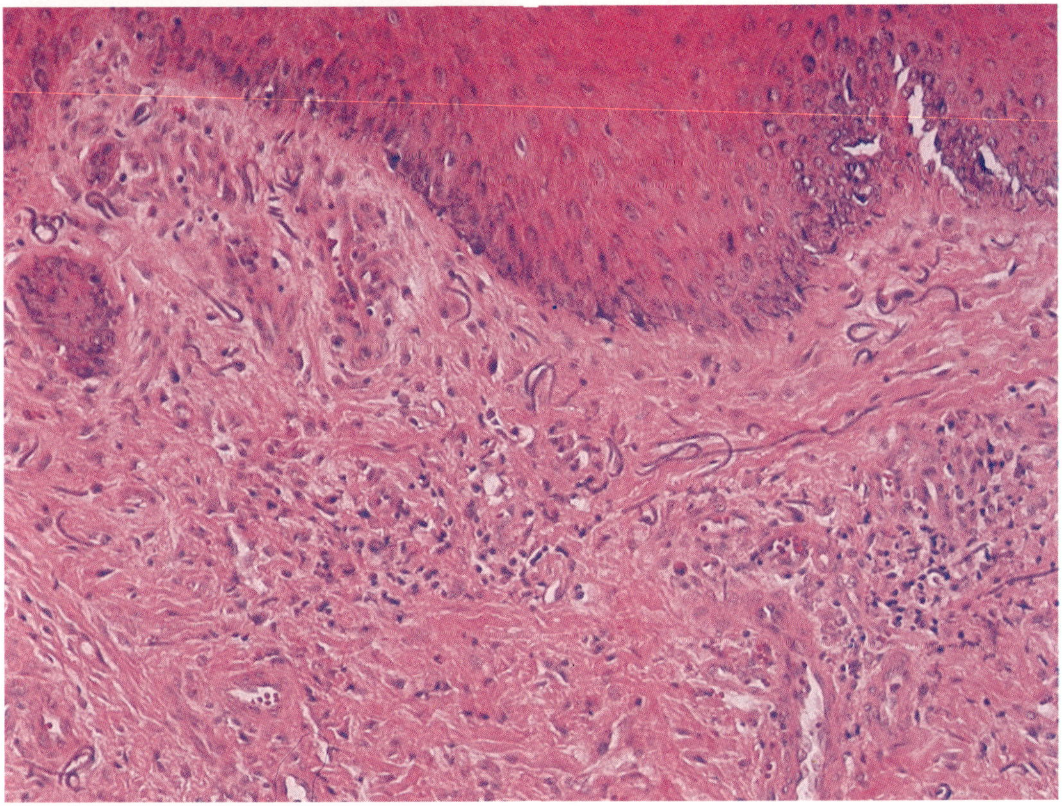

Onchocerciasis

A 7-year old Chestnut crossbred mare was admitted for treatment of an increasingly troublesome skin problem that had spread from the ventral abdomen, breast, and neck up over the shoulders and withers. Some irritation was also apparent about the face and eyes.

Clinically, the patient was affected by a dermatitis consisting of erythema, scaling, marked lichenification and some peripheral papules. The involved area as represented by the withers appeared edematous and hard (Fig. A).

Histopathologically, hyperkeratosis, acanthosis, and a chronic upper dermal inflammatory infiltrate were conspicuous. In addition, the upper dermis was populated by a large number of microfilariae (Fig. B).

Ophthalmologically, funduscopy revealed a small, coiled larva presumptively identified as *Onchocerca cervicalis,* seen in the 8 o'clock position of Fig. C. Invasion of the horse's eye is known to occur by at least 3 species of nematode parasites: *Thelazia californiensis* of the suborder, Spiruvata, and *Setaria equina* and *Onchocerca cervicalis* of the suborder, Filariata, all belonging to the same order, Spirurida (GEORGI, 1974). Thelazia has been incriminated as causing chronic conjunctivitis (GELATT, 1972). Setaria has been found occasionally in the anterior chamber of the eye. Onchocerca, on the other hand, has been ascribed etiologic importance for the keratoiridocyclitis seen commonly in periodic ophthalmia. The microfilariae have been isolated from all tissues of the eye, and identified with acute and chronic inflammatory reactions attributed to the release of antigens by the dead microfilariae. In a survey of 100 cases of cutaneous onchocerciasis, invasion of the eye with microfilariae occurred in 60% of the infected horses (STANNARD and CELLO, 1975). In an earlier study of diseased eyes from 100 horses, 88 demonstrated microfilariae present in cornea or conjunctiva; whereas in 100 normal horses, only 26 showed microfilariae, and these were present without apparent lesions. Three lesions were noted to be characteristic of the disease: multiple white nodules in the pigmented conjunctiva at the limbus, irregularly-shaped areas of depigmentation immediately adjacent to or surrounding the optic disc, and extra ocular dermatitis on the eyelids, face, withers, or ventral abdomen--the skin in these areas showing hyperpigmentation, hair loss and scurf, with skin biopsis yielding many microfilariae of *O. cervicalis* (CELLO, 1962, 1971).

Treatment (see Cases 37 and 39) is directed at 1) killing the microfilariae with diethylcarbamazine, 2) suppression with adrenocorticosteroid of the intense allergic reaction that attends release of antigen upon the death of the microfilariae, and 3) control of the insect vector. Recognizing the importance of prevention, it is of great benefit and no small savings to provide protection for the susceptible horse by such means as a screened stall (with the screen wire on the *outside* of the stall), stabling during the late afternoon and night hours, especially if Culicoides and Aedes species are the vectors, use of space sprays (pyrethrins, piperonyl butoxide, etc.) in the barn, black light insect electrocutors, topical repellants on the horse's coat, or, perhaps most simply, moving the horse some distance to a new location away from the principal source of the insect vector.

CELLO, R. M.
Recent Findings in Periodic Ophthalmia. Proc. of 8th Ann. Convent. of AAEP, 123–133, 1962.
CELLO, R. M.
Ocular Onchocerciasis in the Horse. Equine Veterinary Journal. 3:148, 1971.
GELATT, K. N.
The Eye, Chapter 15, 399–432. Equine Medicine & Surgery American Veterinary Pub., Inc., Wheaton, Il 1972.
GEORGI, J. R.
Parasitology for Veterinarians 2nd Ed., W. B. Saunders Co., Philadelphia, 1974.
STANNARD, A. A. and CELLO, R. M.
Onchocerca cervicalis Infection in Horses from the Western United States. Am. Journal of Vet. Research, 36–7, 1029–31, 1975.
RIEK, R. F.
Studies on Allergic Dermatitis (Queensland Itch) of the Horse. Australian Vet. Journal, 29, July 1953. Australian Journal of Agricultural Research, V6, 161–70, 1955.

A

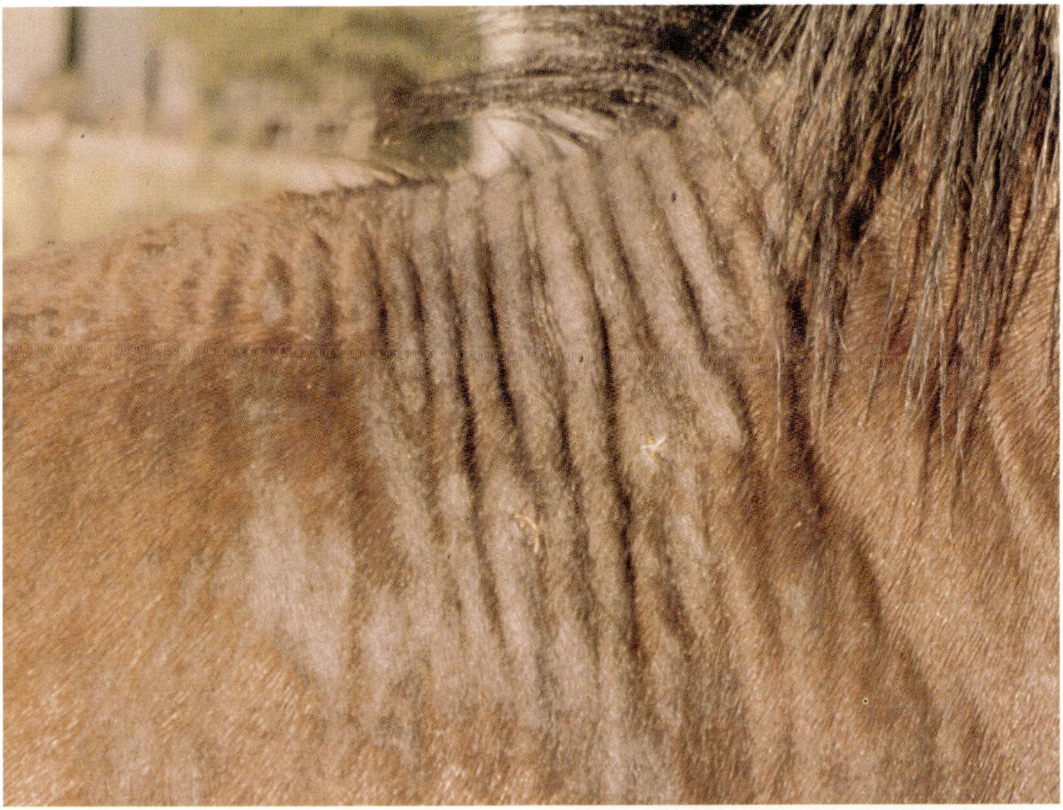

B

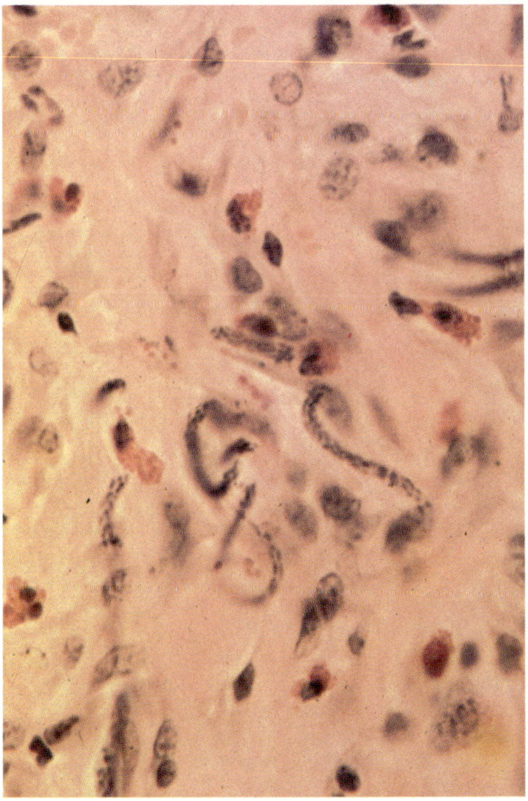

C

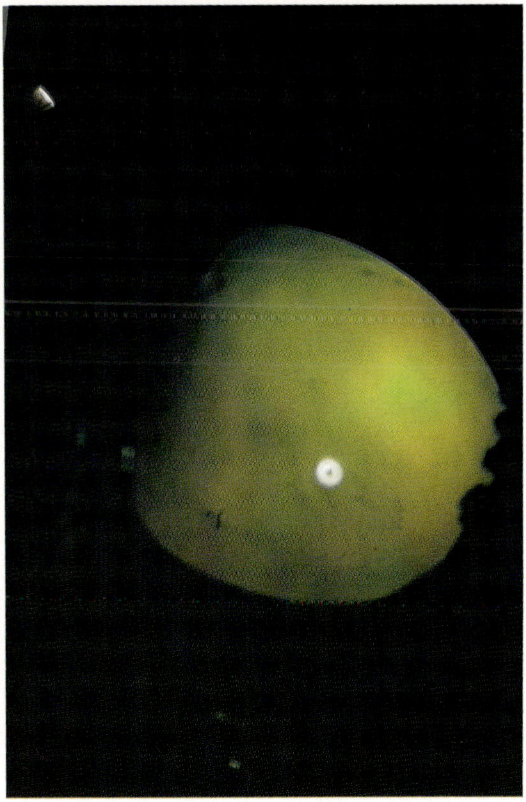

Onchocerciasis

A 4-year-old male Quarter Horse was referred because of a 1-month history of a generalized eruption which was first noticed during the late spring.

Clinically, there were numerous papules, nodules and slightly raised scaly plaques. Some of the lesions were also characterized by partial hair loss (Fig. A).

Histopathologically, the study of 3 different biopsy specimens (kindly performed by Dr. R. Crawley, Auburn University School of Veterinary Medicine) showed the following features:

Biopsy #1: The epidermis was intact and normal. The adnexa were normal. The dermis was edematous and contained an exudate of eosinophils, mast cells, and lymphoreticular cells. The dermal exudate was prominent around dermal vessels which had hypertrophied endothelium. There were several microfilaria in the involved areas of the dermis (Fig. B).

Biopsy #2) The changes were similar to #1 but the dermal edema was more marked. Also, the dermal exudate was more marked. There were microfilaria in inflamed areas.

Biopsy #3: There was focal ulceration and dried exudate on the surface. There was moderate acanthosis and hyperkeratosis. There was active fibroplasia in the superficial dermis. The deeper dermis contained a multifocal exudate of eosinophils and lymphoreticular cells. There was focal lymphoid follicle formation in the deep dermis. There were degenerated microfilaria within an inflammatory focus in some places.

Treatment was carried out by oral administration of diethylcarbamazine citrate (D.E.C.), 6.6 mg/kg daily mixed with feed for 3 weeks, in conjunction with dexamethasone administered on feed, 10 mg total daily dose for 3 days and 5 mg. total daily dose for 4 days of the first week of D.E.C. treatment. Clearing was rapid initially, but the condition regressed somewhat after discharge, and the entire schedule had to be repeated. The owners were cautioned to continue the D.E.C. treatment for 21 days out of each month, and to exercise rigorous fly control.

In horses, onchocerciasis does not have a geographic predilection, and it may occur in cold as well as warm climates. For example, MARCOUX et al (1977) described 3 patients observed in Quebec. As in many of our patients, hair loss was a conspicuous clinical feature. The diagnosis was also confirmed by histopathological studies. On the other side of the North American continent, McMULLAN (1975) reported findings on a much larger series (38 cases) observed in Texas. In Colombia, a study performed by EBERHARD and ORIHEL (1978) demonstrated microfilariae in 16 (53%) horses believed to be infested with *Onchocerca cervicalis*.

EBERHARD, M. and ORIHEL, T.C.
Equine and Bovine Onchocerciasis in Colombia Journal of Parasitology 64:191, 1978.
MARCOUX, M., FRECHETTE, J.L. and MORIN, M.
Infection par Onchocerca cervicalis au Quebec: signes Cliniques et Method de Diagnostique. Canadian Veterinary Journal 18:108, 1977.
McMULLAN, W.C.
Filarial Dermatitis in the Horse. Journal of the American Veterinary Medical Association 167:9, 1975.
(Grateful acknowledgement to DR. DAVID HARRINGTON, School of Veterinary Medicine, Auburn University.)

A

B

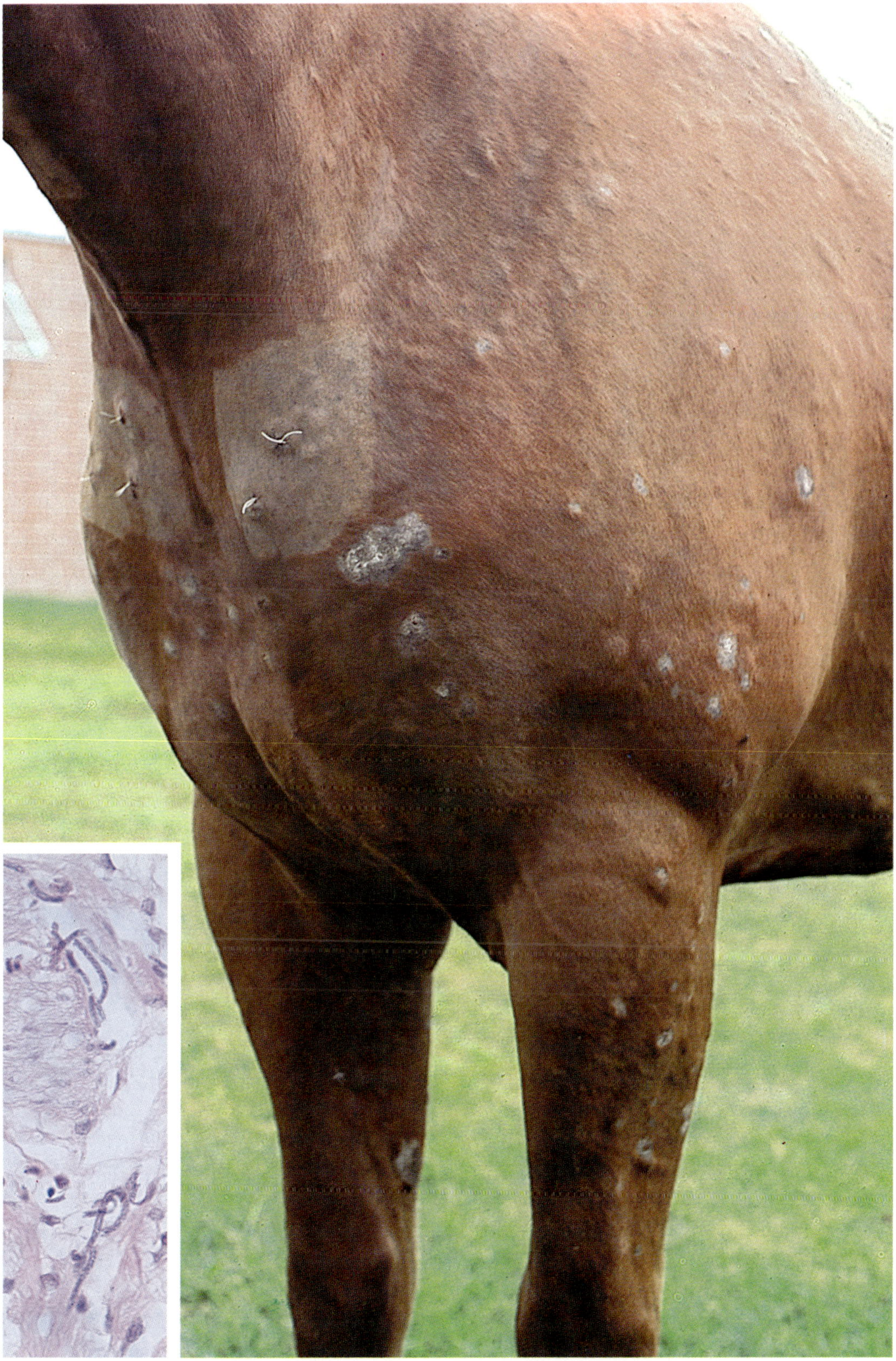

Tumors

If one wishes success with tumors, early diagnosis must be achieved.

Histopathological study of serial sections from different areas of any tumor is always advisable.

Some tumors can be cytologically benign but behave aggressively in a destructive fashion. Other tumors can be cytologically malignant but have a rather protracted course. In any event, treatment better be radical.

Sarcoid

A 4-year old grey Arab mare was referred for evaluation and management of a lesion that had started to develop on the right eye one month earlier and was growing quite rapidly.

Clinically, a raised, granulomatous sore, 4 cm in diameter, distorted the architecture of the eyelid. A culture of the ulcerated surface yielded *Staphylococcus* and *Streptococcus* sensitive to gentamicin and cephalothin. A biopsy of the surgical specimen provided the diagnosis of sarcoid, one of the most common of tumors that occur anywhere on the skin surface of equidae irrespective of sex, breed or geographic region. The cause is attributed to a virus similar to that incriminated in bovine papilloma, and experimentation has demonstrated that it can be transferred from site to site on the same animal as well as transmitted to other animals of the same species. Within limits, the bovine papilloma virus has evoked sarcomatous-like growths in horses. Despite its classification as a benign skin tumor, and, as such, has not been identified internally, sarcoid does display a doggedly persistent recurrence following surgical excision. (Fig. A demonstrates a later recurrence in the scar from the surgical excision.)

Histopathologically, a 4 mm punch biopsy was removed in order to establish a diagnosis prior to a decision regarding the best therapeutic procedure. Study of serial sections showed complete disappearance of the epidermis at the surface of the tumor where there was an admixture of fibrin and large numbers of leukocytes. Immediately under that superficial layer there was a zone of highly cellular and loose connective tissue with many dilated capillaries (Fig. B). The deeper part of the tumor was formed by newly-formed capillaries surrounded by proliferating spindle-shaped cells and thin connective tissue fibers mostly arranged in parallel fascicles but in places forming whorls (Fig. C).

Treatment consisted of surgical excision. The postoperative course was complicated by dehiscence of the wound closure, and healing occurred by second intention. The lesion recurred in the bed of the scar within 30 days and was excised the second time in conjunction with the local infiltration of bovine transfer factor. In less than 60 days the tumor had grown back in the lateral canthus (Fig. A) and was injected 3 times at weekly intervals with tuberculin, hoping to avoid further cicatricial distortion of the palpebral fissure and function of the upper lid. One month later, the tumor was reinjected with tuberculin, and by the end of the next month had begun to regress. Complete remission followed, and 5 years later there has been no evidence of regrowth.

Resistance to treatment is characteristic of sarcoid, particularly the rapidly growing or multiple lesion, as opposed to the solitary, slowly growing one. Modalities of treatment used include chemical cautery with escharotic agents such as podophyllum, 25 to 50% in Compound Tincture of Benzoin, electrofulguration, cryosurgery, topical antimetabolites such as 5-fluorouracil (following surgical excision), radiation therapy, and local immunotherapy by injection of BCG (bacille Calmette Guérin) vaccine, tuberculin, or bovine transfer factor. Cryosurgery has enjoyed a widely-acclaimed reputation recently for having some immunotherapeutic effect, bolstering its initial action of physiologic inhibition and tissue destruction.

HABER, H.
in Systemic Pathology, p. 1566. Edited by G.P. Wright and W. St. Clair Symmers. Longmans, London, 1966.
(Grateful acknowledgement to Dr. K.W. Harris, Birmingham, AL, and Dr. E.C. Firth, U. of Utrecht, The Netherlands.)

A

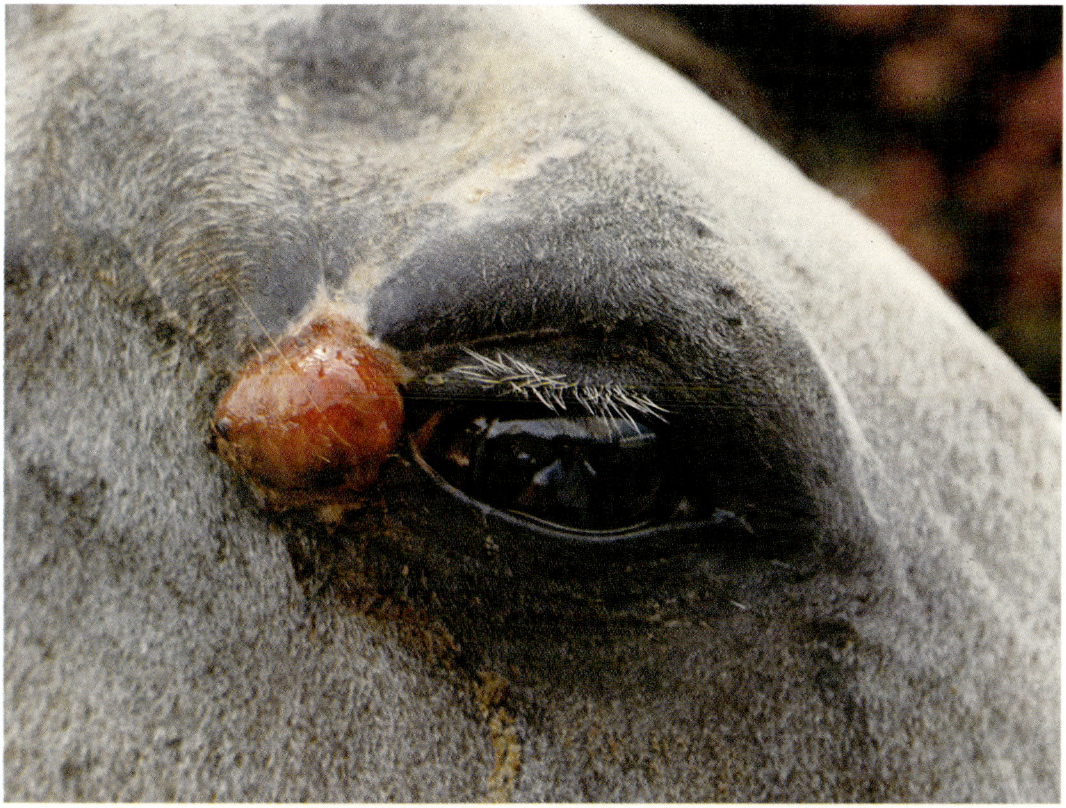

B

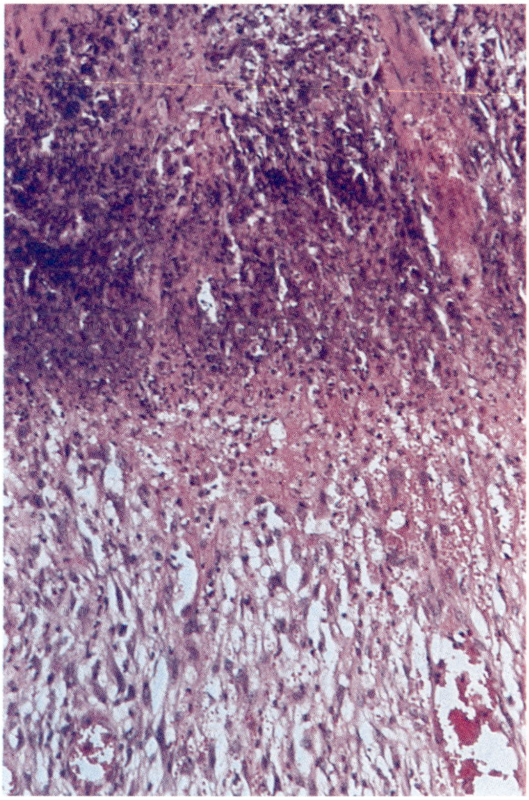

C

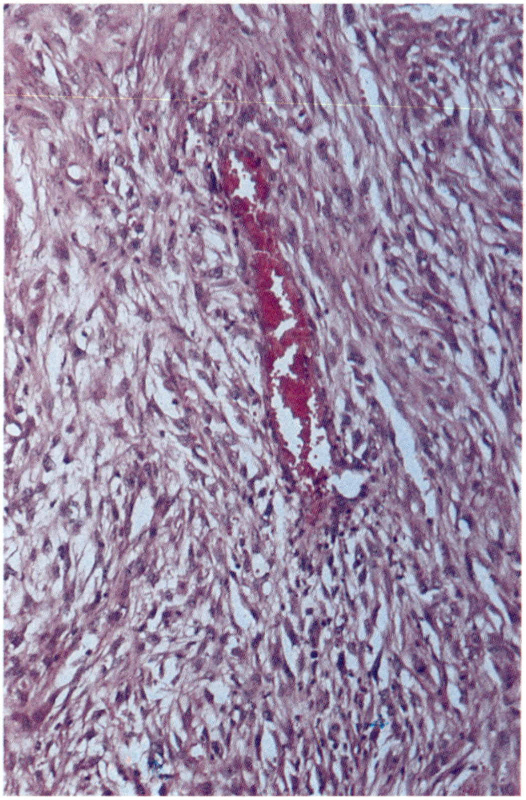

Sarcoid

A 6-year old bay Quarter Horse gelding was admitted for a lesion in the skin bordering the medial canthus and invading the upper and lower lids of the right eye.

Clinically, an ulcerated, nodular mass at the canthus was continued laterally by similar, sessile lesions undermining an intact epidermis. The lesions were particularly larger over the lower palpebral furrow where some of them had become confluent forming a multilobulated tumor. In some parts the surface of the lesions was eroded (Fig. A). This appearance is typical of sarcoids that border the eye. Nonmalignancy notwithstanding, invasion of the deeper tissues, including the musculature of the lids, contributes to the difficulty of surgical management and can be likened in this respect to deep-seated basal cell epitheliomas and facial squamous cell carcinomas in the human. It is for this reason that surgical revision of scars that interfere with function of the eyelids is not infrequently required following removal of the sarcoid. Of course, this judgement should not be made in less than 6 months if possible to defer plastic surgery that long without undue injury to the eye.

Histopathologically, a 3 mm punch biopsy taken from one of the nodules with intact skin showed a number of interesting features. The epidermis was atrophic with keratotic plugging of some of the follicular orifices (Fig. B). There was a diffuse dermal proliferation of spindle-shaped cells forming fascicles or whorls. Numerous capillaries were also present throughout the tumor and appeared compressed by the massive growth of the neoplasm (Fig. C).

Treatment consisted of surgical excision following by a course of 5-fluorouracil administered topically to the tumor bed as a solution of 500 mg (10 ml) in 90 ml propylene glycol, q.d. for 30 days. A border of petrolatum was used to protect the normal skin areas and care was exercised to avoid accidental contact with the eye proper. Healing by second intention followed cessation of the drug, and the case was lost to followup. This antineoplastic agent is also available as a 2% or 5% cream or solution (5% strength recommended) SERRI (1970).

Alternative methods that have demonstrated merit and should be considered for use in such areas are the repeated injections of B.C.G., Bovine Transfer Factor, or tuberculin and the use of cryosurgery. Both techniques reportedly share an immunotherapeutic effect (see Cases 40, 42, and 43).

SERRI, F.
International Conference on 5% Fluorouracil Ointment in Dermatology. Dermatologica 140 (Supplementum I), 1970.

A

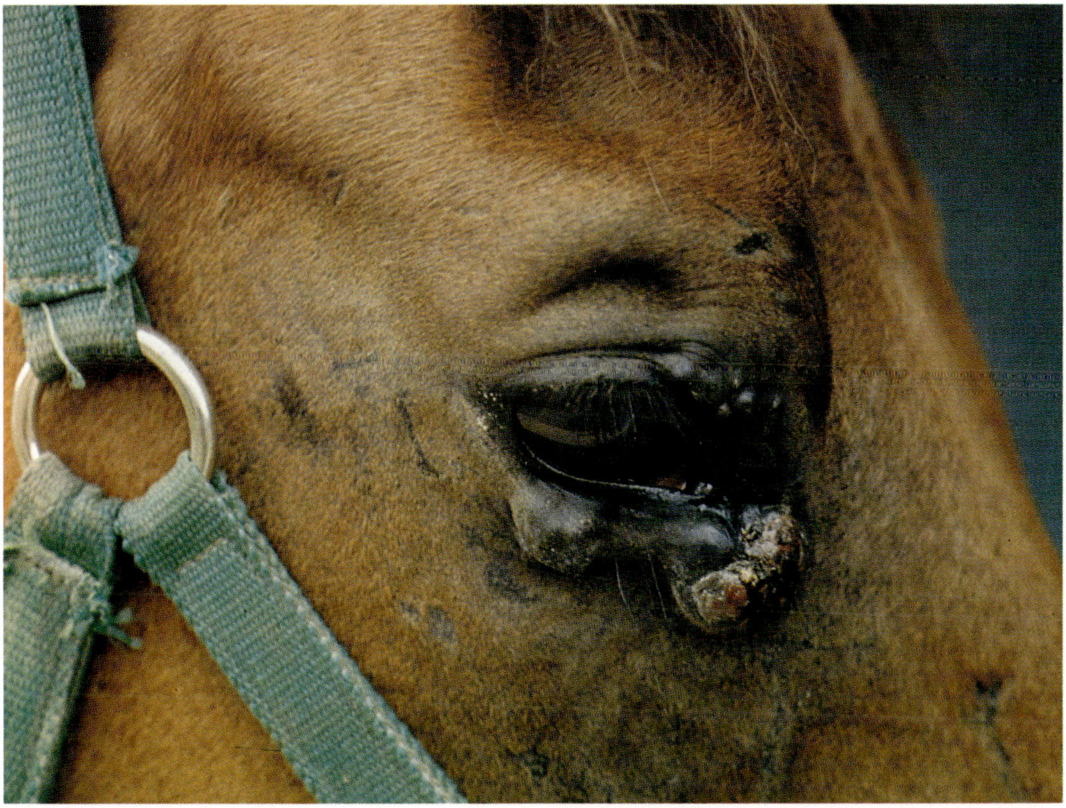

B

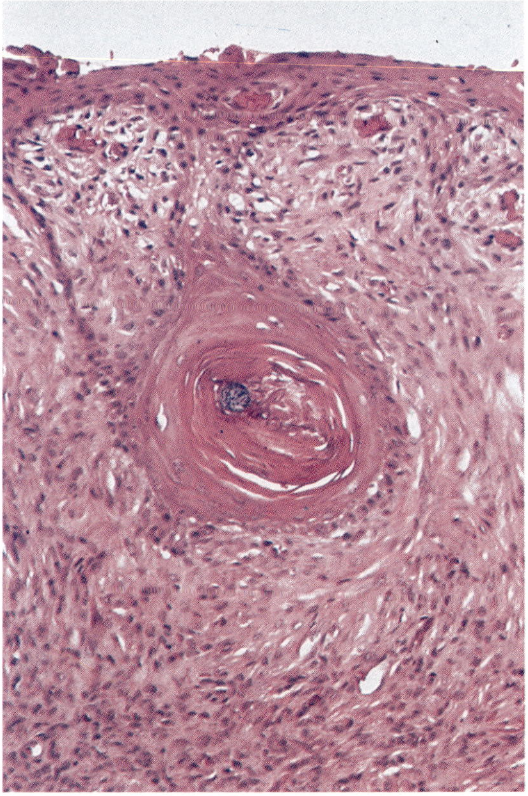

C

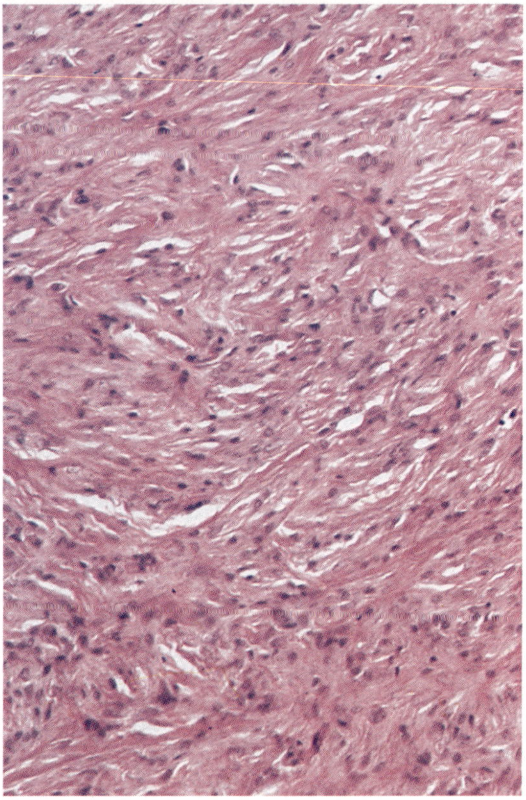

Sarcoid

A 6-year-old bay Thoroughbred mare, 5 months pregnant, was examined during a consultation in a large breeding farm because of an orbital tumor which had been growing steadily since its onset about 18 months earlier.

Clinically, the entire right orbit was filled by a multilobular tumor that had already advanced beyond the borders of the orbit and was extending itself in all directions. The surface had a red-yellowish color in some parts and was covered with dark crusts of coagulated blood. Each large lobule was formed by a multitude of smaller nodules (Figs. A and B). No signs of secondary infection were obvious and the tumor was not particularly malodorous. Further examination of the horse disclosed another much smaller tumor over the external aspect of the left hock.

Histopathologically, serial sections were performed on pieces of the tumor obtained from 6 different areas at various levels. There was absence of epithelial structures. The tumor displayed various stages of growth according to the area that was studied. There was vascular proliferation throughout the neoplasm. In some areas, surrounding the vessels, were polymorphonuclear leukocytes including numerous eosinophils and loose connective tissue with thin collagen bundles and wide spaces of ground substance. In other areas, the vessels were tightly surrounded by a more dense connective tissue including thick collagen bundles, fibroblasts and little ground substance; there was some tendency for the collagen bundles to interweave and to radiate in a cartwheel-like fashion.

Treatment. This patient was not under the authors' care thus it was only possible to offer advice as to the course of action. An important consideration, prior to treatment, was to differentiate between sarcoid and squamous cell carcinoma. When the latter was ruled out and the diagnosis of sarcoid became established as a result of the histopathological diagnosis, the following immediate measures were suggested: 1) complete resection of the tumor; 2) subsequent enucleation of the entire eye if indeed there were any structures not yet destroyed by the tumor; 3) careful exploration of the bony structures of the orbit. It was further recommended that the smaller tumor on the leg be completely excised. The value of the case lies in the extreme example provided, and serves well to illustrate how locally invasive and destructive a "benign" tumor can be. Issue can scarcely be taken with the opinion that the prognosis in this case was grave indeed.

It has been proposed by WYMAN et al (1977) that equine sarcoid may be caused by a virus. These investigators infiltrated lesions of two patients with BCG before excision; and, at regrowth, BCG and sonicated, fourth passage autogenous tumor cell cultures were injected with successful result. Interestingly, SOM et al (1976) found sarcoid to be rather frequent in racehorses in India. From a comparative standpoint the clinical and microscopic resemblance of equine sarcoid with human dermatofibrosarcoma protuberans (DEGOS 1960) are remarkable.

(Grateful acknowledgement to Dr. PEDRITO BLAQUIER of *Haras La Biznaga, Islas, Argentina.*)

DEGOS, R.
Fibrosarcome de la Peau de Darier-Ferrand. Dermatologie. P. 875. Editions Medicales Flammarion. Paris, 1960.

SOM, T.L., DEB, P. and NANDJ, S.N.
Incidence of Sarcoid in a Race-Horse Progeny. Indian Journal of Animal Health 15:75, 1976.

WYMAN, M., RINGS, M.D., TARR, M.J. and ALDEN, C.L.
Immunotherapy in Equine Sarcoid: A Report of Two Cases. Journal of the American Veterinary Medical Association 171:449, 1977.

A

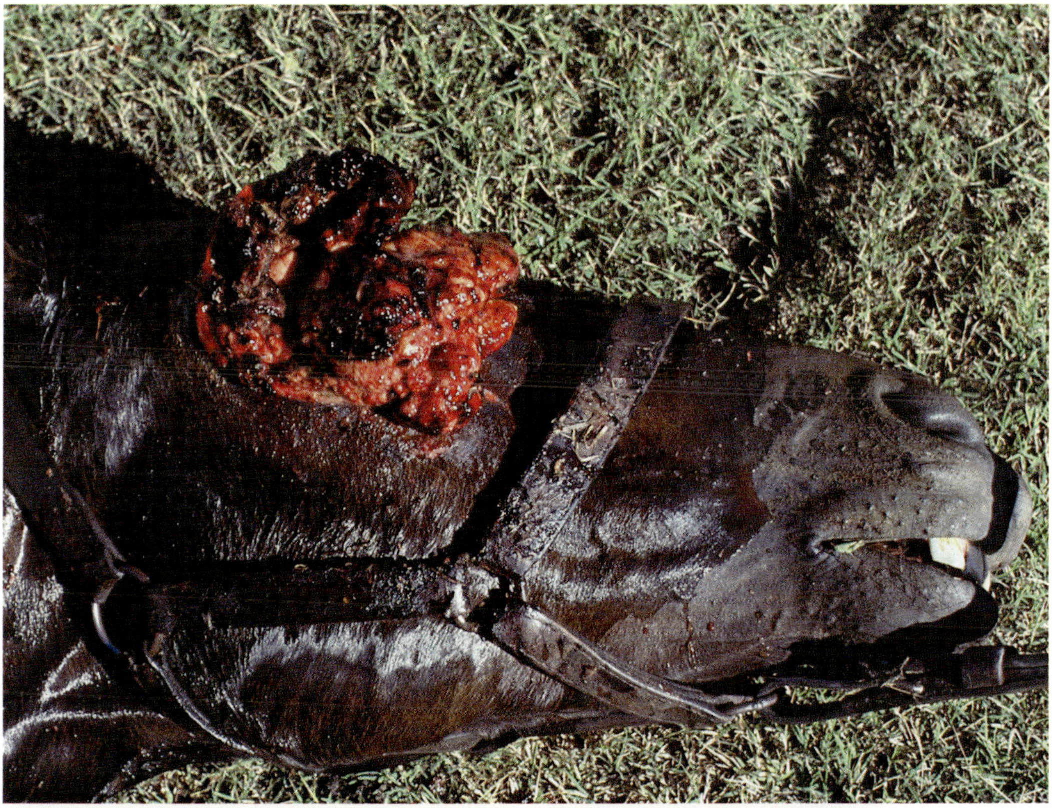

B

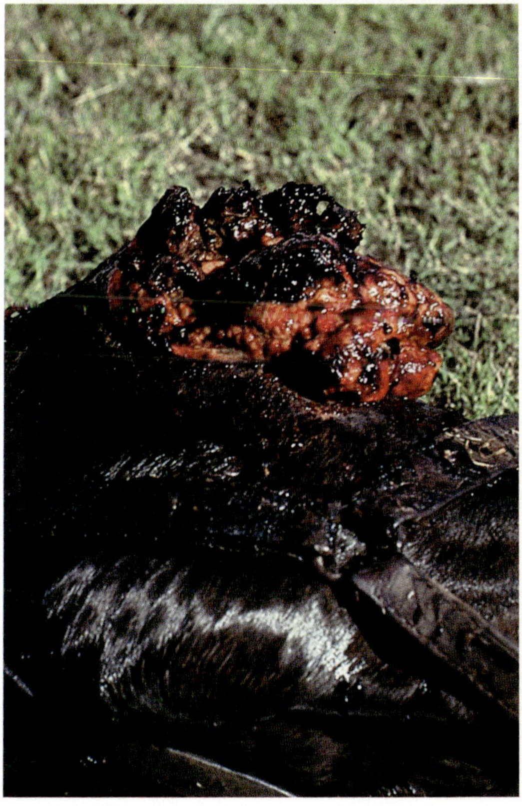

C

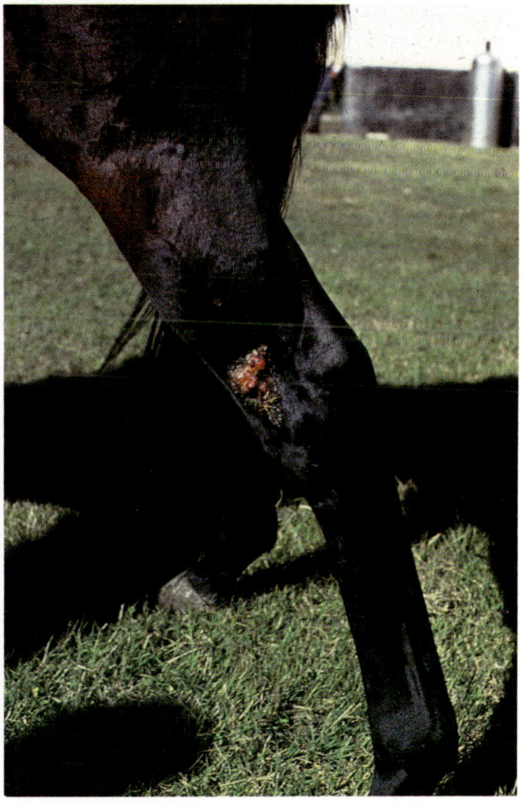

Sarcoid

A 9-year-old bay crossbred gelding was admitted because of a tumor of rapid growth that had first been noticed under the right axilla six months earlier.

Clinically, a multilobulated, cauliflower-shaped tumor composed of numerous hard nodules was found. The majority of the nodules had a red color and a glossy surface. A few of the nodules were darker suggesting that hemorrhagic changes were taking place inside those parts of the tumor (Figs. A and B). The vascularity could be attributed to the proximity of the major brachial supply.

Histopathologically, serial sections of different nodules provided an overall view of various stages of growth in the neoplasm. There were places where general proliferation of many dilated capillaries, thin connective tissue fibers, wide spaces of ground substance and fusiform cells were the main features. In other places vascular spaces were narrow and fewer and the main components were fibroblast – like cells with a storiform pattern (Fig. C) (STOUT and LATTES 1967).

Treatment was by surgical excision under local anesthesia. Postoperative medication consisted of topical application of 5% fluorouracil q.d. for 30 days, taking precautions to protect the surrounding skin surfaces with petrolatum. Healing by contraction and epithelialization followed discontinuation of the antimetabolite. Although protracted study was not done, no return of tumor growth was evident on the last inspection.

FRETZ and BARBER (1980) employed cryosurgery in fifty horses with sarcoid. Twenty-six horses had single and 24 horses multiple sarcoids for a combined total of 204 tumors. Two methods were used: 1) one consisted of 2 rapid-freeze, slow-thaw cycles to −20°C; 2) the second included 3 rapid-freeze, slow-thaw cycles to −30°C. The first method resulted in the recovery of 8 of 13 horses (63%) with sarcoids after the initial treatment; whereas, the second method produced recovery of 26 of 37 horses (70%) after the initial treatment. These authors believed that, when used with proper precautions, cryosurgery was an effective and safe treatment for sarcoids. The following precautions were considered important: preparation for aseptic surgery, use of local or general anesthesia, use of thermocouples to determine the rate and depth of freeze, protection of surrounding skin with insulators, routine preoperative tetanus prophylaxis, application of pressure bandage where possible for the first 24 hours after surgery to control hemorrhage or prophylactic presurgical ligation when a sarcoid was directly over a large superficial vein.

FRETZ, P.B. and BARBER, S.M.
Cryosurgery as the Sole Treatment for Equine Sarcoids. The Veterinary Clinics of North America, 10:847, 1980.
STOUT, A.P. and LATTES, R.
Tumors of the Soft Tissues. Fascicle I. Atlas of Tumor Pathology, p. 44. Armed Forces Institute of Pathology, Washington 1967.

A

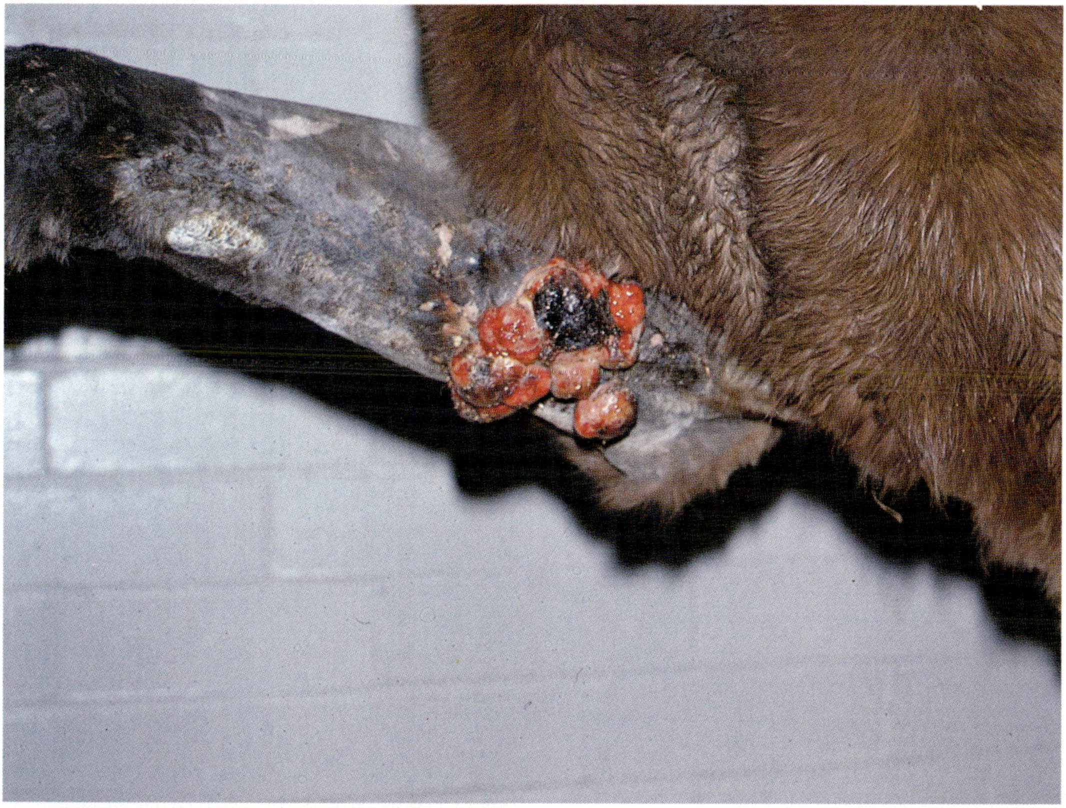

B

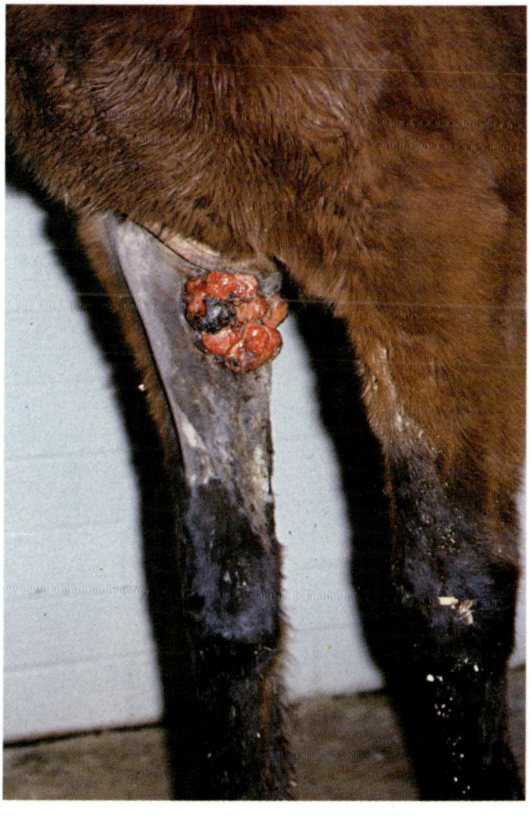

C

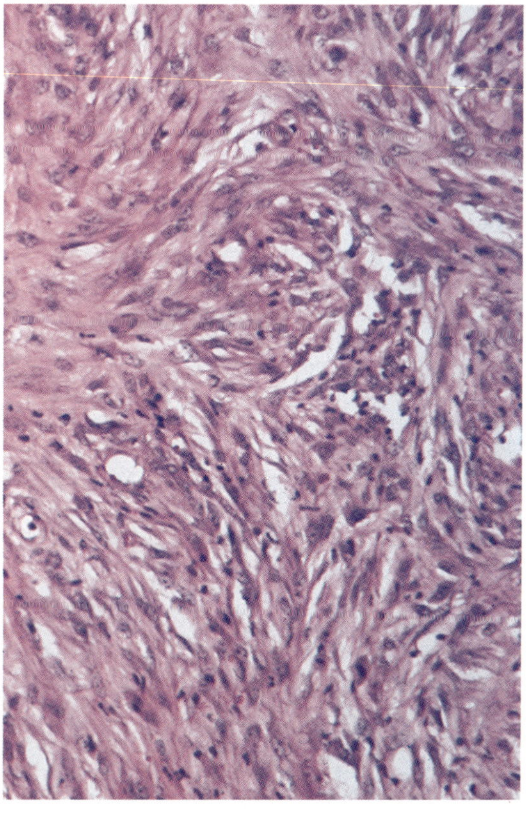

Melanoma

A 4-year-old grey Trakehner mare was referred because of multiple, rapidly enlarging, tumors.

Clinically, an oval tumor measuring approximately 3.0 cm × 1.5 cm was observed over the right parotid region (Fig. A). Although anchored to the dermis and visibly displacing the skin, the tumor was also fixed to the underlying layers. This suggested invasion of the parenchyma of the parotid salivary gland and, possibly, adjacent structures. Also numerous, rounded, fairly hard nodules, 1–5 cm in diameter (Fig. B), were seen in different areas of the skin, particularly in the perineal region.

Histopathologically, the large as well as the small tumors presented the same characteristic picture of metastatic melanoma. The epidermis was slightly atrophic with resulting disappearance of the rete pegs. The basal cell layer displayed large amounts of melanin but no junction activity. Beneath a narrow subepidermal grenz zone, the dermis contained massive amounts of melanin which obscured most details of other components. Interestingly, the pilary muscles appeared free of pigment (Figs. C and D).

Treatment. Due to the characteristic behaviour of malignant melanomas and to the fact that palpation indicated preexisting invasion of the parotid region of the throat, surgery would have required a radical neck dissection at the least. Nor would this have precluded contamination of the field with exfoliated tumor cells. For these reasons, it was decided to resort to radiation therapy. Treatment of the large tumor with cobalt irradiation produced negligible reduction in size. Notice the depigmented area under the halter (Fig. A) resulting from the irradiation. The mare was 6 months pregnant at time of treatments, and gestation was completely uneventful resulting in a live, healthy foal. The foal was weaned at 4 months, and the mare was rebred.

Melanomas develop in horses regardless of their breed, with even mules sometimes being affected (Runnells & Benbrook 1941). For reasons not well understood, they develop more frequently in old grey horses. Melanomas may appear without any premonitory symptoms but may also be heralded by vitiligo (Lerner & Cage 1974). In grey horses from the Vienna Spanish Riding School, Gebhart & Niebauer (1977) observed melanomas in 20 out of 31 horses older than 10 years, whereas none of 23 younger than 10 years showed melanomas.

GEBHART, W. and NIEBAUER, G. W.
Beziehungen Zwischen Pigmentschwund und Melanomatose am Beispiel des Lippizanerschimmels. Archiv für Dermatologische Forschung 259, 29–42. 1977.

LERNER, A. B. and CAGE, G. W.
Melanomas in Horses. Yale Journal of Biology and Medicine 46, 646–649. 1974.

RUNNELLS, R. A. and BENBROOK, E. A.
Malignant Melanomas of Horses and Mules. American Journal of Veterinary Research 2, 340–344. 1941.

A B C D

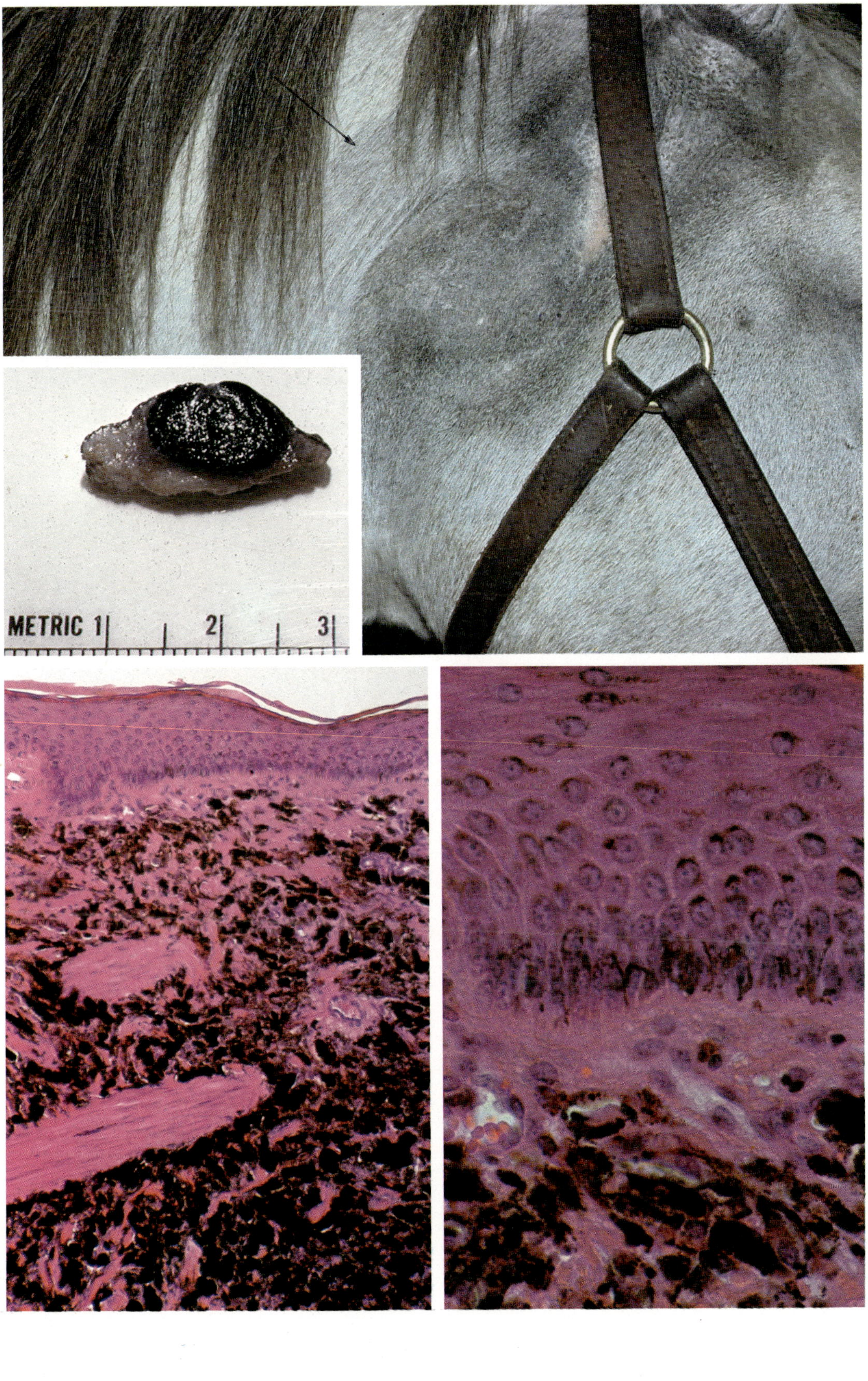

Melanoma

A 12-year old grey mare was referred because of a perianal lesion of unknown duration.

Clinically, a sharply demarcated, somewhat oval ulcer, with a flat border was found in a 9 o'clock position about 2 cm to the left of the anal orifice (Fig. A). The ulcer measured approximately 2 cm × 3 cm. While the external part of the ulcer showed a yellowish-red granulation surface, the center was deeply black with the pigment spreading centrifugally towards the lower edge of the ulcer (Fig. B).

Histopathologically, the ulcer revealed complete absence of the epidermis and papillary dermis that were replaced by granulation tissue. The epidermis surrounding the ulcer was moderately acanthotic. The mid dermis showed a chronic inflammatory infiltrate. The deeper dermis and subcutaneous tissue were completely invaded by cells displaying great pleomorphism, many mitotic figures and massive amounts of melanin which obscured the cytological details. Some of the cells were very large and confluent with one another. There were many histiocytes and some lymphocytes surrounding the neoplastic cells. There were large amounts of melanin throughout the specimen. The pigment was even found within secretory tubules of sweat glands and among fat cells (Fig. C).

Treatment was by liberal surgical excision including a wide margin of normal skin and fascia down to the sphincter ani medially and the origin of the semimembranosus muscle laterally. The tumor was well encapsulated and dissection was unhampered. Dead space was packed with 5% iodoform gauze and the skin closed with mattress sutures. The gauze was removed apace with granulation of the deeper layers and the skin incision healed by first intention. No evidence of recurrence existed on last report 6 months later; however, perineal melanoma is too prevalent in aging grey horses to warrant a favorable prognosis for more than a short time.

As previously pointed out (HAYES 1968) it seems that by far the most common site of equine melanoma is the perianal region. STANNARD (1972) feels that equine melanomas develop in one of 3 different ways. The most common is a very slow growth over several years without metastases. The second most common is an apparent benign tumor which suddenly becomes malignant. Finally, some melanomas behave clearly in a malignant fashion from the start. The tumor in this patient appeared to belong to the first group, although a more prolonged follow-up would be required to determine if it later fell into the second category. Because of the already ulcerated nature of the lesion it was not possible to study the epidermodermal junction, an indispensable piece of information in the evaluation of any melanoma (LOPANSRI and MIHM 1979).

HAYES, M.H.
Veterinary Notes for Horse Owners p. 341. Arco Publishing Co., New York, 1968.
LOPANSRI, S. and MIHM, Jr., M.C.
Clinical and Pathological Correlation of Malignant Melanoma. Journal of Cutaneous Pathology 6:180, 1979.
STANNARD, A.A.
Melanoma, Equine Medicine and Surgery. Edited by E.J. Catcott and J.F. Smithcors. p. 395. American Veterinary Publications, Wheaton, Illinois, 1972.

A

B

C

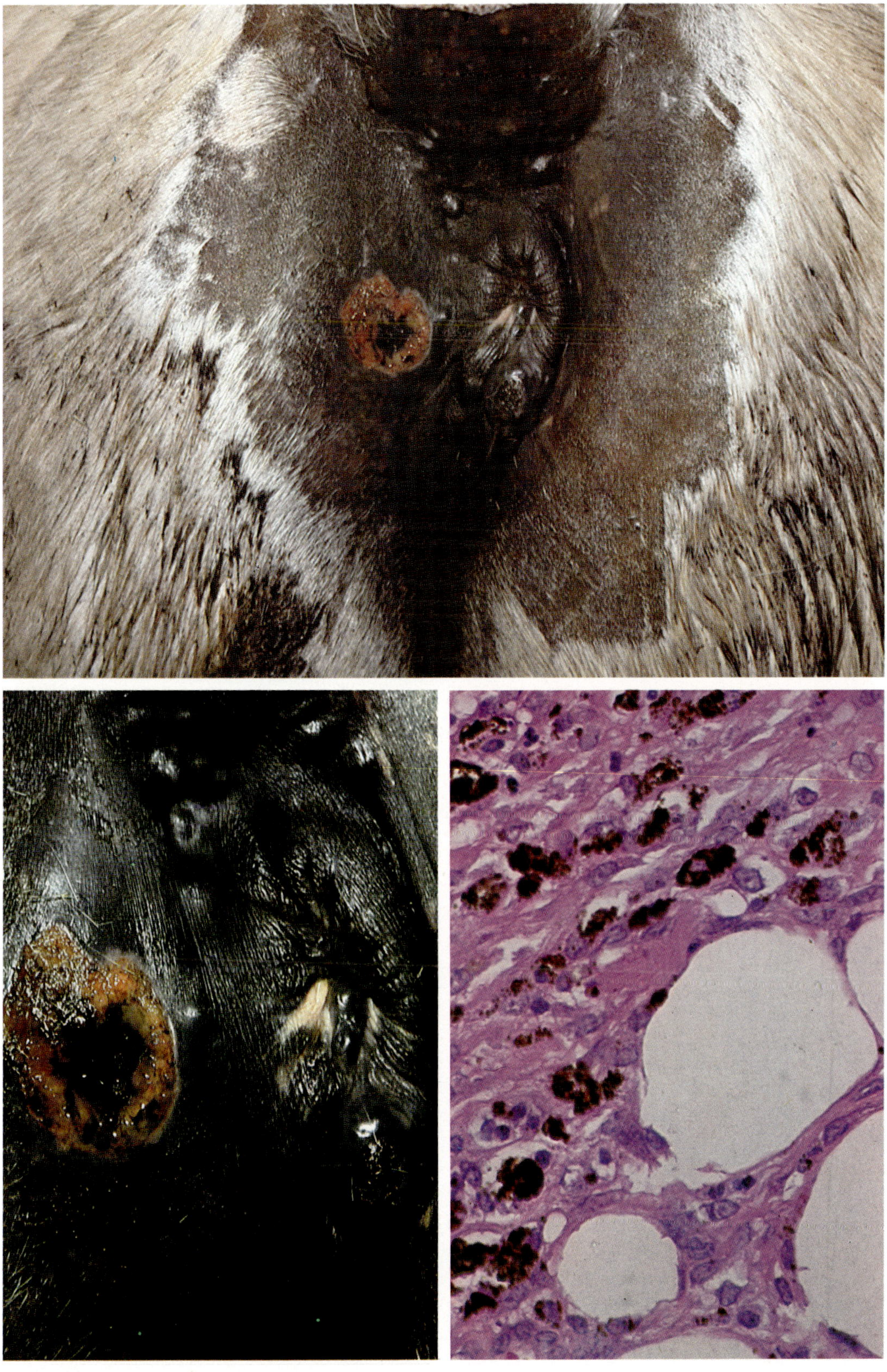

Squamous Cell Carcinoma

A 5-year-old Appaloosa mare was admitted for the recent complaint of a milky-white growth on the left eye.

Clinically, a raised, leucomatous plaque approximately 2 cm in diameter occupied an area of the lower cornea and adjacent bulbar conjunctiva from the 5 to 7 o'clock positions (Fig. A). The lesion had a pinkish color with visible vascular infiltration from the conjunctiva, a gelatinous appearance, and outward displacement. Photophobia, tearing and interference with vision were not features of this case.

Histopathologically, a Grade I squamous cell carcinoma with well-keratinized islands was found. There were many horny pearls and individual cell keratinization. Some of the keratinized cells appeared multinucleate. A prominent inflammatory infiltrate mainly composed of lymphocytes and plasma cells were found surrounding the neoplasm and also within the tumor between the islands of keratinized cells (Figs. C and D).

Treatment consisted of surgical excision by lamellar keratectomy done under general anesthesia with exposure extended by medial canthotomy (Fig. B). Postoperative irradiation by ^{90}strontium beta ray applicator was done twice at an interval of one week for treatment periods of approximately 6 minutes (determined by calibration of the source) to give a total dose of 10 to 20 thousand rads. No history of recurrence was known.

In a parallel case reported by Gelatt (1974) superficial keratectomy was repeated before recurrence was controlled. According to Morgan (1969) when the cornea is involved, there is less downward invasion because of the resistance of Bowman's membrane, Descemet's membrane and the substantia propria, lending some currency to the use of split-thickness keratectomy.

However, others warn that the impression that the invasive and destructive propensities for the adnexa and orbit do not apply to the globe may be false assurance stemming from mainly superfical examinations; and that invasion does occur either through the cornea or the sclera in 10–15% of the cases (JUBB and KENNEDY, 1970).

Cook (1966) has pointed out that multinucleate tumor cells are commonly found in intraepithelial carcinoma of the conjunctiva. In humans, squamous cell carcinomas of the conjunctiva at the corneoscleral limbus occur particularly in compromised hosts (NEWELL).

In horses, the tumor arises most frequently from the membrana nictitans (MORGAN, 1969; GELATT, et al, 1974) and predisposing factors include the lack of pigmentation in the lids as well as solar radiation. This claim is supported by the higher incidence of the disease in geographic regions of greater sunlight (AKEREJOLA, et al, 1978; MISDORP, 1967).

AKEREJOLA, O.O.; AYIVOR, M.D.; and ADAMS, E.W.
The Veterinary Record. 103:336, 1978.
COOK, C.A.
Systemic Pathology. p. 1069. Edited by G. Payling Wright and W. St. Clair Symmers Longmans, Green and Co., Ltd., London, 1966.
GELATT, K.N.; MYERS, V.S., JR.: PERMAN, V.: JESSEN, C.
Journal of American Veterinary Medical Association 165:617, 1974.
JUBB, K.V.F. and KENNEDY, P.C.
Pathology of Domestic Animals. Second Ed., V.2:542. Academic Press, New York & London, 1970.
MISDORP, W.
Journal of Comparative Pathology 77:211, 1967.
MORGAN, G.
Journal Small Animal Practice 10:563, 1969.
NEWELL, F.W.
Ophthalmology, p. 228. C.V. Mosby Company, St. Louis, 1978.

Grateful acknowledgement to Dr. R.A. Albert, Jr., and Dr. W.R. Brawner, Jr., School of Veterinary Medicine, Auburn University, AL 36849.

A

B

C

D

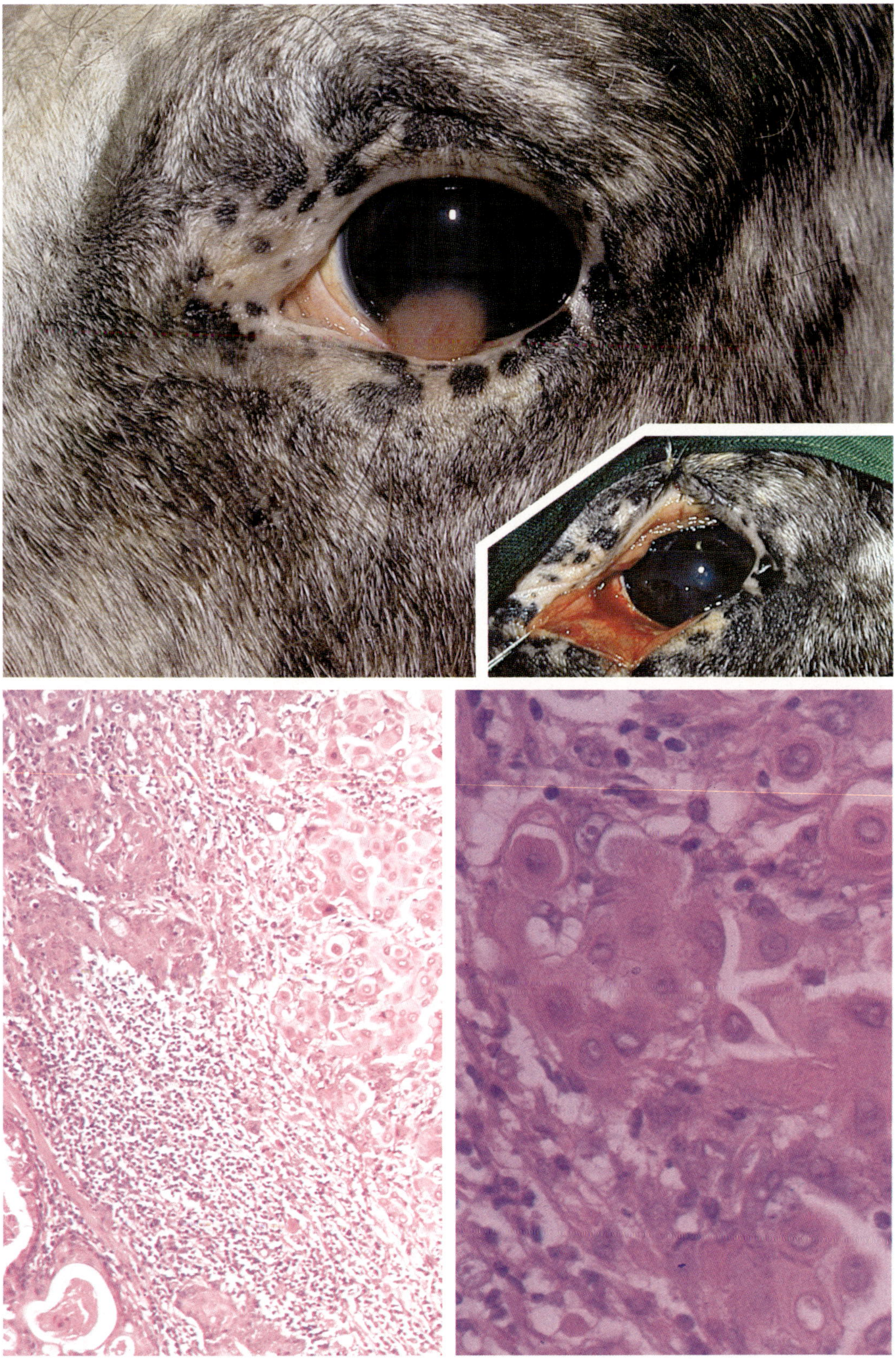

Squamous Cell Carcinoma

Two different patients were presented for evaluation of ulcerated areas involving the left eyelids.

Clinically, one of the patients (Fig. A) showed a very small superficial ulceration of the central portion of the lower lid. The lesion had a duration of about 3 months. The other patient (Fig. B) had more extensive invasion of both upper and lower lids by an ulcerated process, with partially indurated borders and a red denuded surface. The ulcer was beginning to spread into the skin surrounding the medial canthus. This patient's problem had started to develop about 6 months earlier. The skin surrounding the eye was entirely white in the first patient (Fig. A) and predominantly white in the second patient (Fig. B). In both cases there were signs of actinic damage such as thinning, hardening, wrinkling and mild erythema of the periorbital skin.

Histopathologically, the two patients demonstrated similar squamous cell carcinomas. Because of the large number of keratinized cells, little atypicality and only partial invasion of the dermis by the tumoral masses, these neoplasms were rated as Grade I Squamous Cell Carcinomas. An interesting feature of both tumors was the presence of a rather intense inflammatory infiltrate in the dermis surrounding the neoplastic masses. The infiltrate was predominantly composed of lymphocytes and some plasma cells (Fig. C).

Treatment of Grade I carcinomas of the lids that are characterized by slowly progressing ulcers (as opposed to granulomatous lesions) may be approached by fulguration or by ionizing radiation. In both instances, but primarily in the first, periodic checkups for recurrence is needed. The advantages of fulguration lie in its simplicity and availability, placing the modality in access to a larger number of patients. The disadvantages are that its effects are superficial, often necessitating repeated treatments, which in turn are attended by cicatricial entropion and eventually constriction of the palpebral fissure. The alternatives are the same ones that apply to the granulomatous lesions, namely surgical excision and/or ionizing radiation, in this case the implantation of radon seeds or the equivalent (BISTNER, et al, 1977). Mindful of the invasive nature of the neoplasm and of the surgical principles that apply, excision may involve full thickness resection of the eyelid lesion and blepharoplasty by such means as a sliding vertical flap of skin and orbicularis muscle backed with conjunctiva elevated from the uninvolved lower recesses of the eyelid and fornix. Irradiation used in conjunction with blepharoplasty should be done preoperatively to reduce the size of the lesion and postoperatively to treat recurrence (BISTNER, 1977; GELATT, 1972).

These two patients demonstrate very well what LEVER (1975) has been teaching for many years, namely that in squamous cell carcinoma Grade I (BRODERS, 1932) the dermal inflammatory reaction is much more pronounced than in the more advanced forms of squamous cell carcinoma. It seems that the host, when initially invaded by the tumor cells is able to react, thus offering a better prognosis at that early stage.

BISTNER, S.I., AGUIRRE, G. and BATIK, G.
Atlas of Veterinary Ophthalmic Surgery. W.B. Saunders Company, Philadelphia, 1977.

BRODERS, A.C.
Practical Points on the Microscopic Grading of Carcinoma. New York State Journal of Medicine 32:667, 1932.

GELATT, K.N.
Chapter 15, The Eye. Equine Medicine and Surgery, Second Edition, edited by E.J. Catcott and J.F. Smithcors, American Veterinary Publications, Inc., Wheaton, Illinois, 1972.

LEVER, W.F.
Histopathology of the Skin, p. 477 J.B. Lippincot Co., Philadelphia, 1975.

A

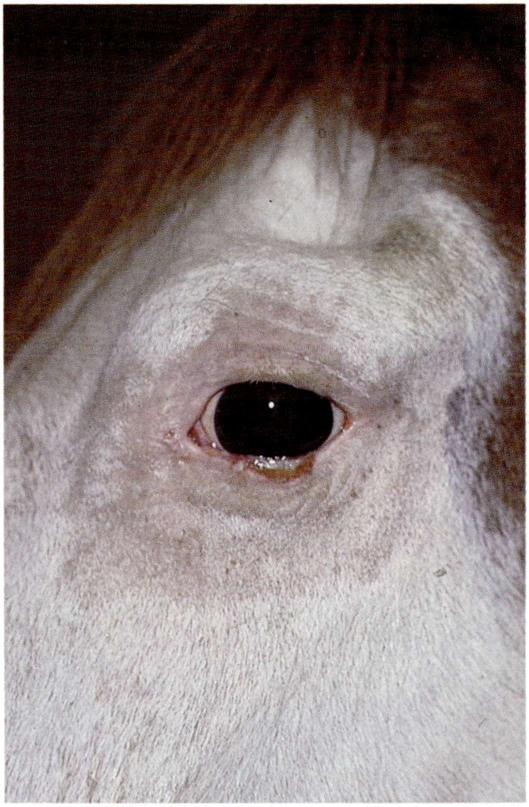

B

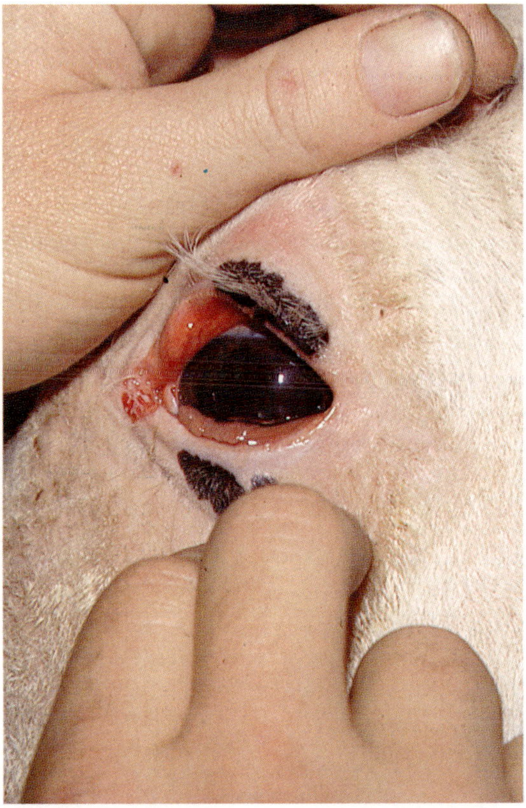

C

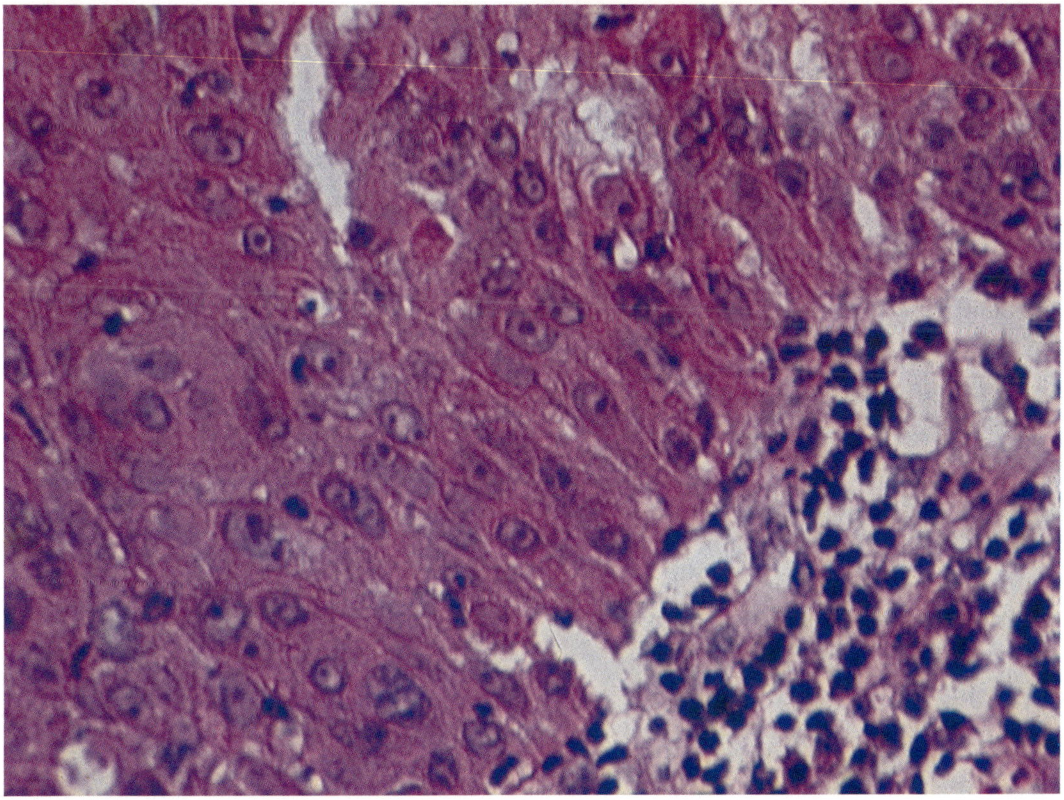

Squamous Cell Carcinoma

A 9-year-old bay Quarter Horse gelding was admitted for the complaint of a tumor of the left eye which had been noticed several months earlier as a small growth on the third eyelid. In recent weeks, its character had changed and the rate of growth accelerated.

Clinically, the lesion had displaced the visible architecture of the globe and protruded through the palprebral fissure, completely obscuring sight in that eye (Fig. A). Chronic lacrimation had altered the dependent area of the face. Remarkably, the primary eyelids and canthi appeared to be unaffected.

Histopathologically, the tumor showed some keratinization but in general it was poorly differentiated. A prominent feature were cells with a clear, almost vacuolated cytoplasm as mentioned by SANDERSON and MACKIE (1979). These vacuolated cells were often forming islands demarcated by a cellular infiltrate of lymphocytes, histiocytes and plasma cells (Fig. C).

Treatment. The tumor was injected with a 0.5% solution of cycloheximide using a total of 1 cm^3 for each treatment that was applied three times a week. The solution was injected into five different areas of the tumor each one receiving 0.2 cm^3. A very significant reduction in the size of the neoplasm, estimated as about 40% was accomplished after 4 weeks on this program.* Owing to the aggressive nature of the tumor and its known propensity for metastasis, the lesion was subsequently removed by en bloc (transpalpebral) enucleation (BISTNER, 1977; GELATT, 1972). Although the orbit appeared free of invasion and the superficial lymph nodules of the parotid region palpably normal, long-term survival was given a guarded prognosis. Although radon implants were unavailable for use in this case, they would have been indicated (see Case 47).

As mentioned in Case 46, ocular squamous cell carcinomas in the horse see highest incidence in the nictitating membrane. Although initially of low malignancy, in due course they do invade the orbit and destroy the eye. Metastasis is seen first in the superficial lymph nodes of the parotid region but remote spread has been observed in the heart, lungs, liver and kidneys (JUBB and KENNEDY, 1970; MORGAN, 1969).

GRAHAM and JOHNSON (1972) have published in their description of Bowen's disease with carcinoma, a picture quite similar to Fig. B.

BISTNER, S.I., AGUIRRE, G. and BATIK, G.
Atlas of Veterinary Ophthalmic Surgery. W.B. Saunders Company, Philadelphia, 1977.
GELATT, K.N.
Chapter 15, The Eye. Equine Medicine and Surgery, Second Edition, edited by E.J. Catcott and J.F. Smithcors. American Veterinary Publications, Inc., Wheaton, Illinois, 1972.
GRAHAM, J.H., JOHNSON, W.C. and HELWIG, E.B.
Dermal Pathology, p. 591 Harper and Row, New York, 1972.
JUBB, K.V.F. and KENNEDY, P.C.
Pathology of Domestic Animals. Second Ed., V.2:542 Academic Press, New York & London, 1970.
MORGAN, G.
Journal Small Animal Practice 10:563, 1969.
SANDERSON, K.V. and MACKIE, R.
Tumours of the Skin in Textbook of Dermatology Edited by A. Rook D.S. WILLKINSON and EBLING, F.J.G., p. 2187. Blackwell Scientific Publications. Oxford, 1979.

* See Case 30 on Warts for action of cycloheximide

A

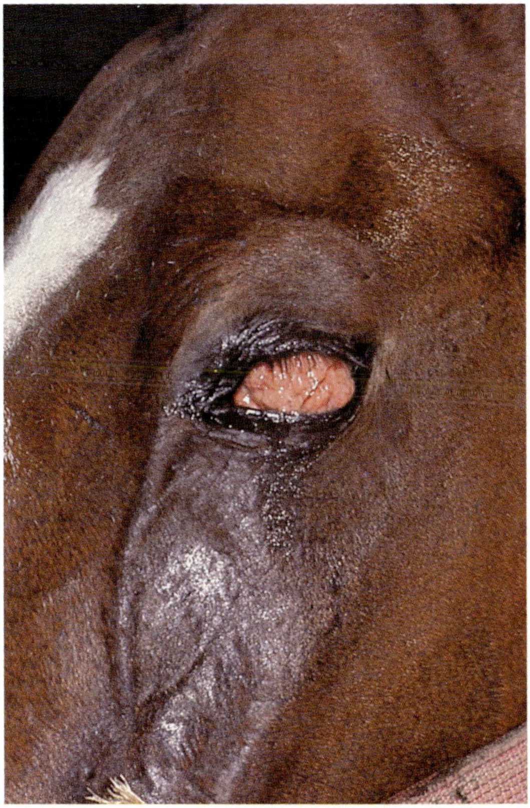

B

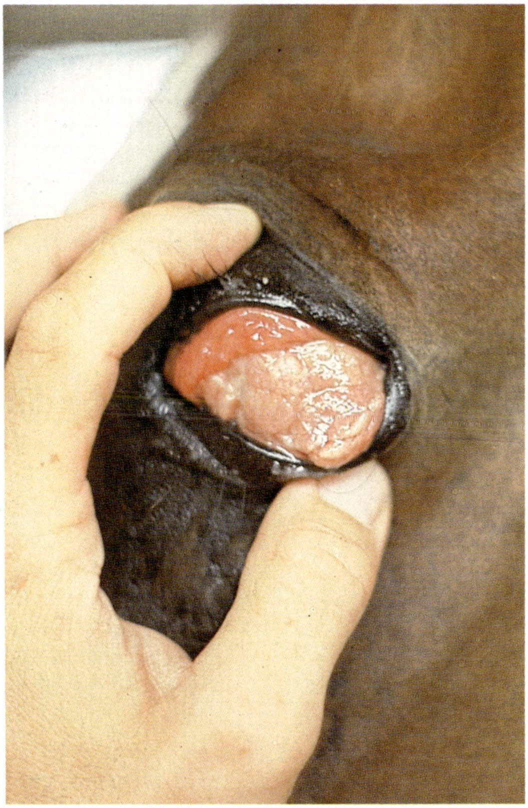

C

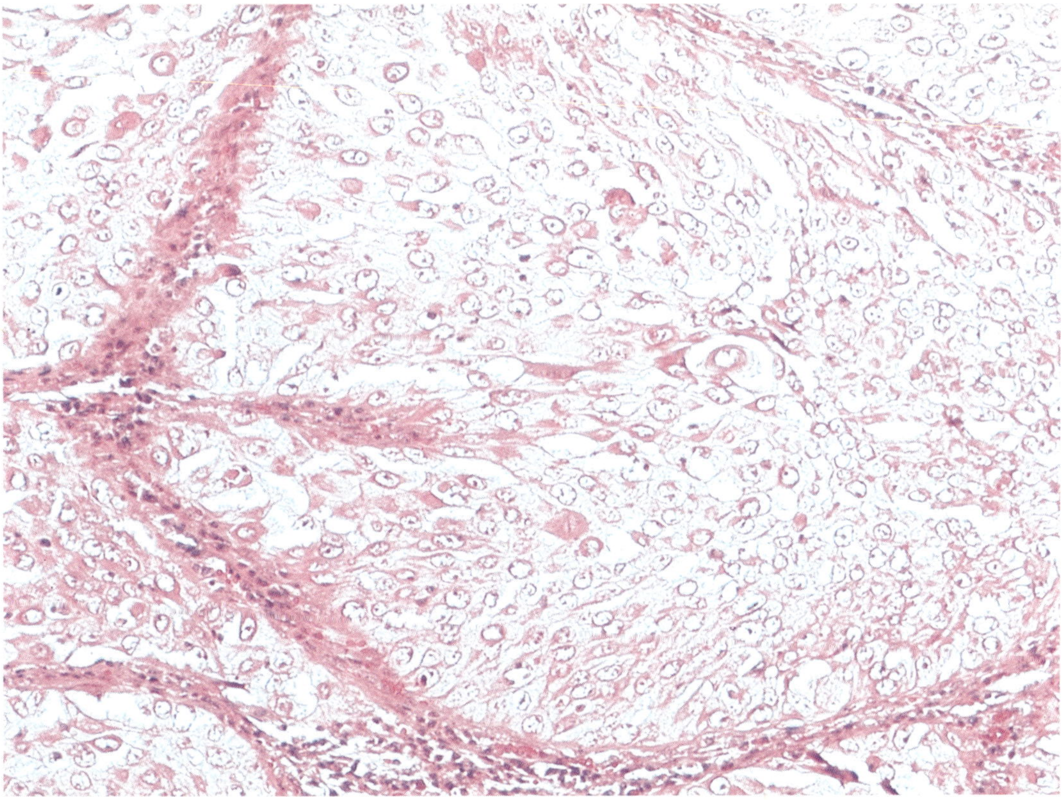

Squamous Cell Carcinoma

A 20-year-old Appaloosa horse was referred for evaluation and treatment of a chronic ulcer on a white skin area of the left nostril.

Clinically, an oval ulcerated crater, approximately 14 cm × 12 cm, with an erythematous moist surface covered a large portion of the left nostril (Fig. A). A left submandibular lymph node was distinctly enlarged and could be easily palpated.

Histopathologically, the same picture of a Grade III squamous cell carcinoma was seen in both the ulcerated skin and the lymph node. Invasion of the dermis by the tumor mass was striking. There was minimal keratinization. A large number of the tumor cells were atypical and mitoses were numerous (Figs. C and D).

Treatment consisted of radical surgical excision with primary closure of the surgical wound. The results were very satisfactory at the surgical site (Fig. B). The tumor, however, had already metastasized and the horse was subsequently euthanatized.

In the management of squamous cell carcinoma it must be kept in mind as summarized by GRABB and SMITH (1968) that this tumor has the capacity for rapid and wide local spread and for distant spread by blood stream and lymphatics. Besides prolonged exposure to sunlight other factors play a role in ultraviolet radiation injury. FREEMAN and KNOX (1964) found that the rate of development of skin tumors was higher in mice exposed to ultraviolet light and kept in a hot environment than in similarly exposed mice kept at room temperature. Later OWEN and KNOX (1978) showed that wind accelerates cutaneous carcinogenesis induced by ultraviolet radiation. Their data suggested a similar effect produced by high humidity.

This may be further supported by the reports of squamous cell carcinoma in the equidae of Northern Nigeria (AKEREJOLA, et al, 1978) and Queensland, Australia (MURRAY, et al, 1978).

AKEREJOLA, O.O., AYIVOR, M.D. and ADAMS, E.W.
The Veterinary record, 103:336, 1978.
FREEMAN, R.G. and KNOX, J.M.
Influence of Temperature on Ultraviolet Injury, Archives of Dermatology, 89:859, 1964.
GRABB, W.D. and SMITH, J.W.
Plastic Surgery, p. 592. Little Brown and Co., Boston, 1968.
MURRAY, D. R., LADDS, P.W. and CAMPBELL, R.S.F.
Australian Veterinary Journal, 54:338, 1978.
OWENS, D.W. and KNOX, J.M.
Influence of Heat, Wind, and Humidity on Ultraviolet Radiation Injury, International Conference on Ultraviolet carcinogenesis, p. 161.
Dept. of Health, Education and Welfare, Publication No. 78-1532, 1978.

A

B

C

D

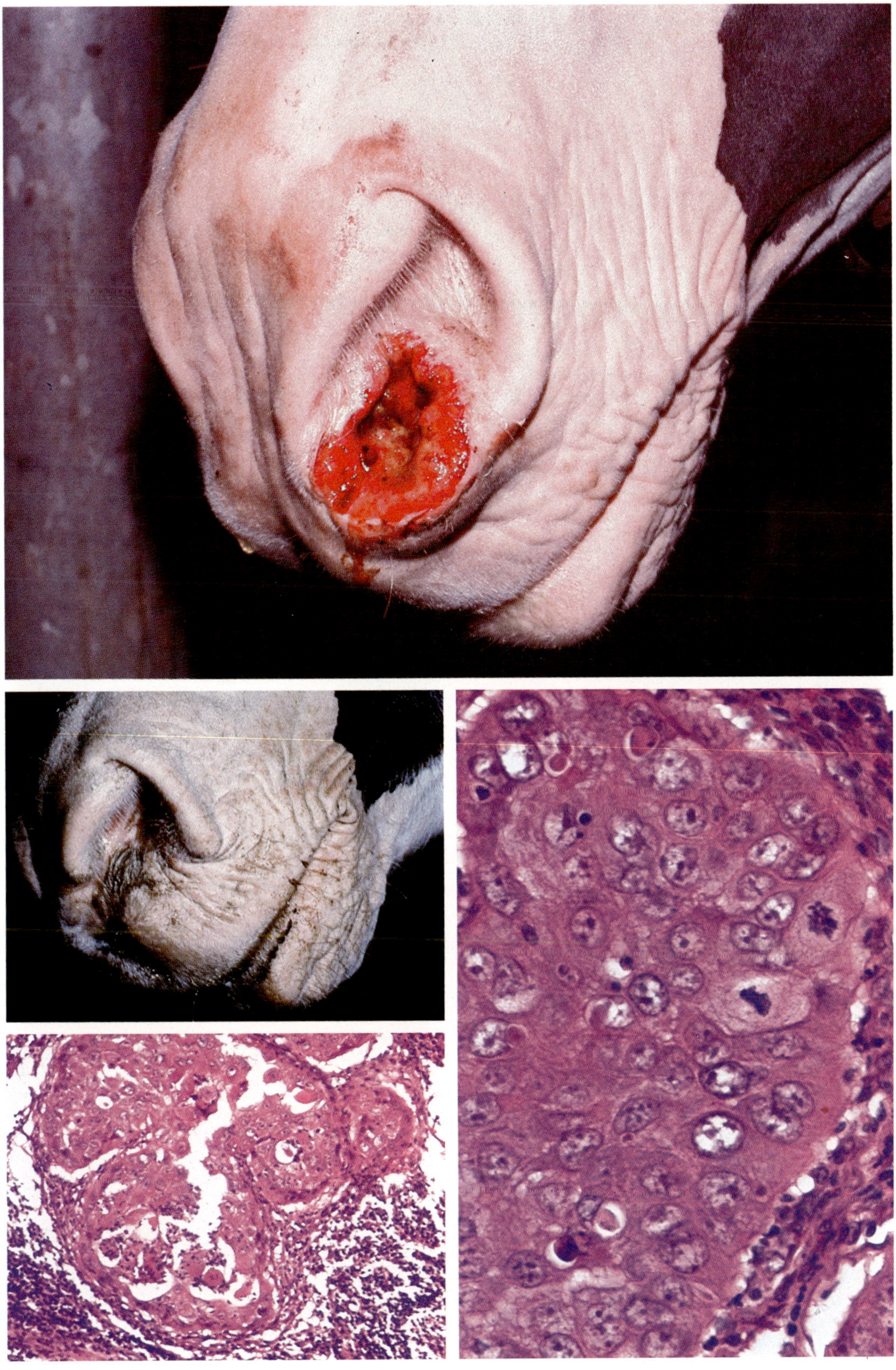

Squamous Cell Carcinoma

A 12-year-old bay pony was presented for treatment of a chronic skin disease of the penis. The condition had been noticed for some time but had only recently become sufficiently objectionable to the owner to precipitate a visit to the clinic.

Clinically, the shaft of the penis, the prepuce and the glans were involved by a process composed of flat, verrucous or superficially ulcerated lesions that were confluent in many areas forming plaques (Fig. A). The urethral meatus was entirely involved and more ulcerated than the rest of the penis. Ulceration was most severe in the dorsal aspect of the fossa glandis (Fig B).

Histopathologically, the tumor was a well-differentiated Grade I squamous cell carcinoma with many horn pearls, little penetration into the dermis, and a prominent inflammatory reaction mainly composed of lymphocytes and plasma cells (Fig. C).

Treatment of such an extensive lesion requires radical resection of the entire prepuce (including both inner and outer laminae) and amputation of the penis (balanoposthectomy). If there is no evidence of spread to the superficial inguinal lymph nodules, en bloc resection is not required, and urethrostomy can be made just caudal to the site of the natural external preputial orifice. Longitudinal as well as transverse spatulation of the transected urethra will prevent the postoperative stenosis due to cicatricial constriction.

Tumors of the penis and prepuce include commonly the squamous papillomas as well as squamous cell carcinomas, and further clouding the diagnosis are the frequent granulomas of cutaneous habronemiasis. For this reason, diagnosis should always be confirmed by histopathologic examination. The gross appearance of the lesions in this case closely parallel JUBB and KENNEDY's description (1970) of keratinized and ulcerated tumors; however, the following Case 51 better displays the fungating characteristics of growth.

JUBB, K. V. F. and KENNEDY, P. C.
Pathology of Domestic Animals. First Ed., V.1:481. Academic Press, New York & London, 1970.
WALKER, D. F. and VAUGHAN, J. T.
Bovine and Equine Urogenital Surgery, p. 136. Lea & Febiger, Philadelphia, 1980.

A

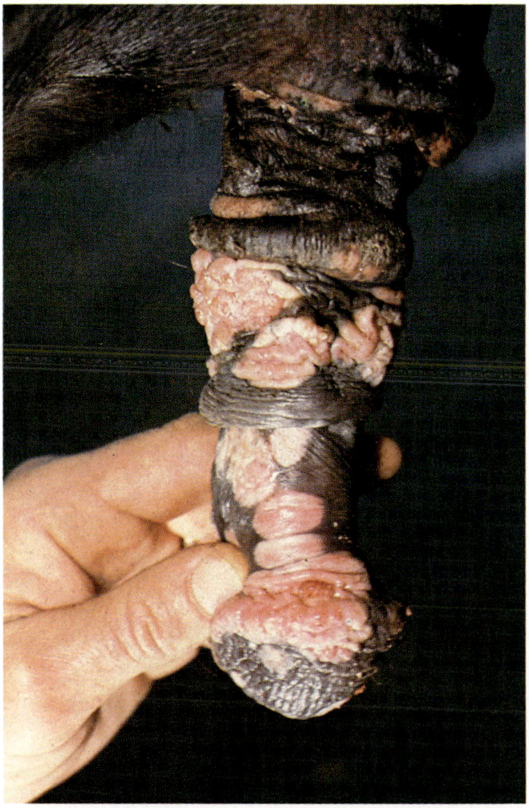

B

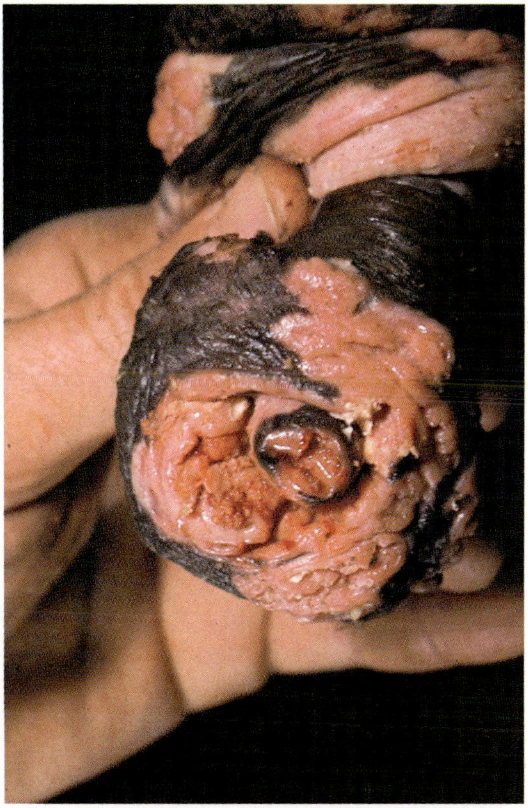

C

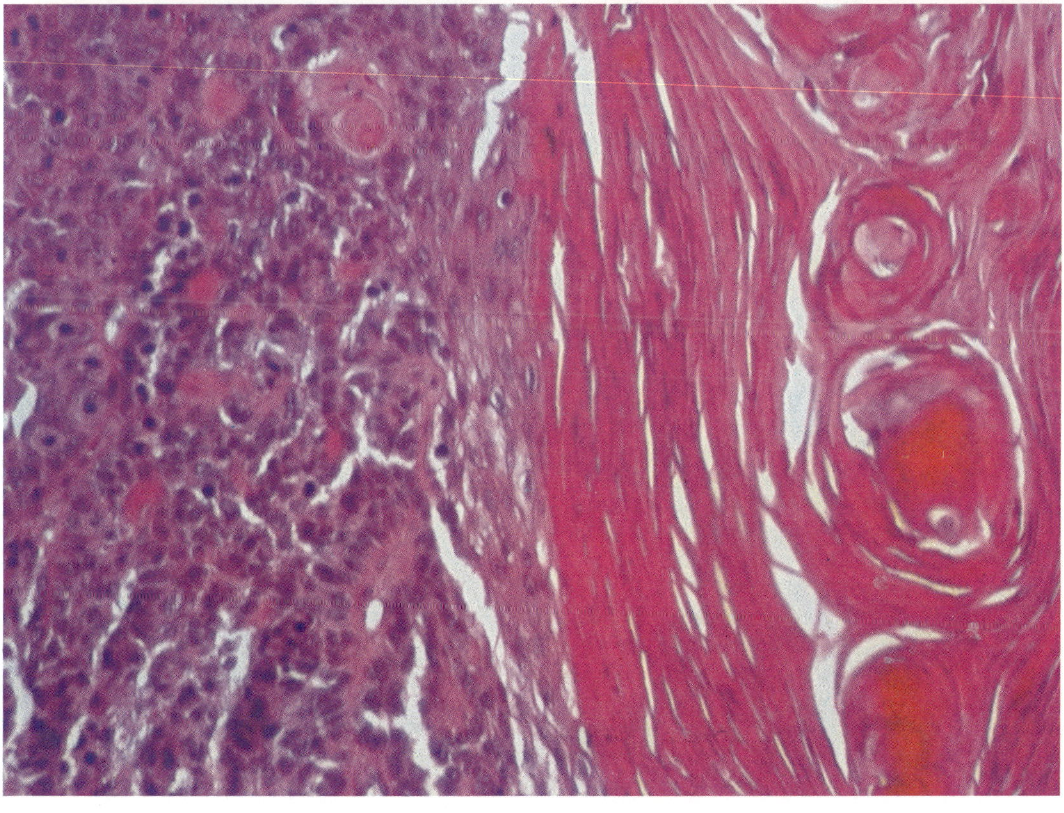

Squamous Cell Carcinoma

A 7-year-old bay half-bred gelding was admitted for surgery to remove a large, ulcerated mass on the penis. The owner had become alarmed at the tumor's rapid increase in size during the last few weeks.

Clinically, a vegetating, multilobulated tumor with a yellowish-red color, hard consistency, moist surface and numerous fine telangiectasiae was growing posteriorly from the mid-portion of the shaft of the penis proximally to the preputial attachment. The entire tumor had a tendency to grow towards the outside rather than to invade the surrounding or the deeper layers of the skin (Fig. A).

Histopathologically, the tumor was a Grade II squamous cell carcinoma with relatively little keratinization and a good number of mitoses. Many of the tumor cells appeared vacuolated and atypical (Figs. B and C).

Treatment was by amputation of the penis (phallectomy). This decision was based on the biopsy Grade II and the tumor's history of rapid growth. Alternatively, circumscribed carcinoma in situ that is slow-growing and has not invaded the tunica albuginea of the penis can be excised with a generous margin of normal skin and subcutaneous adventitia without amputation of the penis, the technique being of obvious value in the entire male used for breeding purposes. In this case, the tumor also impinged on the corpus spongiosum, and limited dissection would have most assuredly breached the urethra.

An interesting histological survey of 244 tumors from 155 horses revealed the external genitalia as second in incidence only to the skin in the systemic distribution of lesions. In percentage of horses with tumors, 57.1% involved skin, 17.4% external genitalia, and 10.3% eye and orbit. Of the 19 squamous cell carcinomas in the series, 8 involved the epithelium of the penis and prepuce, 8 affected the eye, 2 the clitoris, and 1 the hard palate. (BAKER and LEYLAND, 1975.)

In AKEREJOLA's series of 11 cases of squamous cell carcinoma (1978), 5 involved the penis or prepuce and 5 the eyelids. Accumulation of smegma with age and the lack of pigmentation were advanced as possible predisposing influences for the occurrence of carcinomas in an area unexposed to direct sunlight.

AKEREJOLA, O. O., AYIVOR, M. D., and ADAMS, E. W.
The Veterinary Record, 1978.

BAKER, J. R. and LEYLAND, A.
The Veterinary Record, 96:419, 1975.

A

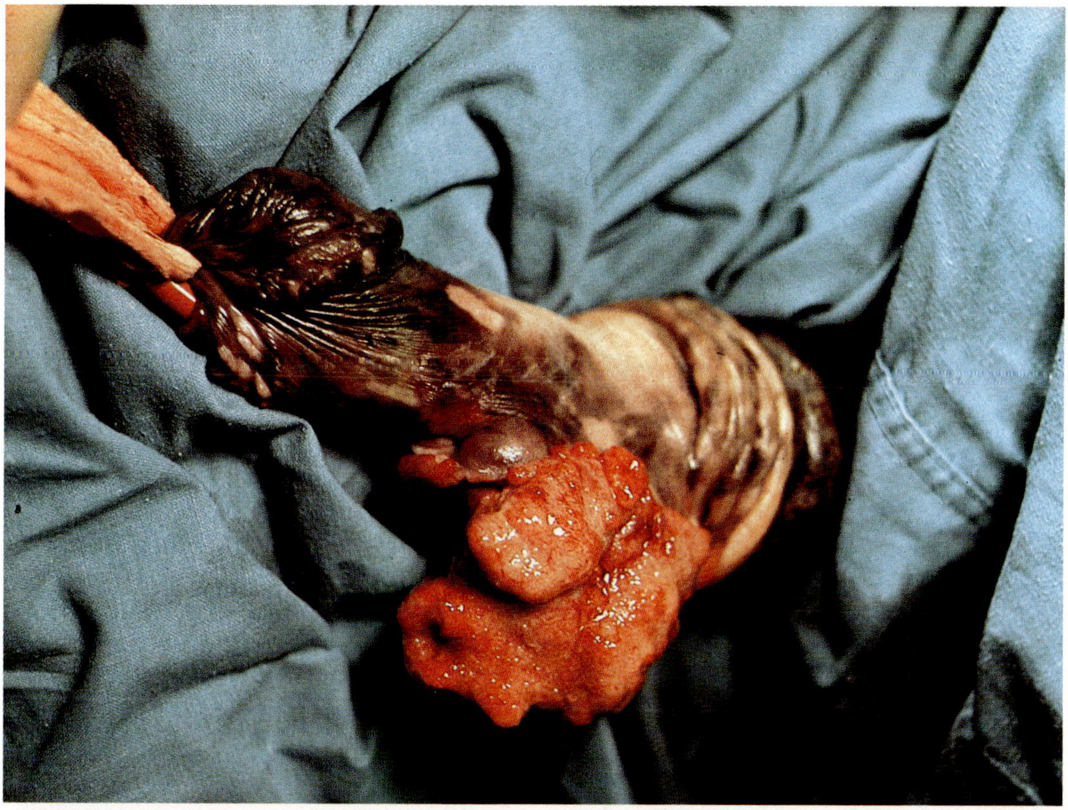

B

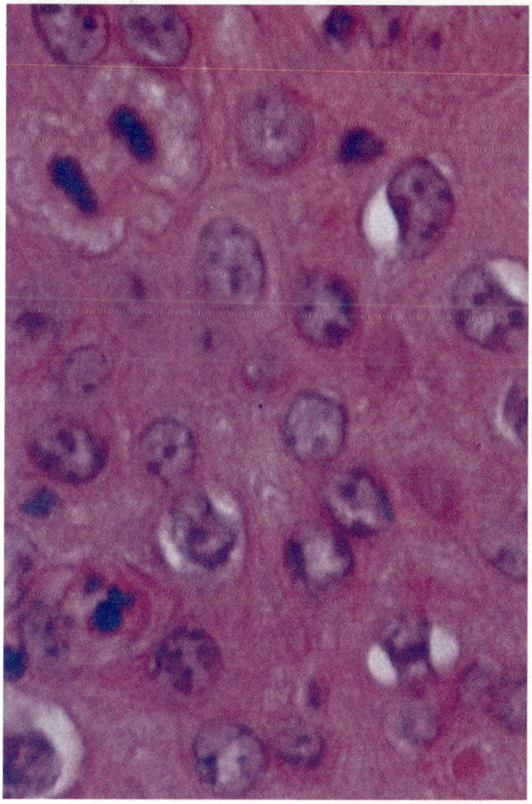

C

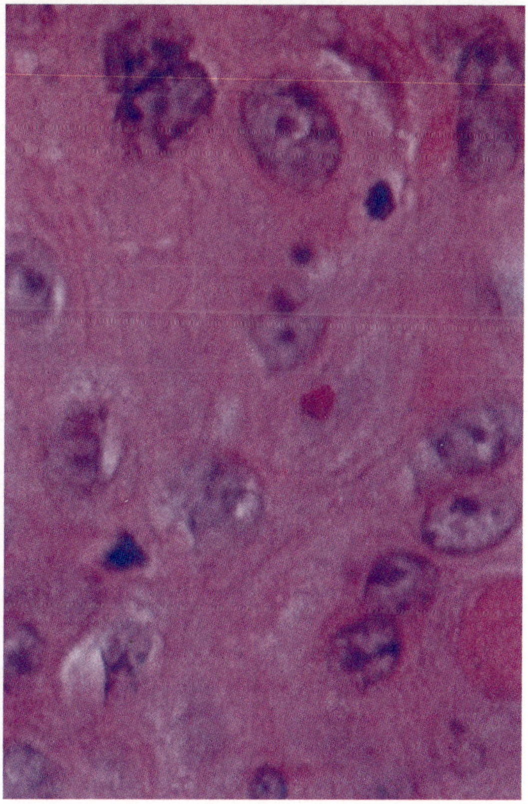

Squamous Cell Carcinoma

A 10-year-old female Paint horse was examined because of a large mass that had been growing in the genital region over the past 6 months.

Clinically, a rounded pedunculated tumor, approximately 20 cm in diameter protruded outside the vulva. It had a firm consistency, and was covered in part by dark crusts of coagulated blood under which the tumor itself showed red and yellowish areas alternating with some islands of epidermis. Multiple nodules partially covered by yellowish crusts and some small ulcers were also present at the edges of the vulva. The entire process involved areas of white skin (Fig. A).

Histopathologically, many of the tumor cells were atypical and there were very few keratinized areas. There were numerous mitoses, many vacuolated cells and occasional acantholysis. The epidermodermal junction was indistinguishable (Figs. B and C).

Treatment was by unilateral vulvectomy and excision of the satellite lesions closed under suture and followed with orthovoltage x-ray therapy, 4,000 rads total dose administered in 6 equal fractions, twice weekly for 3 weeks. There was no recurrence during the year the case was available to inspection. However, even in the case of carcinoma in situ, when neglected as long as this case had been, optimistic prognosis is unwarranted.

JUBB and KENNEDY (1970) asserted that squamous cell carcinoma of the vulva is well-known in the mare and the cow, and McMULLAN (1976) associated a frequency of the vulval tumors in areas close to natural body openings and particularly on unpigmented skin.

STANNARD (1972) presented a patient with extensive involvement of the vulva and perivulvar region also developing in white skin. The tumor was mostly ulcerated. He described another tumor in the external genitalia of an aged gelding with a cauliflower-like morphology.

JUBB, K. V. F. and KENNEDY, P. C.
Pathology of Domestic Animals. Second Ed. V.I:548 Academic Press, New York & London, 1970.

McMULLAN, W. D.
Equine Dermatology. Proceedings of the American Association of Equine Practitioners, p. 318, 1976.

RUNNELLS, R. A. and BENBROOK, E. A.
Epithelial Tumors of Horses. American Journal of Veterinary Research, 3:176, 1942.

STANNARD, A. A.
Equine Medicine and Surgery. Edited by E. J. CATCOTT and J. F. SMITHCORS, p. 397. American Veterinary Publications, Wheaton, Illinois, 1972.

A

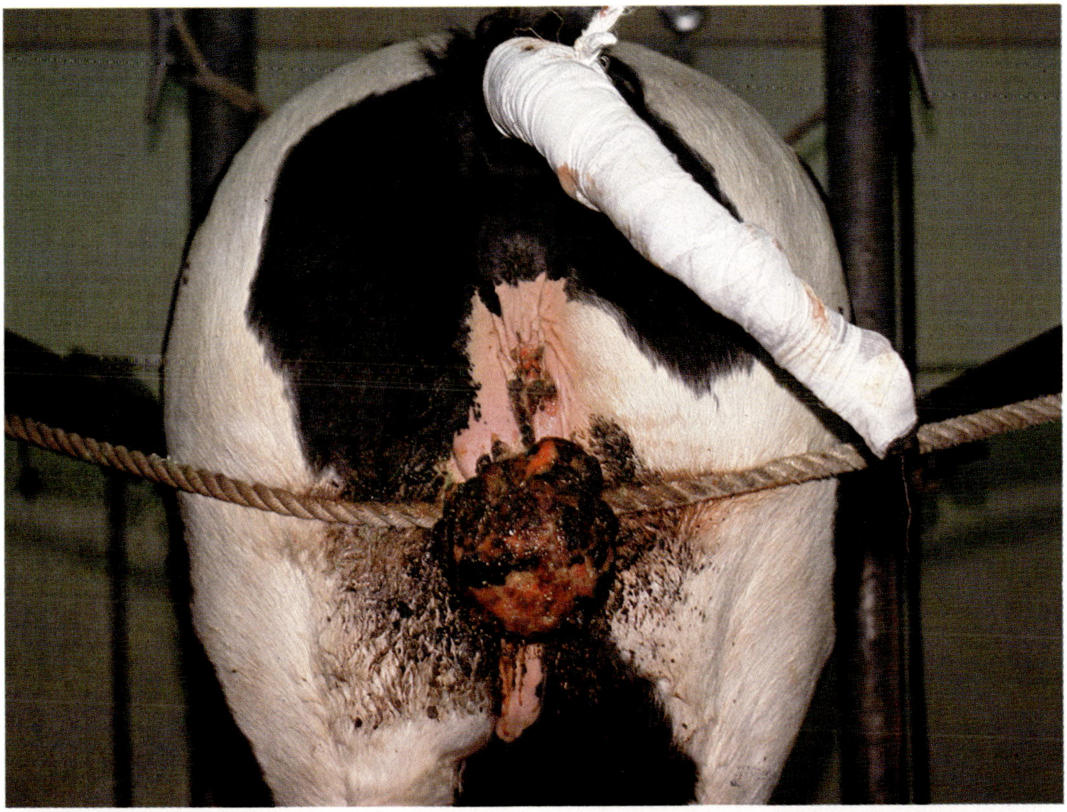

B

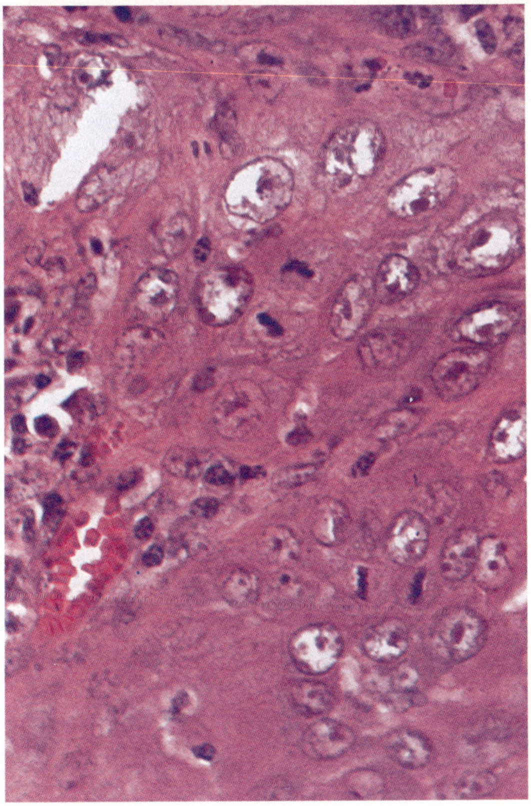

C

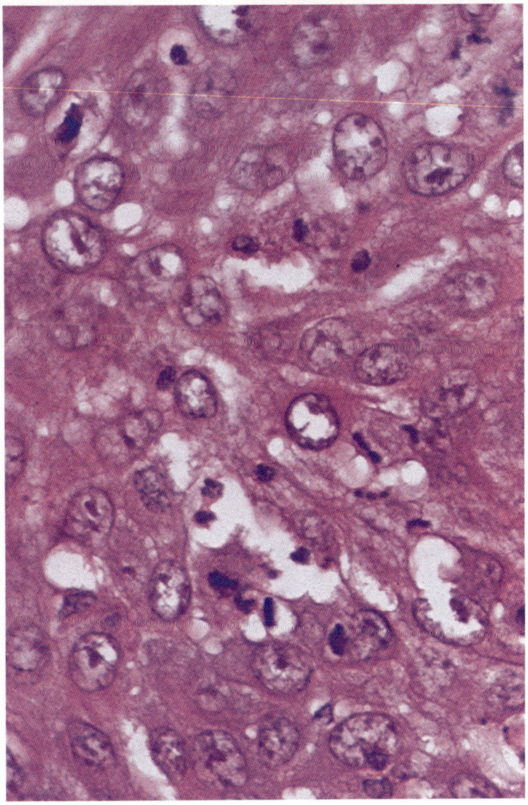

Squamous Cell Carcinoma

A mature paint mare was presented for the complaint of a large, suppurating mass occupying the region of the udder and medial aspect of the left thigh. The mare had been a patient a year previously at which time a unilateral vulvectomy had been done for squamous cell carcinoma of the left labium. The wound had healed with local recurrence.

Clinically, a large, indurated mass extended from just below the vulva ventrally and cranially to occupy or displace the udder, primarily the left half, and appeared to invade the muscles of the medial aspect of the left thigh. There was an overlaid plaque of edema that was penetrated in multiple sites by draining abscesses and ulcers producing a malodorous discharge (Fig. A).

Histopathologically, a biopsy confirmed squamous cell carcinoma Grade IV, interpreted to be a recurrence of the previous lesion.

The mare was euthanatized, and upon necropsy remote metastasis to the lung was discovered (Fig. B). Cut surface of the left mammary gland revealed complete replacement of the normal architecture by neoplasm (Fig. C). There was also extensive invasion of the gracilis muscle of the left thigh.

The vulva and vagina of the mare are drained by the caudal group of the anorectal lymph nodes situated at the dorsolateral border of the anus, on the levator ani and external anal sphincter muscles; and also by the superficial inguinal (mammary) lymph nodes between the ventral abdominal wall and the udder in the region of the external pudendal vein as it exits the abdominal wall. Some of the nodes extend to the ventral pelvic wall and lateral face of the udder. These constitute the natural routes of spread for carcinomas of the vulva in the mare (SAAR and GETTY, 1975).

The tumor in this case illustrates the aggressiveness of recurrent lesions and their propensity for spread, which argues well the defense for early and accurate diagnosis and effective management of the primary tumor upon first encounter.

SAAR, L. I. and GETTY, R.
Chapter 23, Equine Lymphatic System. Sisson and Grossman's The Anatomy of the Domestic Animals, Fifth Edition, p. 626. W. B. Saunders Company, Philadelphia, 1975.

(Grateful acknowledgement to Dr. Denise S. Jones, Sadieville, Kentucky.)

A

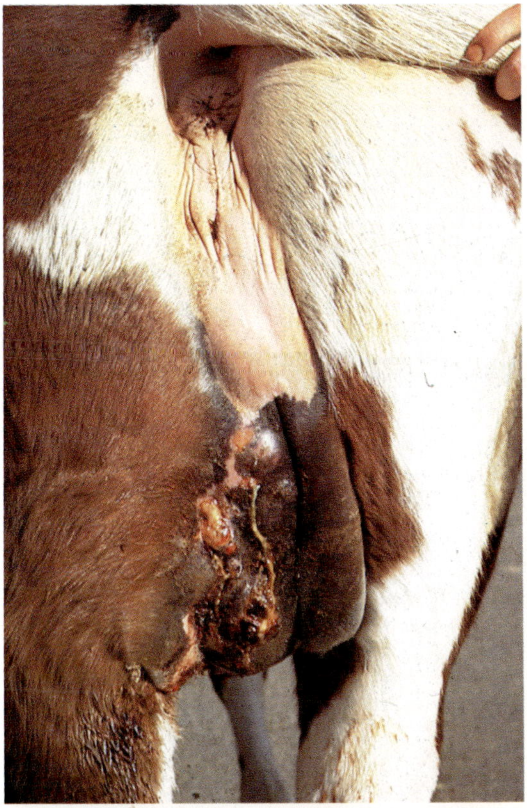

B

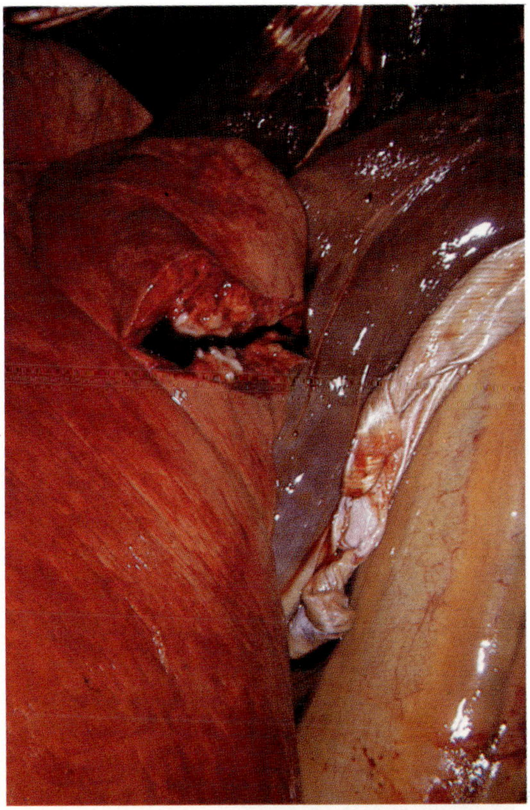

C

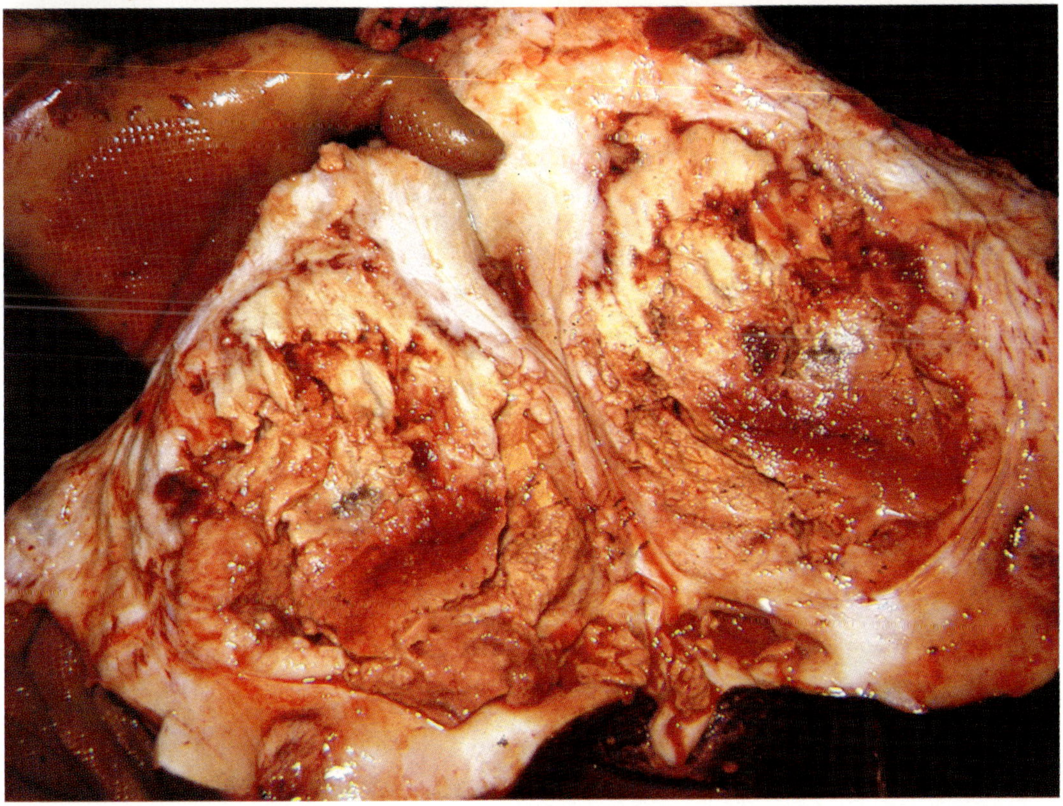

Inflammatory Dermatoses

Diseases described in this chapter are of varied etiology. Multiple factors usually act together to produce the cutaneous changes.

Histopathological features are not always diagnostic but biopsies are helpful to understand the disease process.

If properly treated patients like these will heal without serious cutaneous sequelae.

Chronic Dermatitis

A 7-year-old male Quarter Horse required dermatological management because of a cutaneous problem over the left hip.

Clinically, the central part of the affected area showed a superficial excoriation partially covered by small dark crusts. Incompletely surrounding the excoriations, the skin was hypopigmented and had partial hair loss. In places the skin had a cigarette paper-like appearance. There were also some excoriations in the periphery (Fig. A).

Histopathologically, a 6 mm punch biopsy was removed from the hypopigmented zone which showed a number of changes. There was acanthosis, hydropic degeneration of the basal cell layer and a chronic inflammatory infiltrate in the upper dermis. In addition considerable incontinence of pigment was found in many parts of the upper dermis and the mid-dermis. (Fig. B).

Treatment. The patient was treated using 1% hydrocortisone acetate in an ointment base (PHYSICIAN's DESK REFERENCE 1979) twice daily. The response was immediate and very rapid so only two weeks' treatment was needed. Hydrocortisone acetate (hydrocortisone 21-acetate) is a white crystalline powder insoluble in water, as a matter of fact considerably less soluble than hydrocortisone (OSOL and PRATT 1973).

In this condition the cutaneous integrity was already broken in certain places. Then it required a type of agent with anti-inflammatory action but at the same time without slowing down healing of the erosions. For this reason, the older, less active hydrocortisone acetate was preferred over the newer, much stronger fluorinated synthetic steroids.

Although clinical inspection suggested some form of minor trauma such as rubbing, the history of the problem was not clear and did not contribute to elucidate the etiology of this dermatitis. The superficial nature of the dermatitis indicated that the skin could heal rapidly and without scarring. This was already suggested by the histopathological findings. The pigmentary incontinence although rather impressive under the microscope was of the magnitude usually seen in dermatoses with hydropic degeneration of the basal cell layer (GRAHAM et al 1972) and has no major diagnostic significance.

GRAHAM, J.H., JOHNSON, W.C., and HELWIG, E.B.
Dermal Pathology, p. 127. Harper and Row, New York, 1972.
OSOL, A. and PRATT, R.
The United States Dispensatory p. 591. J.B. Lippincott Company, Philadelphia 1973.
PHYSICIAN's DESK REFERENCE
P. 1748. Medical Economics Co., Oradell, N.J. 1979.

A

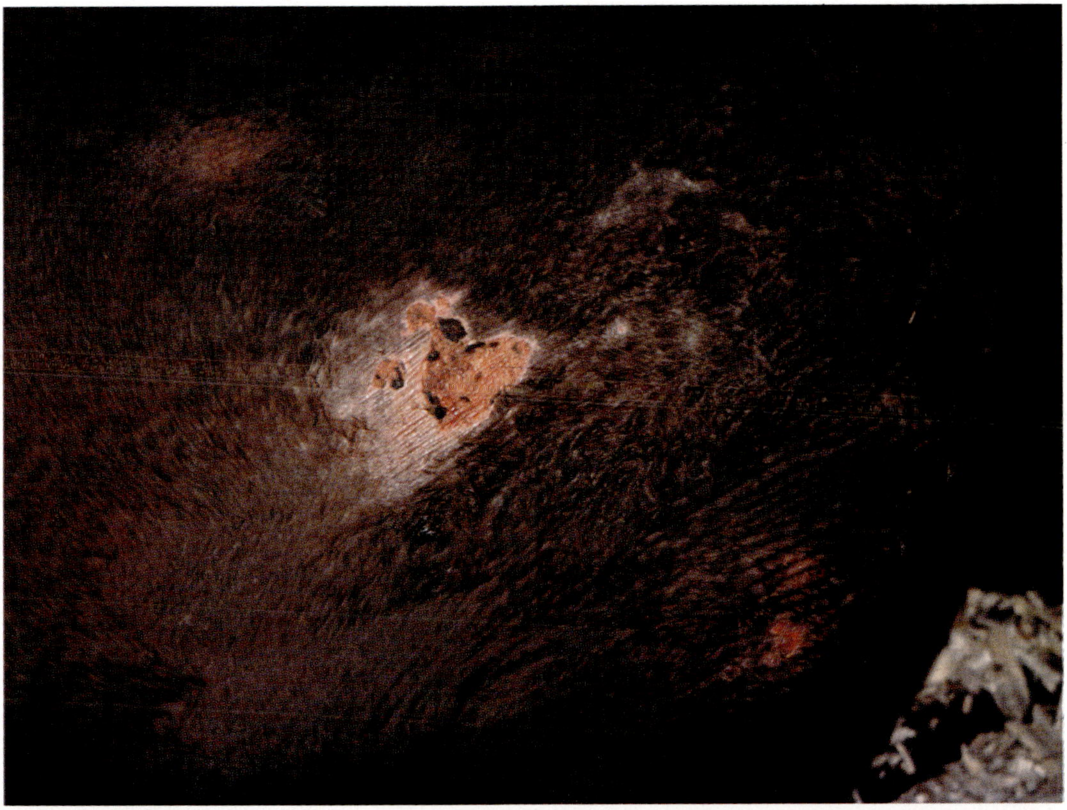

B

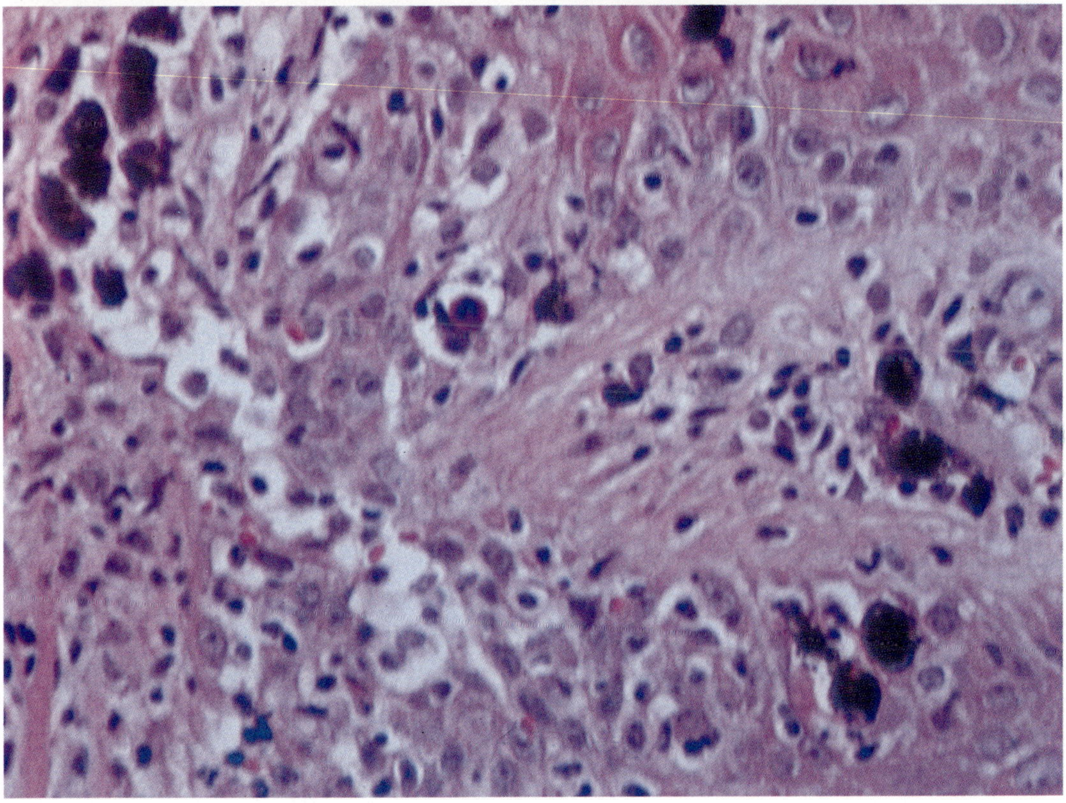

Light Eruption

A 10-year-old female Paint horse admitted to the Isolation Unit due to equine infectious anemia (EIA) required dermatological evaluation because of a generalized rash of two months duration. The condition developed during the middle of the summer.

Clinically, diffuse erythema which faded upon diascopy was specially prominent in the white skin areas while it could not be detected in the pigmented regions of the skin. Many of the erythematous areas showed loss of hair and whitish scales (Figs. A and B).

Histopathologically, the affected areas showed hyperkeratosis and follicular plugging. There was moderate atrophy of the stratum spinosum with disappearance of the rete pegs. The epidermodermal junction appeared intact (Fig. C). PAS stained sections failed to reveal alterations in the basement membrane. The dermis contained a patchy inflammatory infiltrate composed mostly of lymphocytes and erythrocytes (Fig. D). The inflammatory patches were predominantly perivascular and around the pilosebaceous apparatus.

Treatment of the light eruption was achieved by continuous maintenance of the patient in a completely enclosed stall during four weeks. The dermatitis gradually underwent complete clearing. The horse was later euthanatized because of the EIA.

In this patient, the protective role of melanin (LORINCZ 1954) was demonstrated by the fact that the pigmented areas were spared.

The generalized nature of the rash suggests strongly a systemic mechanism rather than a photocontact type of light sensitivity. The possibility of photosensitization induced by a systemically administered drug was seriously considered but the history in this regard was negative.

CLARE (1955) considered four types of photosensitization in domestic animals: a) a primary type; b) a type due to an abnormal pigment synthesis; c) a hepatogenous type and d) a type of uncertain etiology. Because this horse had EIA and in this condition lymphoproliferative changes occur in the liver (KONO and YAMAMOTO 1970), the possibility of a hepatogenous type of photosensitization in our patient was not unlikely.

Clinically and also histopathologically there were many of the features observed in lupus erythematosus. An important change was lacking, namely alterations in the basement membrane of the epidermodermal junction which in this patient's lesions appeared intact.

CLARE, N. T.
Photosensitization in Animals. Adv. Veterinary Science 2:182, 1955.

KONO, S. and YAMAMOTO, H.
Pathology of Equine Infectious Anemia. Proposed Classification of Pathologic Types of Disease. Cornell Veterinary 60:393, 1970.

LORINCZ, A. L.
Pigmentation. Physiology and Biochemistry of the Skin. Edited by S. ROTHMAN p. 520 University of Chicago Press, Chicago, 1954.

PLATE 55

A B

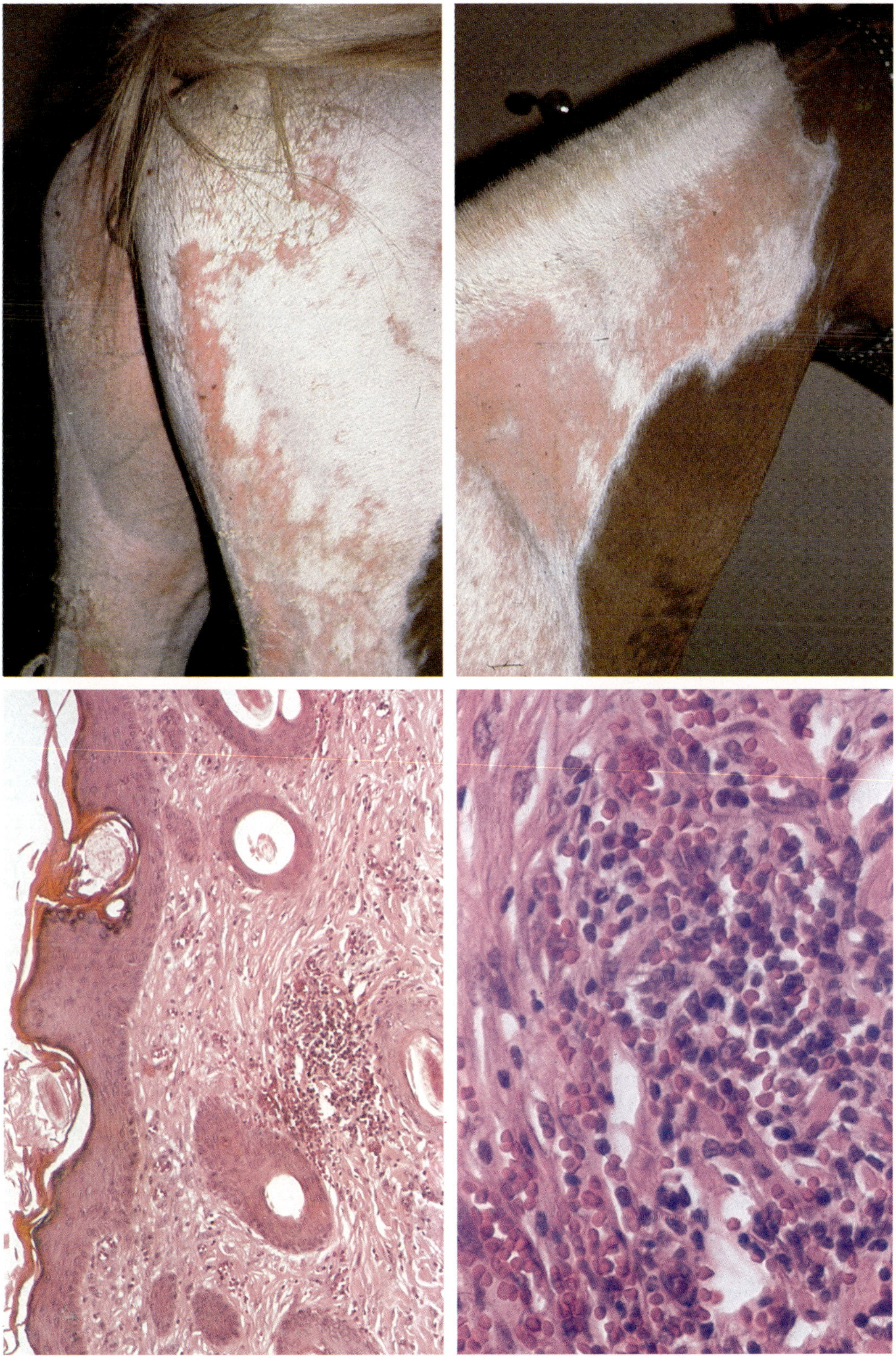

C D

Light Eruption

A 4-year-old Quarter Horse became anorectic and depressed while at the same time developed a dermatitis of the muzzle. He was brought to the hospital in early summer when the condition had become gradually more severe after onset two months earlier.

Clinically, the involved area displayed a diffuse pink erythema. There were also excoriations and crusts of various sizes and small hyperpigmented macules (Fig. A).

Histopathologically, a thin crust composed of fibrin and leukocytes was overlying the skin in the excoriated areas. In the zones of erythema, there were hyperkeratosis and parakeratosis. The infundibula of hair follicles were filled with moderately sized hyperkeratotic plugs (Fig. B). There was focal liquefaction of the basal cell layer. The upper dermis contained dilated capillaries and many extravasated red blood cells. A perifollicular inflammatory infiltrate composed of lymphocytes, plasma cells, histiocytes and some eosinophils was also observed (Fig. C).

Treatment consisted of topical application of 1% hydrocortisone cream twice daily and maintenance of the patient in an enclosed stall continuously for four weeks. Complete clearing of the eruption was obtained. The patient was discharged with instructions to the owner to keep the horse away from the sun avoiding grazing as much as possible for the rest of the summer.

Whether this patient's condition was phototoxic or photoallergic could not be determined although it seems certain that we were dealing with a photocontact rather than a systemic type of photosensitization. The horse had been grazing in a field where several types of pasture were present. No evidence of contact with alsike clover as described by FINCHER and FULLER (1942) could be obtained.

An excellent review of the problem of severe photosensitization involving the nose ("blue nose disease") as observed in Great Britain was presented by TUTT (1973). It was first described as affecting horses in Co. Derry while they were grazing during hot summer weather. The horses had been turned out on a meadow pasture where the plant St. John's Wort was extremely abundant. Some of the horses were so severely affected that they developed facial edema, cerebral symptoms, conjunctivitis and death.

Although it has been recommended as topical treatment of equine skin infections (FENNELL and VASS), trichlorcarbanilide, a common photosensitizer must be avoided if light eruption is to be prevented.

FENNELL, C. and VASS, R.I.
The Treatment of Equine Skin Infections Using Topical Trichlorcarbanilide. Equine Veterinary Journal 18:42, 1976.
FINCHER, M.G. and FULLER, H.K.
Photosensitization-trifoliosis-light sensitization. Cornell Veterinarian 32:95, 1942.
TUTT, J.F.D.
Blue Nose Disease or Photosensitization. Veterinary Notes for Horse Owners. Edited by M.H. Hayes. p. 180. Arco Publishing Company, New York 1973.

A

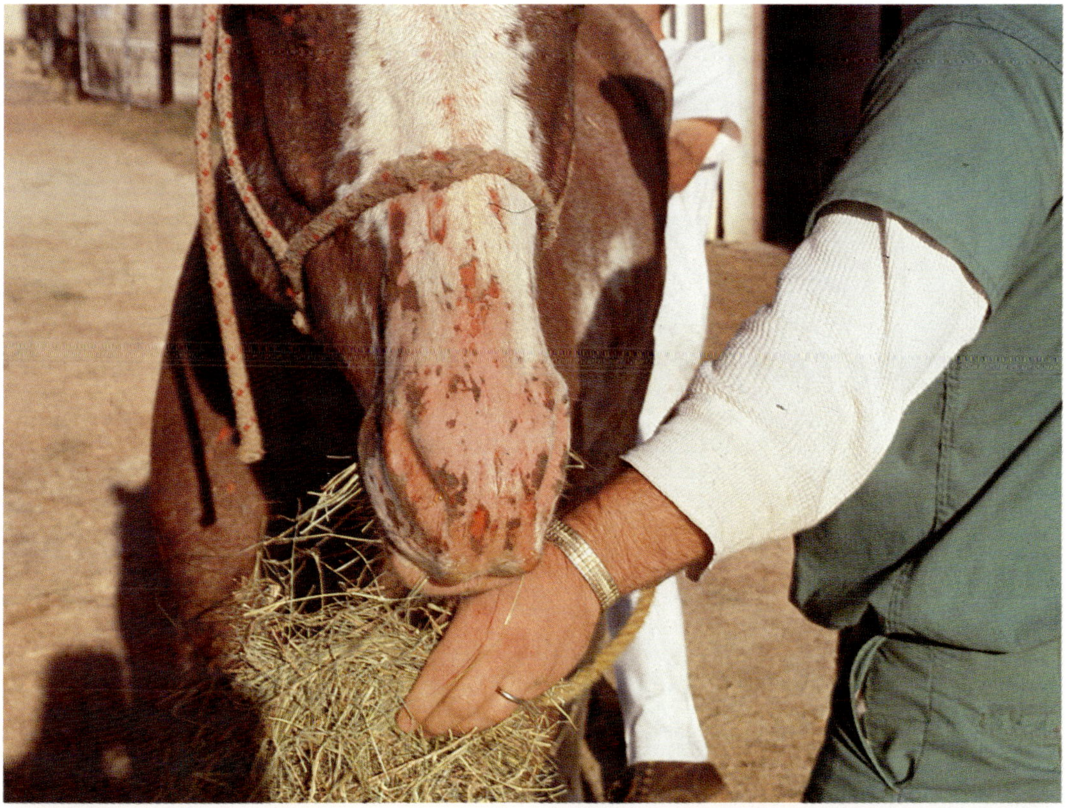

B

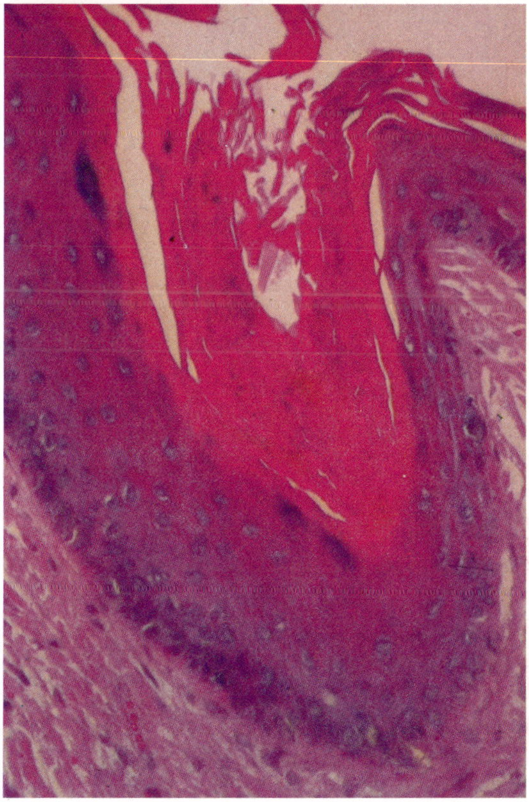

C

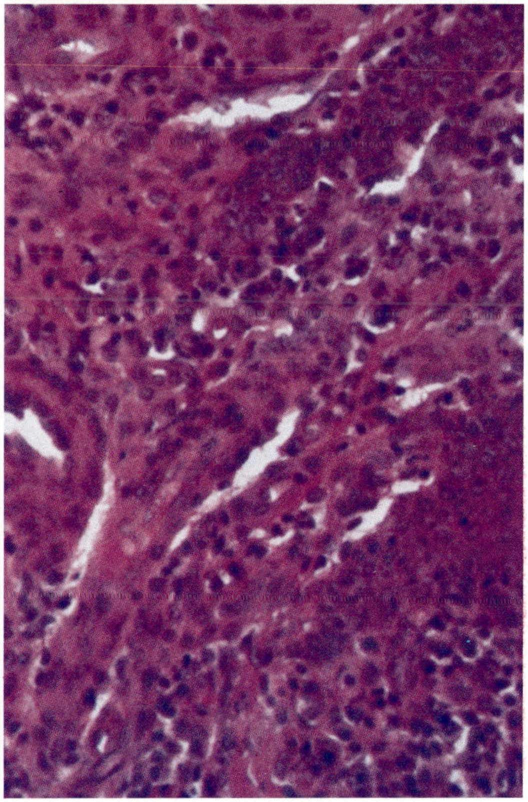

Bullous Eruption

This is the same horse illustrated in Plates 10, 21 and 61, a 13-year-old Tennesee Walking Horse with a perioral problem of approximately two weeks duration.

Clinically, an erythematous, sharply demarcated and somewhat crusted patch was found on the right corner of the mouth, extending more towards the external surface of the lower lip and without involving the oral mucosa (Fig. A).

Histopathologically, there was a clear cut detachment of the epidermis from the underlying dermis with formation of a subepidermal bulla (Fig. C). While the epidermis itself appeared fairly normal, the main pathology was in the dermis. There was an inflammatory infiltrate mostly perivascular and composed of lymphocytes, histiocytes, few plasma cells and some polymorphonuclear leukocytes mixed with erythrocytes. Many of the capillary walls showed cells in process of extravasation. The upper as well as the mid dermis were involved (Fig. D).

Treatment consisted of cleansing of the affected area as described for aural dermatitis. In addition an ointment (PHYSICIANS DESK REFERENCE 1979) combining 1% hydrocortisone, polymyxin B sulfate 5000 units per gram, bacitracin zinc 400 units per gram and neomycin sulfate 5 mg per gram in white petrolatum was applied every twelve hours over six consecutive weeks. Complete clearing was obtained (Fig. B). Despite the fact that over the years warnings have been issued regarding the sensitizing properties of neomycin, we have failed to observe this problem with any significant frequency after using this topical antibiotic in hundreds of patients.

We are aware of the fact that in vitro studies have suggested a better release of neomycin from washable emulsion-type vehicles than from oily bases. However our clinical experience in cases like this patient or in surgical wounds, indicates that better results can be achieved with greasy vehicles.

From a histopathological viewpoint this patient's changes were very similar to human erythema multiforme of the kind showing primarily a dermal component (ACKERMAN et al 1971). Electron microscopic studies by ORFANOS et al (1974) have shown that in the dermal type of erythema multiforme the basement membrane remains attached to the dermis at the floor of the bulla. Furthermore, vascular changes including swelling of endothelial cells, vacuolar degeneration of the vessel wall, thickening or discontinuity of basal lamina and perivascular deposition of fibrinoid material were found.

ACKERMAN, A.B., PENNEYS, N.S. and CLARK, W.H.
Erythema Multiforme Exudativum: Distinctive Pathological Process. British Journal of Dermatology 84:554, 1971.
ORFANOS, C.E., SCHAUMBURG-LEVER, G. and LEVER, W.F.
Dermal and Epidermal Types of Erythema Multiforme Archives of Dermatology 109:682, 1974
PHYSICIANS' DESK REFERENCE
p. 735. Medical Economics Company, Oradell New Jersey 1979.

A

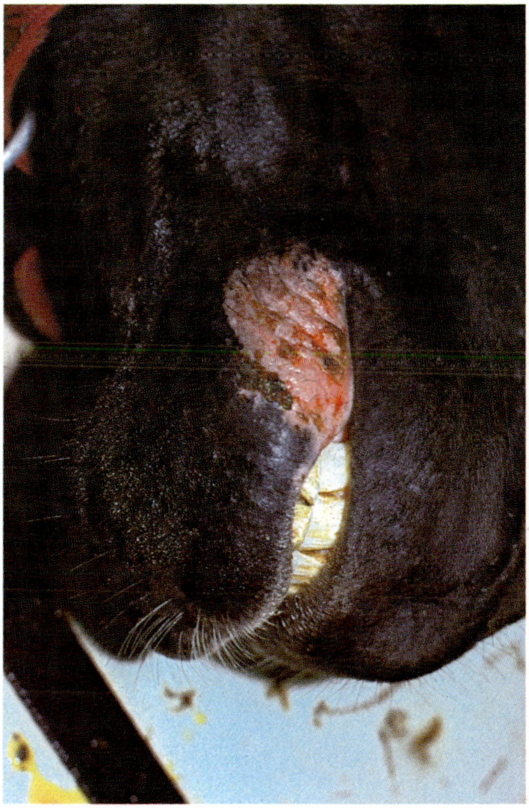

B

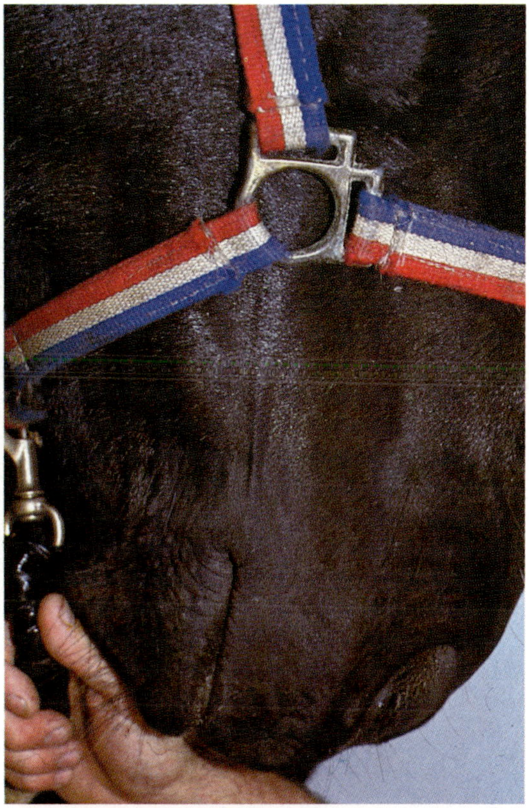

C

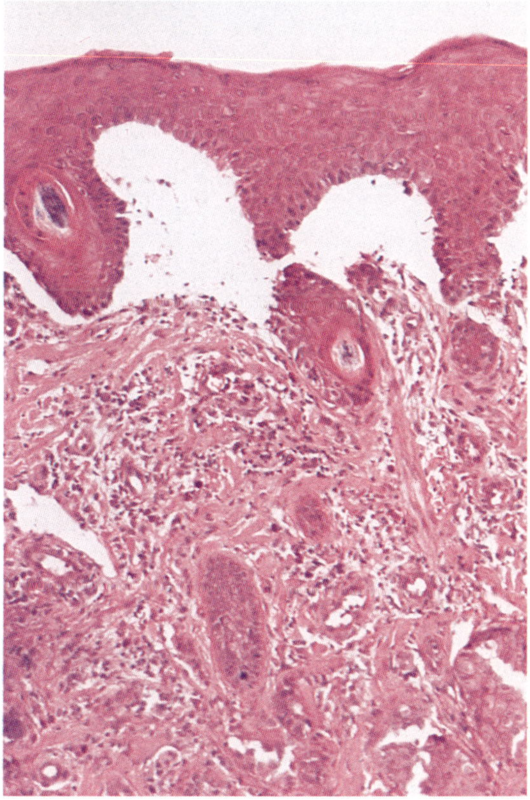

D

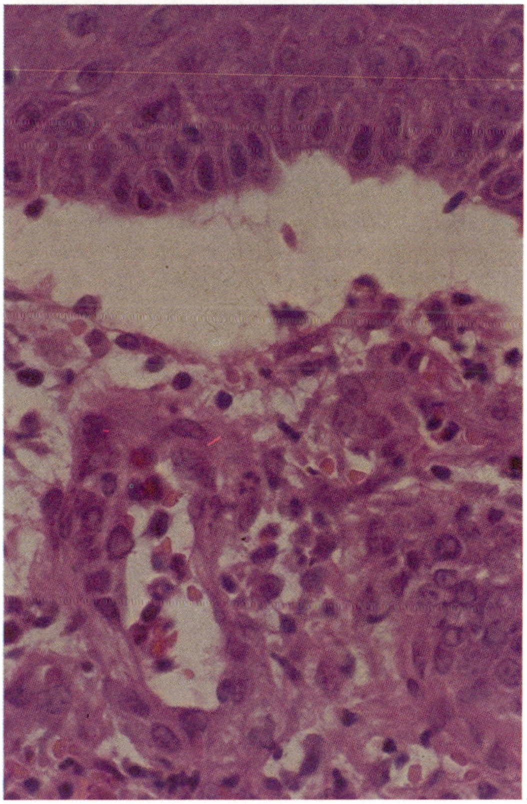

Papular Urticaria

(Fly-Bite Dermatitis)

A 6-year-old Quarterhorse mare was referred for evaluation and treatment of a widespread eruption that developed over a period of two weeks during the summer.

Clinically, numerous generalized round, fairly indurated lesions, papular 1–2 cm to nodular 2–15 cm in size were distributed across the withers, back, loins and croup (Fig. A). Alopecia was not a feature, but the hair overlying the lesions could be easily dislodged by pulling or grooming with a rubber curry.

Histopathologically, the epidermis, although slightly acanthotic, was normal and the epidermodermal junction was intact. The dermis showed dilated capillaries and a very intense inflammatory infiltrate with striking participation of eosinophils. In the superficial dermis the inflammation was focal and perivascular; in the deep dermis it was so diffuse that it even resulted in invasion of the sweat glands (Figs. B and C).

Treatment was carried out with the initial administration of a parenteral antihistamine (doxylamine succinate) followed by maintenance of good grooming and topical use of 0.5% aqueous solution of Methoxychlor as a fly repellant applied lightly over the body and legs with a sponge once daily to several times weekly as needed. Fly control and strict manure disposal in the stabling areas were advised.

Clinically, the lesions of this patient were very similar to human papular urticaria where acquired hypersensitivity to insect bites is accepted as the cause (ROOK 1972). In humans, dog, cat and bird, fleas are regarded as the common cause, but flies, as in this case, can also be involved. In Great Britain, the word "heat bumps" is used to describe this problem. Interestingly, the condition presented by this patient does not seem to be frequent in small animals, at least in connection with fly bites (MULLER and KIRK 1976).

The involvement of the sweat glands by this process, shown so clearly by the microscopic examination, indicates that the function of the sweat gland apparatus was altered. To what degree and for how long this may be a problem it is not possible to establish on the basis of this case alone but it should be kept in mind as a possible pathogenic factor in horses affected by anhidrosis. A histological study by EVANS (1957) showed plugging by keratin in 10% of the ducts in anhidrosis. Further studies of the equine sweat gland apparatus in normal and pathological skin, using modern methods such as scanning electron microscopy, are needed.

EVANS, C.L.
A Histological Study of the Sweat Glands of Normal and Dry-Coated Horses. Journal of Comparative Pathology 67:397, 1957.

MULLER, G. and KIRK, R.W.
Small Animal Dermatology. W.B. Saunders, Philadelphia, 1976.

ROOK, A.J., WILKINSON, D.S. and EBLING, F.J.G.
Papular Urticaria. Textbook of Dermatology 848–849 Blackwell Scientific Publications, Oxford 1972.

A B C

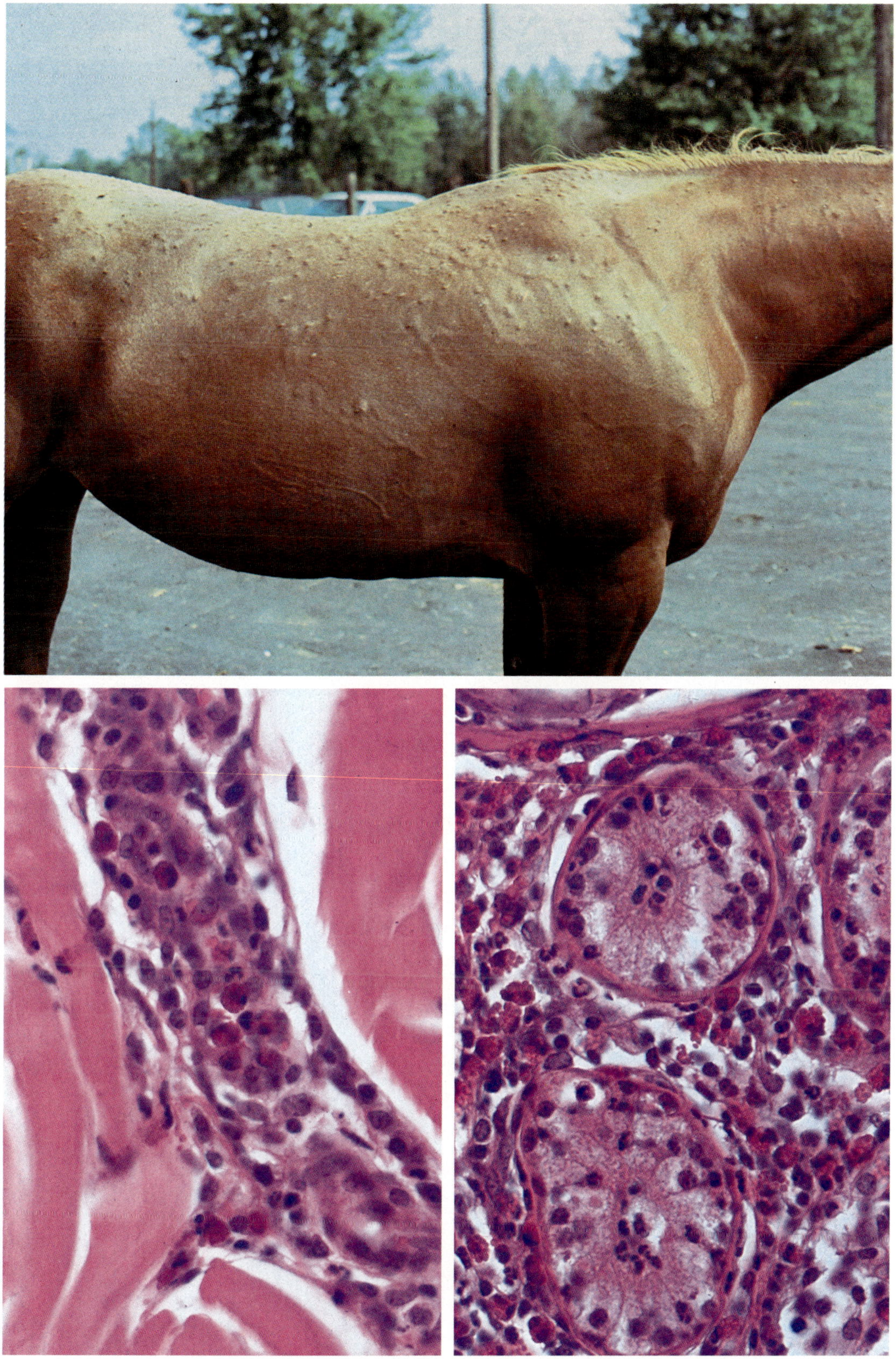

Aural Dermatitis

(Buffalo Gnat Dermatitis)

A 3-year-old bay Thoroughbred gelding presented a rash on the inside of both ears of approximately weeks duration.

Clinically, the middle of the internal surface of the ear lobe (pinna) was involved by a subacute dermatitis characterized by thin scales and crusts of blood and serum covering dried vesicles. The center of the patch had a tendency to form superficial fissures. There was lack of induration both in the affected area and in the surrounding skin. Hair was more sparse than normally but true alopecia was not the main feature (Fig. A). A biopsy was not made.

Treatment. The affected area was carefully treated with 0.025% betamethasone gel applied twice daily (PHYSICIANS' DESK REFERENCE, 1979). The properties of this rapidly penetrating agent are described under eczematoid dermatitis. Prior to the application of the topical steroid every morning, the ear was thoroughly washed employing a superfatted, French-milled overall complexion soap containing refined tallow and coconut oil soaps, refined lanolin and titanium dioxide. The purpose of this cleansing procedure is twofold: first to remove the scales, sebum, crusts and superimposed microorganisms from the surface of the affected ear; second to facilitate penetration of the topical steroid. The patient responded very rapidly and after three weeks on this program complete clearing was obtained. Instructions were given to the owner to continue applying the topical gel three times weekly for three more weeks. The daily use of a fly repellent was also recommended.

This is the type of a problem where the diagnosis can usually be made in view of the history and the clinical features. Because of this, a biopsy is not needed and therefore it was not done in this case.

It is generally agreed that flies (KRAL and NOVAK, 1953) through their feeding on the inner aspect of the ear are the eliciting factor in this condition (BINNINGER 1968). The patient described here had been subject to prolonged exposure to the so-called buffalo gnat or *Simulium pecuarum* (Fig. B) which accounts for the common name given to this condition. Control of these flying insects is difficult because adults are able to fly as far as fifteen kilometers. However, the use of repellants applied directly to the insides of the ears is effective. The volatile organophosphates suspended in a gel base have been used with satisfaction. Also, ear nets are commercially available to protect against certain species of biting flies that are difficult to repel.

BINNINGER, C. E. and PIPER, R. C.
Hyperplastic Dermatitis of the Equine Ear. Journal of the American Veterinary Medical Association 153: 69, 1968.
PHYSICIANS' DESK REFERENCE
p. 1720 Medical Economics Company, Oradell, New Jersey, 1979.
KRAL, F. and NOVAK, B. J.
Veterinary Dermatology, p. 297 J. B. Lippincott Company, Philadelphia, 1953.

A

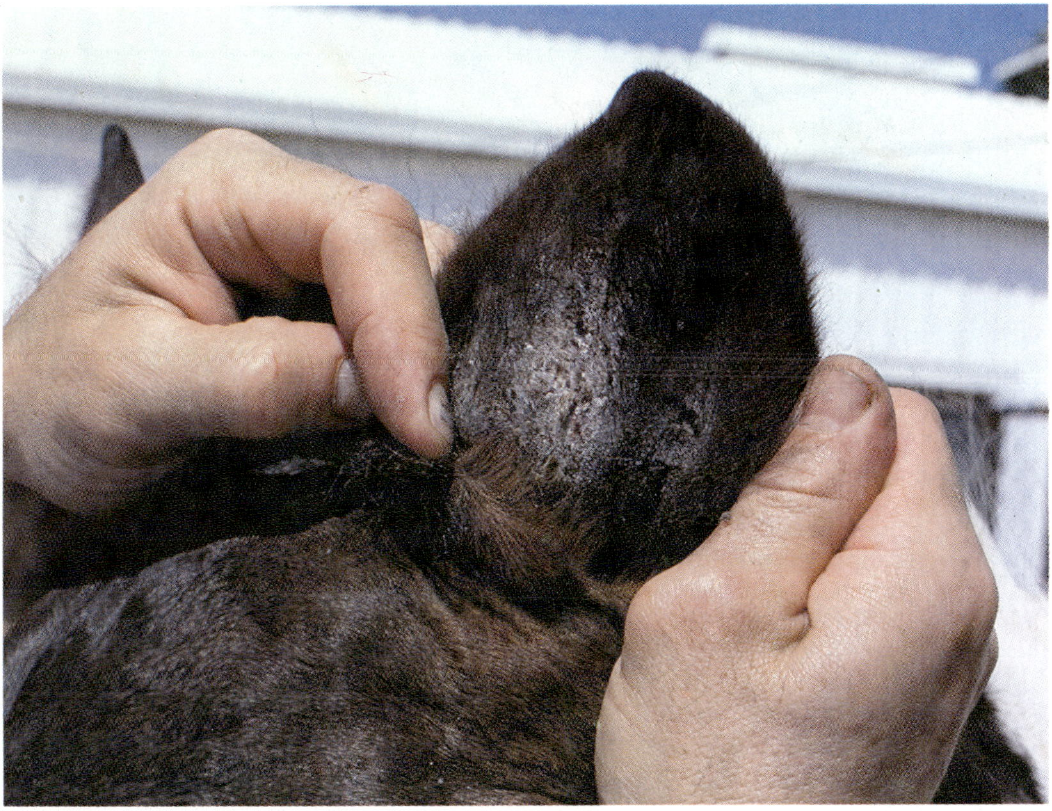

B

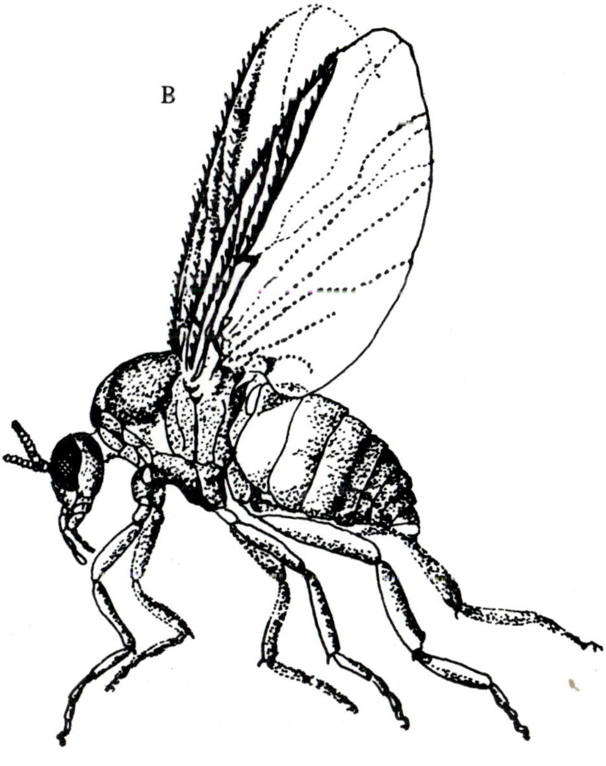

Seborrheic Dermatitis

A 9-year-old Pony gelding had been suffering from a generalized eruption affecting the entire skin for a period of 4 years, becoming milder in the summer and worsening in the winter.

Clinically, when first seen in late summer the skin was dry, scaly and thickened (Fig. A). As the horse started to develop his winter coat, the scales became much more prominent in amounts and in size. In a few areas like above the left jugular groove (Fig. C) there were definite plaques whose features became more apparent after clipping the hair (Fig. D). Close inspection showed lichenification, minor excoriations and a sharply demarcated border. There was no tendency for the plaques to clear in the center.

Histopathologically, a 10 mm punch biopsy was obtained from the center of the plaque and sectioned serially. There was hyperkeratosis, focal parakeratosis, mild acanthosis, an intact epidermodermal junction and a chronic diffuse inflammatory infiltrate in the upper dermis.

Treatment. When the horse reached its worst condition and was referred to us towards the end of a very severe and dry winter it was decided to handle the problem as a case of asteatoic dermatitis or winter eczema (PINKUS and MEHREGAN 1981). Thus the following measures were instituted: 1) clipping of the hair; 2) avoidance of the use of soaps or cleansers with any type of detergent action; 3) topical twice/day application over the entire skin of a water-dispersible antipruritic oil containing as main ingredients mineral oil and lanolin (PHYSICIANS' DESK REFERENCE 1979); 4) very gentle brushing of the scales twice/weekly (Fig. B). Gradual control and final clearing was obtained after this program was carried out for four months. It remained to be seen however, if this was a permanent clearing or a temporary control only. The prolonged follow-up needed for this purpose could not be carried out.

The histopathological study allowed to rule out psoriasis, a disease to our knowledge yet to be described in horses or as a matter of fact in animals. Main features lacking to warrant the diagnosis of psoriasis were the tortuous papillary capillaries and the prominent exocytosis that characterize the lesions of psoriasis (RAMER and MONTES 1980). Although clinically the picture was certainly psoriasiform, the diagnosis of seborrheic dermatitis seems the correct one.

PHYSICIANS' DESK REFERENCE
p. 1835 Medical Economics Company, Oradell, New Jersey, 1979.
PINKUS, H. and MEHREGAN, A. H.
A Guide to Dermatohistopathology. p. 100 Appleton Century Crofts, New York, 1981.
RAMER, G. and MONTES, L. F.
Scanning Electron Microscopy of Psoriasis. Norelco Reporter, 27:1, 1980.

A

B

C

D

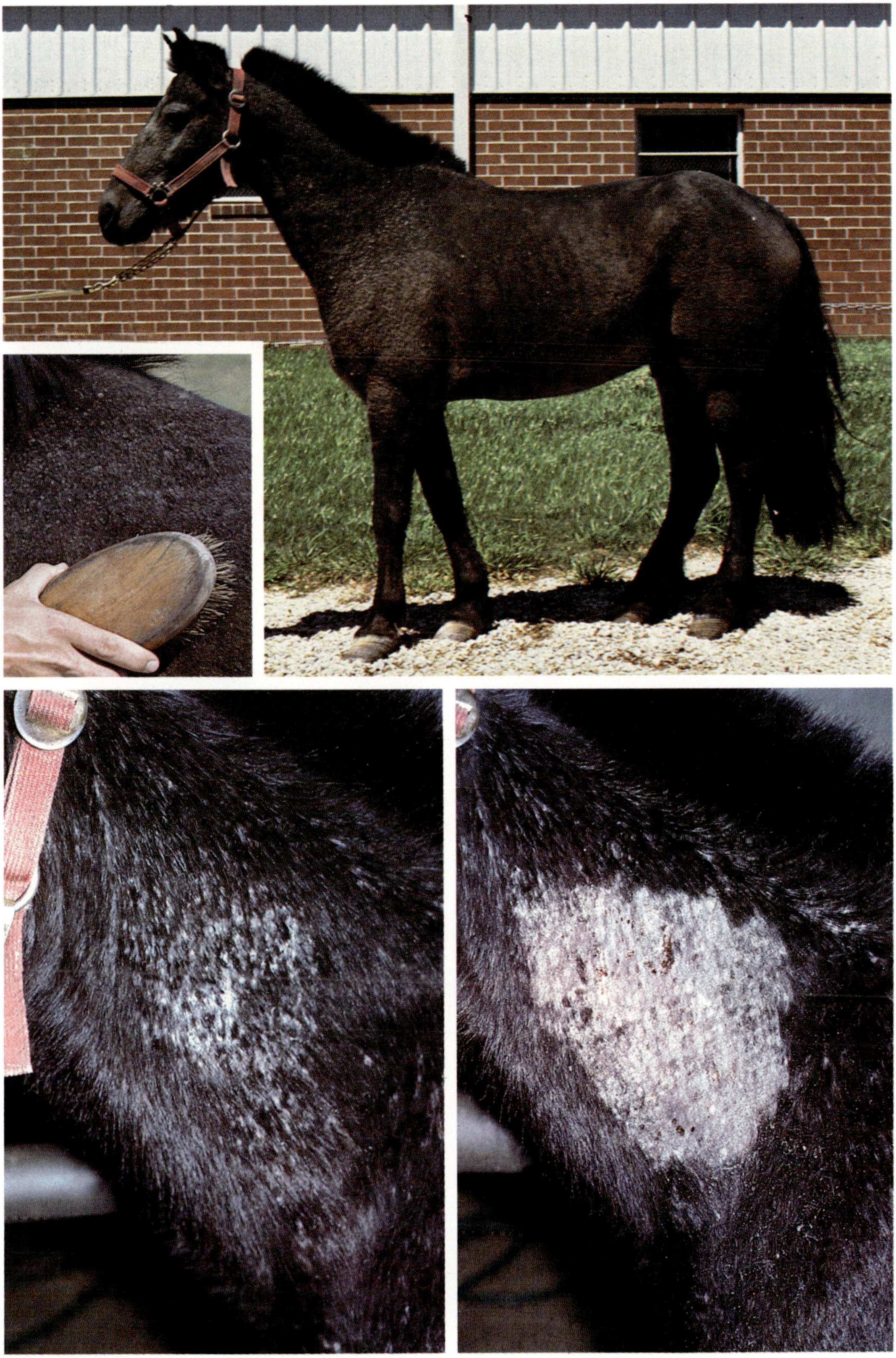

Diseases Affecting Hair

Alterations in growth of hair will change to a variable degree the appearance of a horse.

However, they should not be dismissed as having only cosmetic significance because they may herald a systemic disorder.

Complete evaluation of the patient and microscopic study of the affected hairs must be undertaken.

Alopecia

This patient is the same 13-year-old Tennessee Walking Horse depicted in Plate 10 affected by prurigo nodularis, in Plate No. 21 affected by unguilysis (canker) and in Plate 57 affected by a bullous eruption. The four conditions were found at the time of hospitalization when the hair loss had been present for about 3 weeks.

Clinically, numerous elongated patches of complete hair loss were noteworthy over the back, loins, flanks and croup (Fig. A). The hairs could be easily pulled out from the skin (inset) in areas where the alopecia was starting to develop. The places that were completely bald showed striking depigmentation.

Histopathologically, 8 mm punch biopsies were performed from two of the affected sites. The main finding was the presence of hairs that were either in telogen (resting phase) or in catagen (transitional phase). Very few hairs were in anagen, the active phase of the growth cycle (MONTAGNE and PARAKKAL, 1974). A discrete subacute inflammatory infiltrate was seen throughout the dermis.

Treatment consisted of two main steps that were carried out as follows: 1) daily cleansing of each area of alopecia with a cream containing 2% sulphur, 2% salicylic acid plus a combination of soapless cleansers and wetting agents. PHYSICIANS' DESK REF. 1980. The cream was rubbed for approximately five minutes after which it was thoroughly rinsed with water while acting simultaneously as a shampoo, the purpose for which this preparation was originally designed; 2) following complete rinsing, the areas were treated topically with 0.1% halcinonide cream rubbed well until it disappeared into the skin (MONTES 1977). Regrowth of hair began to occur rather soon with the first clinical evidence in the form of thin whitish shafts appearing on the surface after about two months on this regime. Treatment was continued for another four months at which time complete regrowth of hair was evident (Fig. B). Salicylic acid in the concentration that was used has a definite keratolytic action thus enhancing the penetration of the topical steroid.

The histopathologic study in this patient was of great prognostic value because it allowed to rule out scarring alopecia of any kind, namely permanent loss of the ability to grow hair in the areas involved. Notwithstanding the intactness of the hair bulbs it was risky to prognosticate when and how the regrowth of hair would take place. Another technique of value in patients like this will certainly be the trichogram, the method developed by PECORARO (1964) and his colleagues whereby the density of hair per cm^2, the thickness of hair shafts, the percentage of hair bulbs in anagen and the regeneration time are measured. It is possible that a relationship between the alopecia and the other conditions in this horse may have existed but could not be demonstrated.

MONTAGNA, W. and PARAKKAL, P.
Structure and Function of the Skin. p. 186 Academic Press, New York, 1974.
MONTES, L. F.
Topical Halcinonide in Alopecia Areata and in Alopecia Totalis. Journal of Cutaneous Pathology 4:47, 1977.
PECORARO, V., ASTORE, I. and BARMAN, J. M.
Cycle of the Scalp Hair of the Newborn Child. Journal of Investigative Dermatology 4:427, 1964.
PHYSICIANS' DESK REFERENCE, p. 1837, 1980.

A

B

C

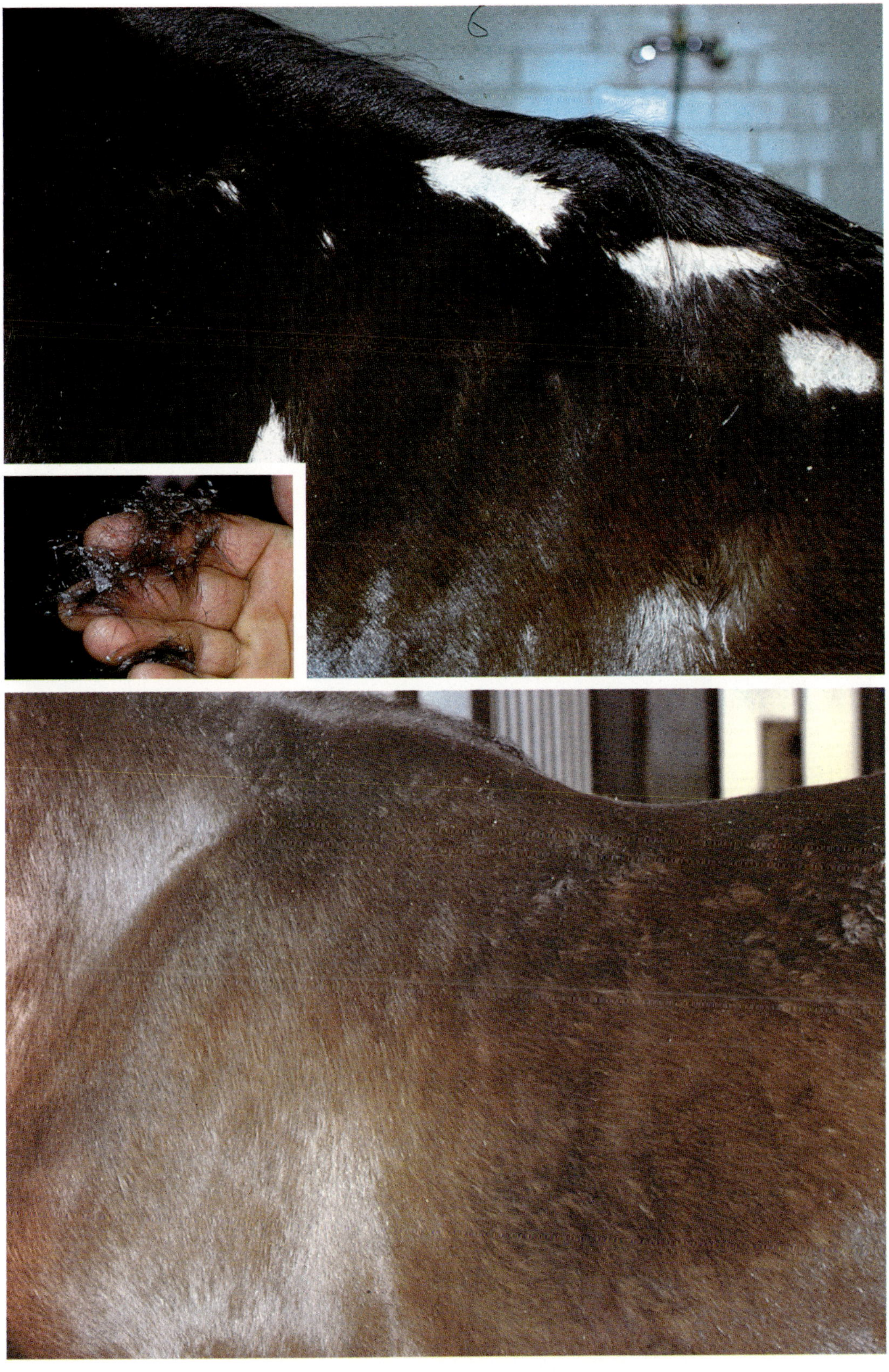

Hirsutism

A 15-year-old pony gelding required dermatological evaluation because of the failure to shed in spring and the unusual persistence of hair through the summer.

Clinically, when examined at the end of the summer, the horse showed long and thick hair over the entire surface of the body (Fig. A). There was a general loss of muscle mass and the horse presented with a swayed back and pendulous abdomen.

Histopathologically, the skin was normal in all its layers. Hairs in various stages of growth cycle were found, although those in anagen were quite predominant. Sebaceous glands were of normal appearance. The sweat glands showed secretory tubules with cells that were predominantly tall and columnar and displayed a luminal border with the characteristic brush appearance indicating secretory activity. Fig. B depicts the general view of the epidermis and dermis in this patient. Hairs are seen in cross sections. Notice the deep location of the secretory coils of the sweat glands. Fig. C illustrates details of the epidermis, upper dermis, including loose connective tissue fibers and many fibroblasts. Sebaceous glands are also shown and appear normal.

The observation of this patient suggested that horses can be excellent material for the study of hair growth. Most of the effects of anabolic-androgenic steroids on the skin, hair and sebaceous glands thus far have included studies on man and on small animals (HOUSSAY 1976). If used in the same degree, the horse could provide data which is still lacking despite the extensiveness of previous studies in other animals.

It has long been known (FLESCH 1954) that the anterior lobe of the pituitary influences hair growth and that pathological hyperpituitarism causes hirsutism. It is generally accepted that in horses with Cushing's syndrome, hirsutism is almost pathognomonic. GRIBBLE (1972) studied 33 horses with tumors from the pars intermedia. Hirsutism was a predominant feature involving all but the mane and tail. In some of the patients the hair was very long up to 12 cm. Our observation of well developed and microscopically very active sweat glands was interesting because GRIBBLE (1972) has seen that some of the affected horses may sweat excessively for no apparent reason.

DEEM and WHITLOCK (1982) report neoplasia of the pars intermedia as being the most common pituitary disease in horses. Expected laboratory findings include: insulin resistant hyperglycemia and glycosuria; relative neutrophilia, lymphopenia and eosinopenia; normal to elevated plasma cortisol but consistently elevated melanocyte-stimulating hormone. Other than the clinical signs observed in this case, lethargy, hunger, polydipsia, and polyuria are frequently described. Immunity is apparently compromised in light of increased susceptibility to infections; and wound healing is impaired.

DEEM, D. A. and WHITLOCK, R. H.
The Pituitary Gland, (from Chapter 17, The Endocrine System), Equine Medicine and Surgery, Third Ed., Vol. II, p. 885-891, American Veterinary Publications, Inc., Santa Barbara, Cal., 1982.

FLESCH, P.
Hair Growth in Physiology and Biochemistry of the Skin. p. 601. Edited by S. Rothman. University of Chicago Press, Chicago, 1954.

GRIBBLE, D. H.
The Endocrine System. In Equine Medicine and Surgery. p. 433 American Veterinary Publications. Wheaton, Illinois, 1972.

HOUSSAY, A. B.
Effect of Anabolic-Androgenic Steroids on the Skin. In Anabolic-Androgenic Steroids. Edited by C. D. Kochakian. Springer-Verlag. Berlin, 1976.

A

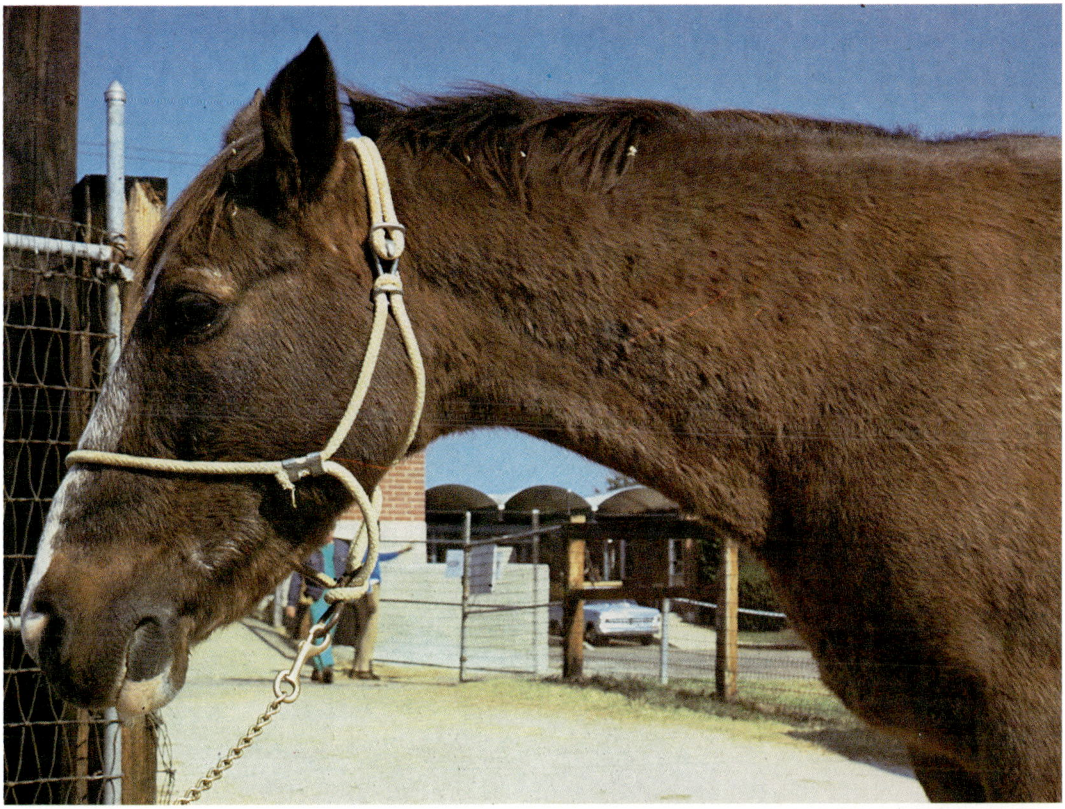

B

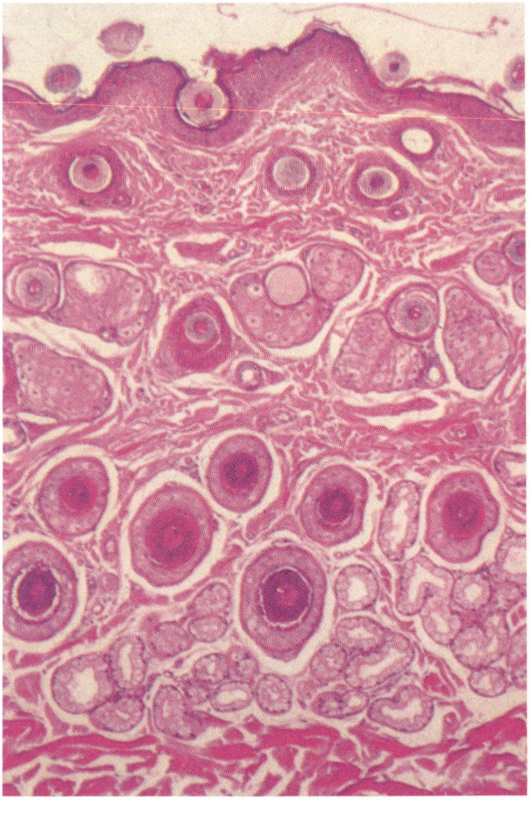

C

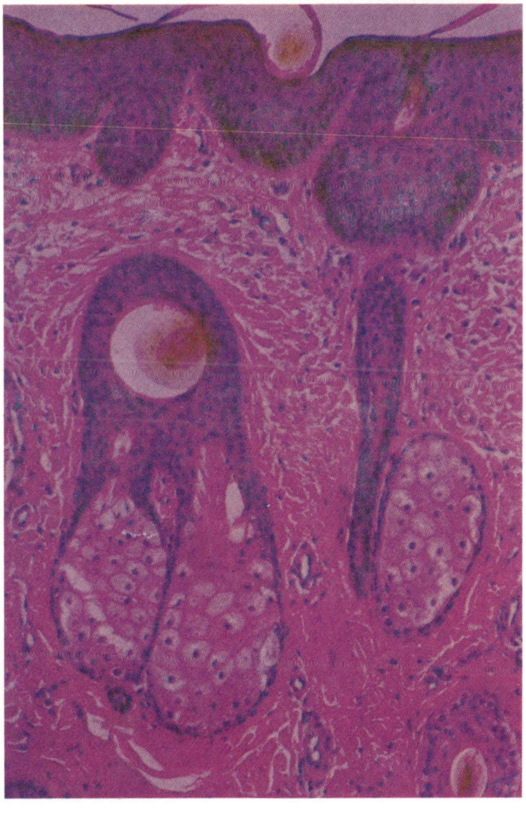

Traumatic Lesions

Horses are continously exposed to a great variety of traumatic agents.

Lesions shown in this chapter are a selection from a wide spectrum of traumatic conditions.

Their management required the combination of surgical, local, and systemic treatments.

Laceration

A 5-year old Chestnut gelding was referred for evaluation of an ulcerated area which resulted from an extensive laceration on the left side of the head that occurred 3 weeks earlier.

Clinically, there was a superficial ulcer extending from the upper part of the muzzle down into the anterior edge of the left nostril and further down onto the upper lip. A biopsy was not performed.

Treatment consisted of topical application once/daily of 1% erythromycin in an ointment base containing mineral oil and white petrolatum (PHYSICIANS' DESK REFERENCE 1979). Although the healing progressed in normal fashion it was felt that the protection afforded by the ointment, in addition to the antibacterial action of erythromycin, would be beneficial in a region subject to both friction and secondary contamination. Erythromycin ointment covers a wide spectrum of action which includes streptococci, staphylococci, pneumococci, propionibacterium acnes and other gram-positive bacteria.

Wounds of the face and head enjoy a remarkable degree of healing by second intention, partly due to the rich blood supply and to the elevation away from common sources of contamination. The time-honored lag phase of 4 to 6 hours between injury and bacterial infection, during which open, contaminated wounds should be converted to clean, closed wounds, can be negotiated for considerably longer periods of time. Reconstruction under suture does benefit from careful debridement and freshening of desiccated tissue surfaces. However, even when the wound heals spontaneously as in this case, approximation of skin edges by rapid contraction of the immature fibroblastic tissue bridging the defect often results in nearly complete hair cover and negligible scarring.

PHYSICIANS' DESK REFERENCE
p. 817, Medical Economics Company, Oradell, New Jersey, 1979.

A

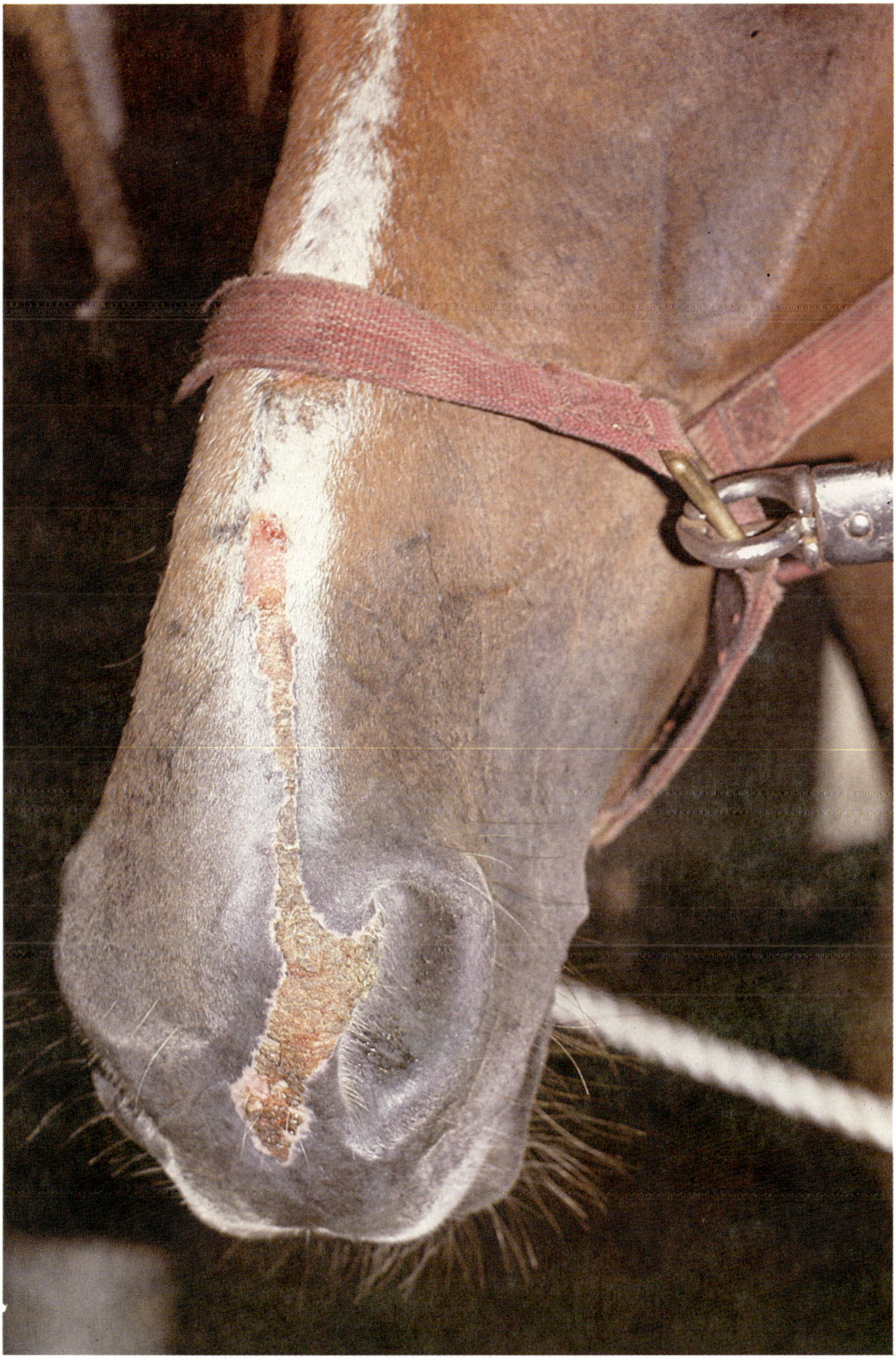

Abrasions and Contusions

A 5-year old bay Quarterhorse mare was admitted for the complaint of an acute central nervous system (CNS) disorder that had resulted in extensive contusions and abrasions to the head from self-inflicted injury.

Clinically, there were many areas of the skin where the epidermis was partially or entirely lost. The skin surrounding the abraded places was markedly swollen and dark brownish in color, indicating subcutaneous extravasation of blood. The forehead was the region most severely injured (Fig. A). The dermatology in this case is but an outward manifestation of a neurologic problem which greatly overshadows the cutaneous lesions. The localized edema of the head can be attributed directly to the effects of trauma and indirectly to edema of stasis resulting from the dependent head carriage, itself another sign of the CNS disorder (Fig. B).

Differential diagnosis would include: 1) trauma to the head; 2) the infectious encephalitides--notably viral encephalomyelitis, rabies, listeriosis, and bacterial abscess (e.g., streptococcus and corynebacterium species); 3) parasitic larval migrations (e.g., *Strongylus vulgaris*) and protozoan (sporozoan) encephalitis, notably toxoplasmosis; 4) toxic encephalitis of chemical origin (e.g., lead, arsenic, mercury, chloriated hydrocarbons, organophosphates, and rodenticides); 5) of plant origin, such as the nigropallidal encephalomalacia due to yellow star thistle, and the hepatic cirrhosis syndrome seen from ingestion of plants containing pyrrolizidine alkaloids (e.g., *Crotelaria spectabilis* and *Senecio jacobaea*); 6) of mycotoxin origin, such as the leucoencephalomalacia seen in moldy corn poisoning; and 7) neoplasia of the brain. This is but a brief list of some important causes of serious CNS disturbances in the horse.

Treatment would be dependent upon diagnosis; and in this case, the reversal of cerebral edema caused by postural congestion of the head as well as the initiating cause. Management of the skin lesions, though decidedly secondary, would simply be a part of good nursing care.

BLOOD, D.C. and HENDERSON, J.A.
Veterinary Medicine, Fourth Edition, The Williams & Wilkins Co., Baltimore, Md., Chapter 11, The Nervous System, 201–225, 1974.

CATCOTT, E.J. and SMITHCORS, J.F.
Equine Medicine and Surgery, Second Edition American Veterinary Publications, Inc. Wheaton, Ill. 1972.

JUBB, K.V.F. and KENNEDY, P.C.
Pathology of Domestic Animals. Second Edition, Vol. 2., Chapter 7, The Nervous System, 341–452, Academic Press, New York & London, 1970.

A

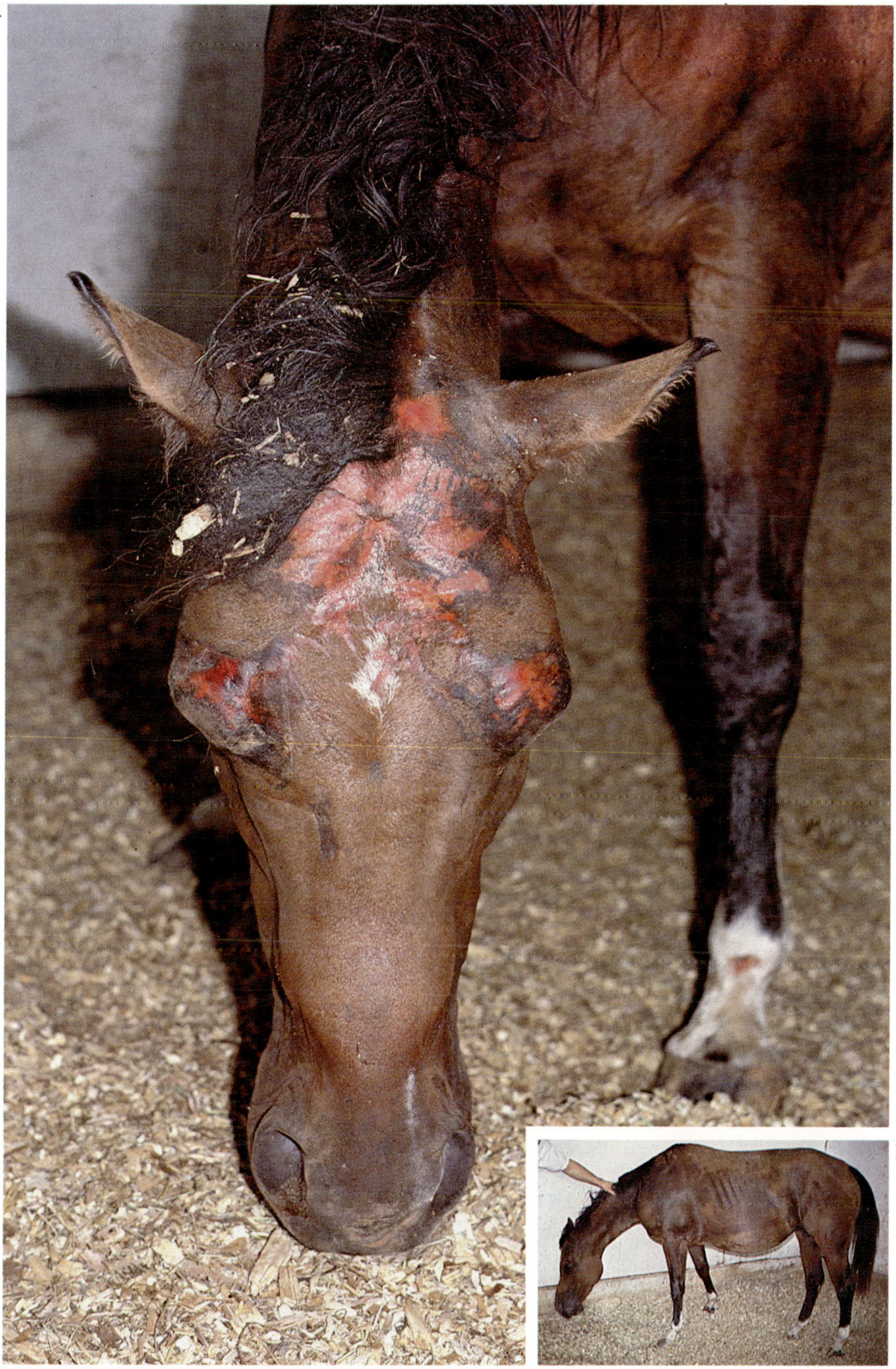

B

Chemical Burn

A 4-year-old Chestnut Thoroughbred gelding was presented because of a slow-healing ulcer of the skin after a cantharides blister two months earlier. The use of this vesicant had been complicated by secondary infection.

Clinically, a very large ulcer was present over the external aspect of the gaskin and hock of the left hind leg. The ulcer was dry, clean and characterized by a healthy looking granulation tissue in the center and a serpiginous border marked by depigmentation. The entire affected area was surrounded by a wide hyperpigmented halo (Fig. A). There were a few smaller ulcers in the same stage of healing posteriorly and on the inner aspect of the gaskin and hock. A comparison of both legs showed only minor swelling of the left leg (Fig. B).

Treatment. This patient was seen in consultation in a large breeding farm at the request of the veterinarian in residence who felt in need of reassurance. The following recommendations were given: 1) application of 1% silver sulfadiazine once/daily; 2) gentle cleansing once/day with complete avoidance of soap and/or cleansers with detergent action.

The certain clinical diagnosis and the obvious normalization of the healing process after a rather turbulent course immediately following the blistering procedure precluded the need for a biopsy. Histopathology has its limitations and this was one instance in which it would not have offered much of a contribution to the diagnosis and management of the problem.

Owing to the absence of proud flesh and to the goodly rate of epithelial ingrowth from the margins, the use of a bandage for protection and counterpressure was not indicated. However, the hock is a notorious producer of proud flesh, and there is the clear need in such cases as this to confine the patient to the barn during the skin healing stages so that movement of the joint is minimized and surveillance of the wound is increased. Also, self-mutilation by licking or chewing can be prevented by the application of a side-stick and surcingle without restricting the patient's liberty in the stall. Control of fly irritation can also be rendered more effectively.

A

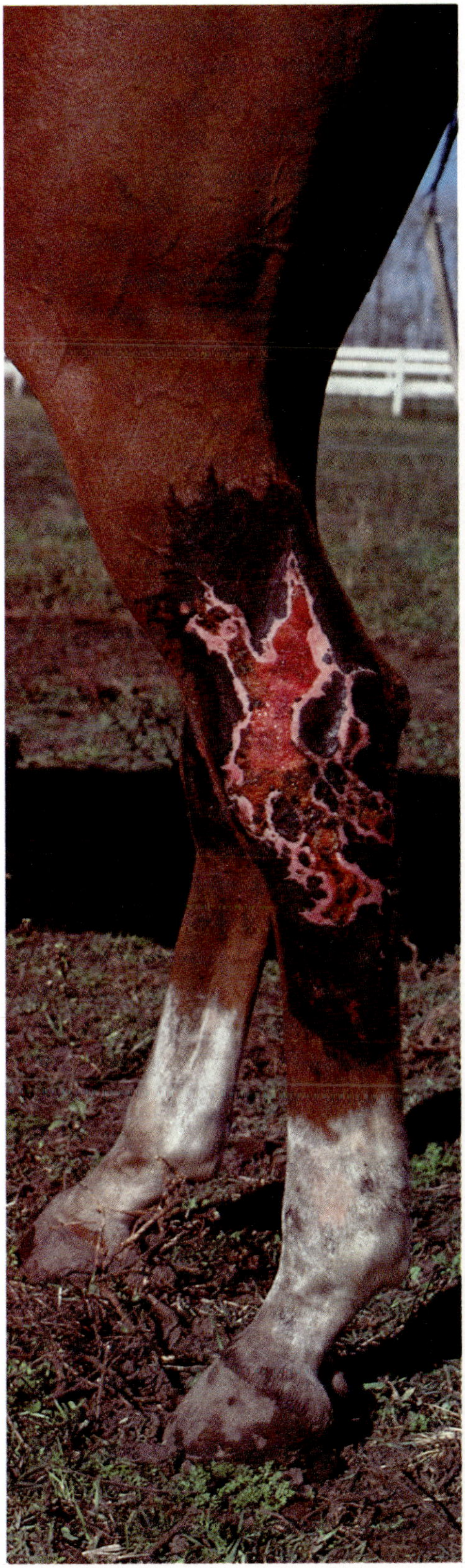

B

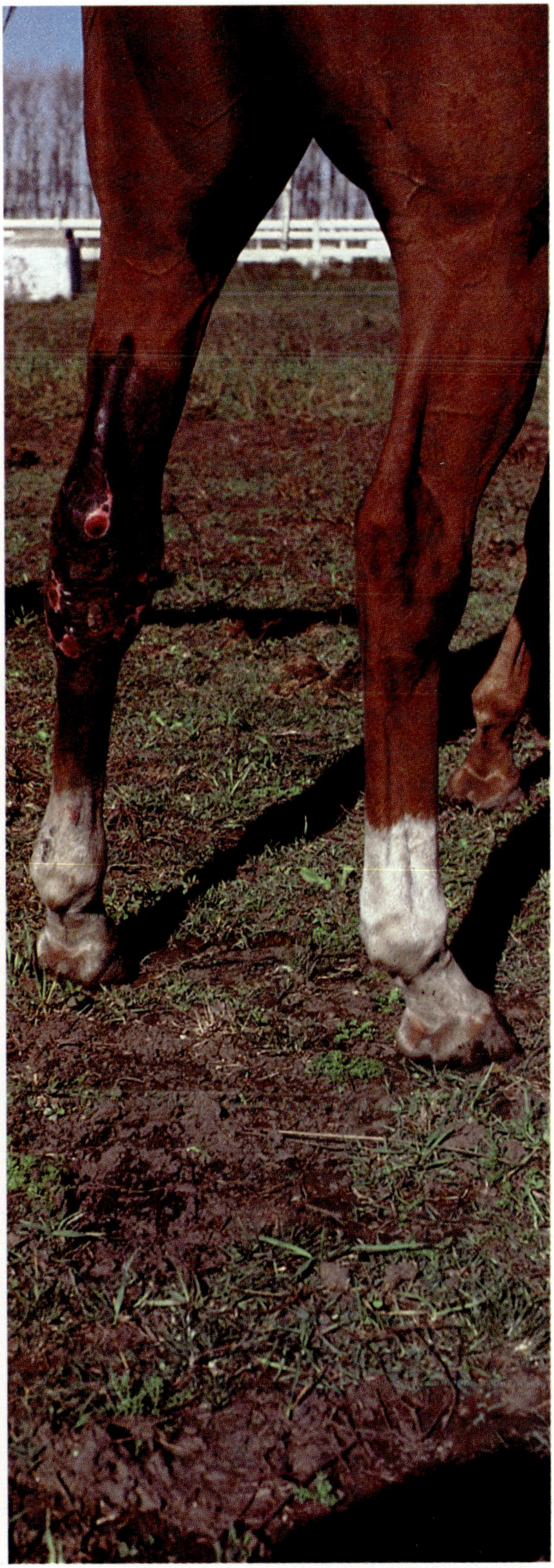

Exuberant Granuloma

A 6-year-old Quarterhorse mare developed an indolent wound of the flexion surface of the left hock which led to an exuberant granuloma uncontrollable by the conservative treatment methods that had been used.

Clinically, a raised ulcerated lesion measuring approximately 15 × 15 cm, with an irregular border, extended across the dorsal surface of the left hock from midway the flexion crease down onto the metatarsus. A raw, red surface covered a thick bed of underlying granulation tissue. The lower limb exhibited edema of stasis. The patient was otherwise asymptomatic. The lesion was similar to those in previous patients such as the one shown in Fig. A.

Histopathologically, there is usually no need to perform a biopsy for diagnostic purposes. If done, however, it will provide at least a view of the connective tissue such as shown in Fig. B. This field demonstrates healthy, wide eosinophilic (mature) collagen bundles together with thinner, slightly basophilic (younger) collagen bundles (LEVER 1967).

Treatment. The lesion was kept under bandage for 10 days to control edema and avoid infection. On the 11th day, the granuloma was excised under general anesthesia with halothane. Topical treatment with nitrofurazone and prednisolone cream under bandage was continued for 11 more days. On the 24th hospital day, the wound was covered with split thickness skin strips harvested from the patient's neck and applied with the tunnel graft technique that threads the grafts just beneath the surface of the granulating recipient site. This method has been used successfully on the leg of the horse where movement and exuberant granulation are difficult to control. Fig. C illustrates the site soon after excision of granulation tissue overlying the grafted strips of skin on the 10th postoperative day. Figs. D and E show nearly complete epithelialization by the 90th postoperative day.

Healing was complicated by purpura hemorrhagica on the 1st postoperative day that required intensive care including adrenocorticosteroids, furosemide, parenteral hemostatic agents, antihistamines, antibiotics, calcium gluconate and transfusions of fresh whole blood. *Pseudomonas aeruginosa* infection of the wound site supervened and was controlled with topical gentamicin (OSOL and PRATT, 1973) (SHELLEY 1974) and daily bandage changes. The strip grafts were reinforced with pinch grafts transplanted in pockets on the 28th day after initial grafting.

Although a hairless, hypertrophic scar was the less than cosmetic result of a turbulent clinical course, function was restored and a long history of constant care ended. The patient was retired as a broodmare.

LEVER, W. F.
Histopathology of the Skin. J.B. Lippincott and Co., Philadelphia 1967.
OSOL, A. and PRATT, R.
The Unites States Dispensatory. p. 545 J.B. Lippincott and Co., Philadelphia 1973.
SHELLEY, W.B.
Consultations in Dermatology, II. p. 114 W.B. Saunders Co., Philadelphia, 1974.
BJORCK, G. and TWISSELMAN, K.:
Tunnel Skin Grafting in the Equine Species. Procs. 17th An. Convent. AAEP, 313–21, 1971.

Grateful acknowledgement: Drs. P.A. Teer, M.F. Vaden-Pierson, and J.M. Humburg.

A B

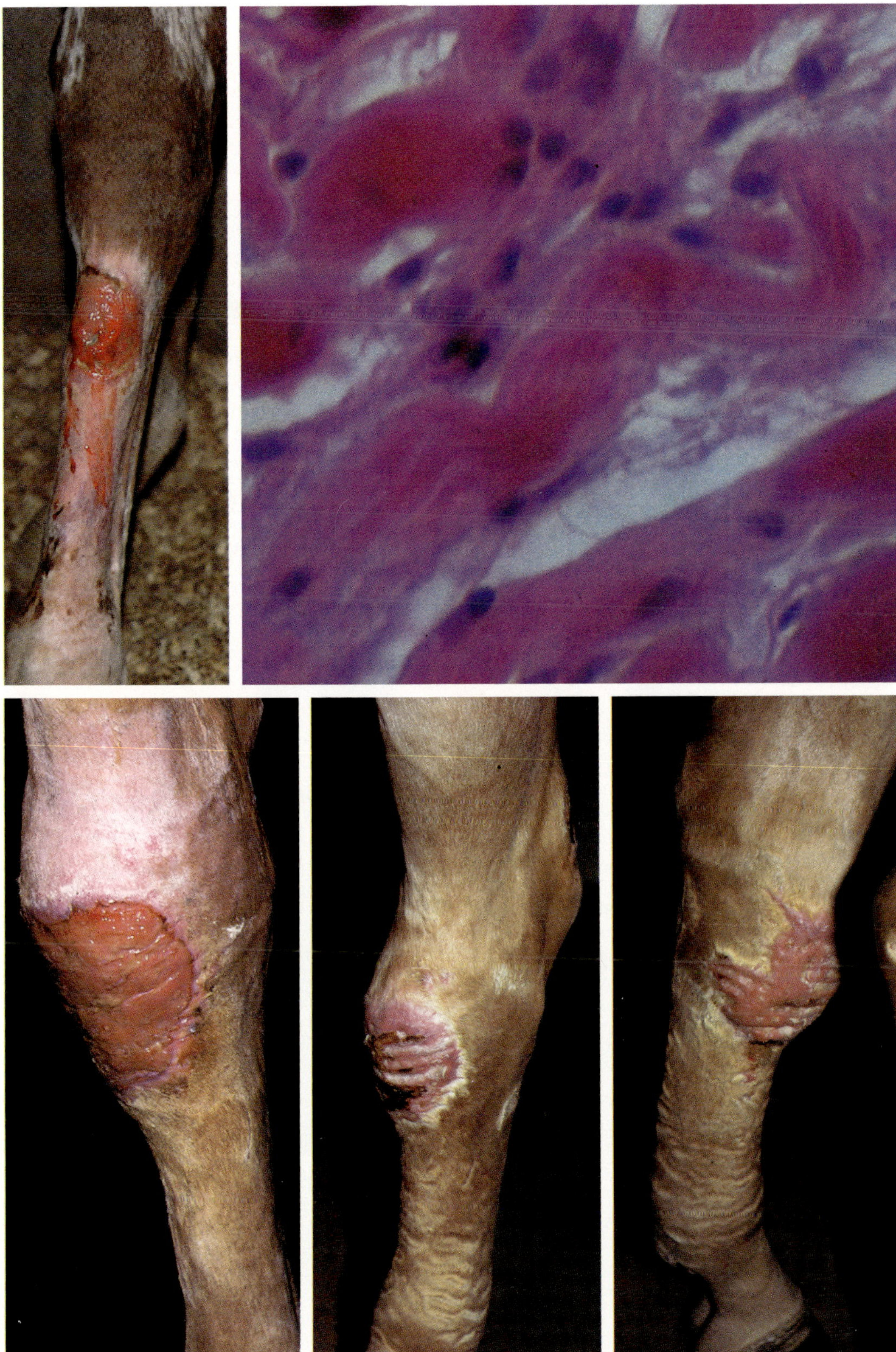

C D E

Indolent Granuloma

A 5-year-old Quarterhorse gelding was admitted with a chronic, nonhealing wound of the left hind leg that had resulted from an injury sustained in a pasture accident several weeks earlier. Treatment of the open wound prior to entry had consisted of miscellaneous topical applications.

Clinically, the left metatarsal region was swollen to twice normal size and the left tarsal joint was puffy with ascending edema. An indolent granuloma, irregularly ovoid in shape and measuring 6 × 9 cm, occupied the lateral aspect of the midmetatarsus (Fig. A). Exuberant granulation tissue was interrupted centrally by a suppurating sinus which was found to extend inward toward the bone when examined by probe.

Radiographically there were two large saucer-shaped bone fragments approximately 6 cm in length that had been fractured from the medial and lateral aspects of the cortex of the diaphysis of the third metatarsal bone (Fig. B).

Treatment: Surgical exploration confirmed the clinical diagnosis of bone sequestrae, which were removed through lateral and medial skin incisions, together with curettage of the underlying bone. The exuberant granuloma and sinus tract were debrided and treated thereafter with 5% iodoform-impregnated gauze packing and B.I.P. under bandages changed daily until suppuration was under control. Penicillin and streptomycin were given intramuscularly for one postoperative week and tetanus immunization was reinforced. Healing was progressive and treatment was discontinued after 6 weeks (Figs. C and D).

This is the kind of problem that should not be regarded initially as a minor condition. The pronounced swelling shown in Fig. A is an indication that all the tissues in the affected area were involved. This may not always be fully apparent during the early management, but becomes striking, when in retrospect, the features depicted in Figs. A and B are compared.

The therapeutic success in this patient was a rewarding result of careful evaluation in the hospital prior to the surgical procedure which was followed by meticulous postperative care.

Differential diagnosis was very important and deep mycoses and related infections were specially considered. Among them, sporotrichosis (MIKKELSEN et al 1957) and maduromycosis (MACKINNON 1962) (MONTES et al 1969), because of their ability to infect bone, were ruled out through proper cultures in special media, all of which were negative.

MACKINNON, J.E.
Mycetomas as Opportunistic Wound Infections. Laboratory Investigation 11:1124, 1962.

MIKKELSEN, W.M., BRANDT, R.L. and HARRELL, E.R.
Sporotrichosis: A Report of 12 Cases Including Two with Skeletal Involvement. Annals of Internal Medicine 47:435, 1957.

MONTES, L.F., FREEMAN, R.G. and McCLARIN, W.
Maduromycosis due to *Madurella grisea*. Report of the Fifth North American Case Archives of Dermatology 99:74, 1969.

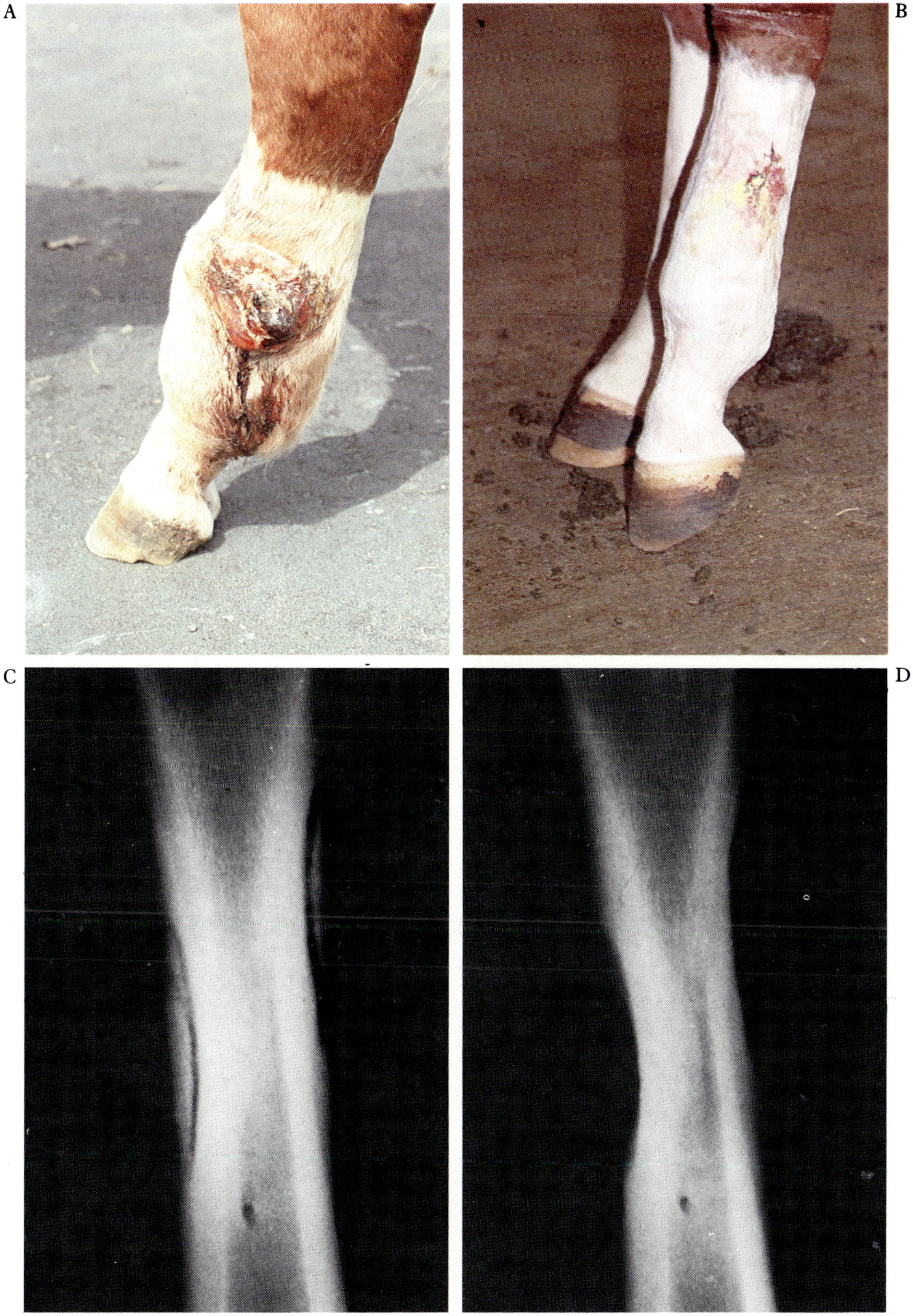
A
B
C
D

Friction Burn

A 9-year-old bay Standardbred gelding was admitted for treatment of an extensive friction burn to the left hip that had resulted when the horse had become cast in the trailer on a trip. The fender over the wheel well was crushed and the horse's hip had lain against the metal rubbing on the surface of the tire.

Clinically, an extensive (more than 15 by 25 cm) third degree burn had resulted in a full-thickness loss of skin, leaving a raw bed of granulation tissue (Fig. A).

Treatment consisted of regular local wound care. The surface of the wound was cleansed with povidone-iodine surgical scrub soap to remove debris and to dislodge any nonadherent scab. Topical antibacterials included povidone-iodine ointment, 0.2% nitrofurazone soluble dressing, and combination antibiotic ointments, e.g., polymixin B-bacitracin-neomycin. One of the most common burn pathogens is Pseudomonas, and it can only be controlled by rigorous, daily treatment. Also of importance is parasite prevention--flies, gnats, midges, etc.-- that aggravate the wound directly and indirectly from incessant tail switching across the wound surface.

Attempted skin grafting by free autogenous transplant was unsuccessful. The enlargement photograph (Fig. C) shows the sites of suture placement around the perimeter of the lesion soon after the graft separated. Healing by contraction and epithelialization continued unabated as is typical of skin healing of upper body surfaces in the horse, especially over deep muscle mass vis a vis bony prominences or flexion creases (Fig. B). Epithelialization was assisted by placement of pinch grafts in the granulating tissue bed.

(Grateful acknowledgement to Dr. M.H. Attleberger.)

A B

C

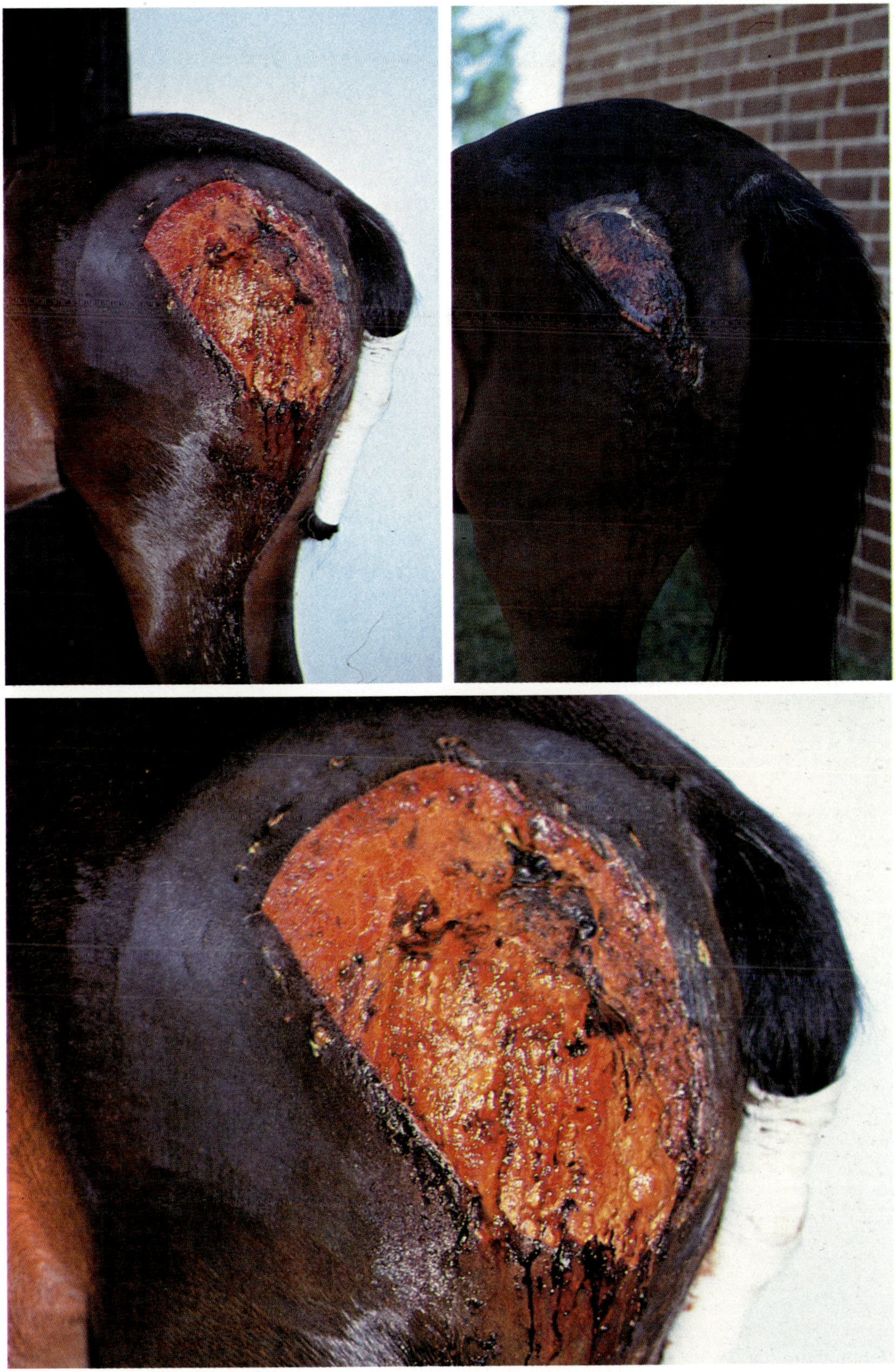

Decubitus Ulcers

An 11-year old Thoroughbred mare was hospitalized with complications of progressively severe chronic laminitis including multiple cutaneous ulcers that had increased in number and size over the past 5 months. The patient suffered from perforation of the soles and abscessed feet. She had great difficulty rising and spent most of the time lying down in the stall (Fig. A).

Clinically, there were ulcers of various sizes located over most of the lateral bony prominences. Some of the ulcers were superficial and covered by crusts; others were deep and filled with exuberant granulation tissue. Skin over the ribs was excoriated and scaly and surrounded by hyper- or hypopigmented skin. Other areas of friction dermatitis were apparent around the ulcers and elsewhere (Figs. D and E, overleaf).

Histopathologically, an 8 mm punch biopsy was obtained from an edge of one of the ulcers including some of the surrounding normal appearing skin. The latter showed hyperkeratosis and focal parakeratosis, an acanthotic epidermis and a superficial dermis with numerous dilated capillaries many of which had a prominent endothelial lining (Fig. B).

The ulcerated skin lacked epidermis. Underneath a thin layer composed of fibrin and blood cells, there was a highly cellular connective tissue including many dilated capillaries with an irregular and sometimes discontinuous endothelial lining, among irregular and thin collagen bundles. Erythrocytes were present in large numbers within the capillaries and in the connective tissue (Fig. C). Beneath the crust of fibrin and blood cells leukocytes were migrating from the superficial capillaries. Many fibroblasts and newlyformed basophilic collagen as well as older eosinophilic collagen surrounded the numerous capillaries in the deeper levels of the specimen.

Treatment of both the ulcers and the underlying problem was unsuccessful, despite intense and varied efforts. The septic process in the pododerm extended to the third phalanx necessitating the decision for euthanasia.

The key to the problem is to avoid prolonged blocking of blood flow by pressure because it interferes with the nourishment of skin and soft tissues (MILLER and SACHS 1974). It must be kept in mind that in this condition the best treatment lies in prevention (ROOK et al 1972). Thus successful management depends upon correction of the primary cause of the debilitating lameness. The use of slings is helpful in selected cases; but, in general, decubitus is best treated by return to the ambulatory state. Deep straw, regularly changed and tossed to prevent fecal contamination and urine scald, makes the best bed. Otherwise, daily wound toilet, application of appropriate protectant and astringent wound dressings, control of the fly population, periodic debridement of necrotic tissues, protective bandages (especially on the lower legs), good grooming and constant nursing care constitute the main course of therapy. If secondary bacterial infection develops, the proper antibiotic following culture and sensitivity studies must be prescribed. In addition, careful attention should be paid to diet and to rule out other constitutional diseases.

A connection between laminitis and decubitus ulcers cannot be postulated. It is appropriate to remember, however, that in the early stages of laminitis (COFFMAN et al 1970) vasoconstriction occurs. This suggests the importance of future vascular studies in patients such as this one.

PINKUS and MEHREGAN (1981) have pointed that decubitus ulcers do not have histologic features that allow a diagnosis. The biopsy was taken in this patient because of continuous interest in equine dermatology and to provide material for studies on decubitus ulcers. As chronic laminitis worsens, the sole of the foot can become infected with *Bacteroides funduliformis* (ADAMS 1974). Although Bacteroides was not identified in these decubitus ulcers, it may be justified to question the role played by possible systemic absorption and circulation of bacterial toxins and tissue degradation products that must have existed in abundance in this patient. Other contributing factors would certainly include general debilitation and cachexia with lowered host resistance affecting the integrity of all systems.

A

B

C

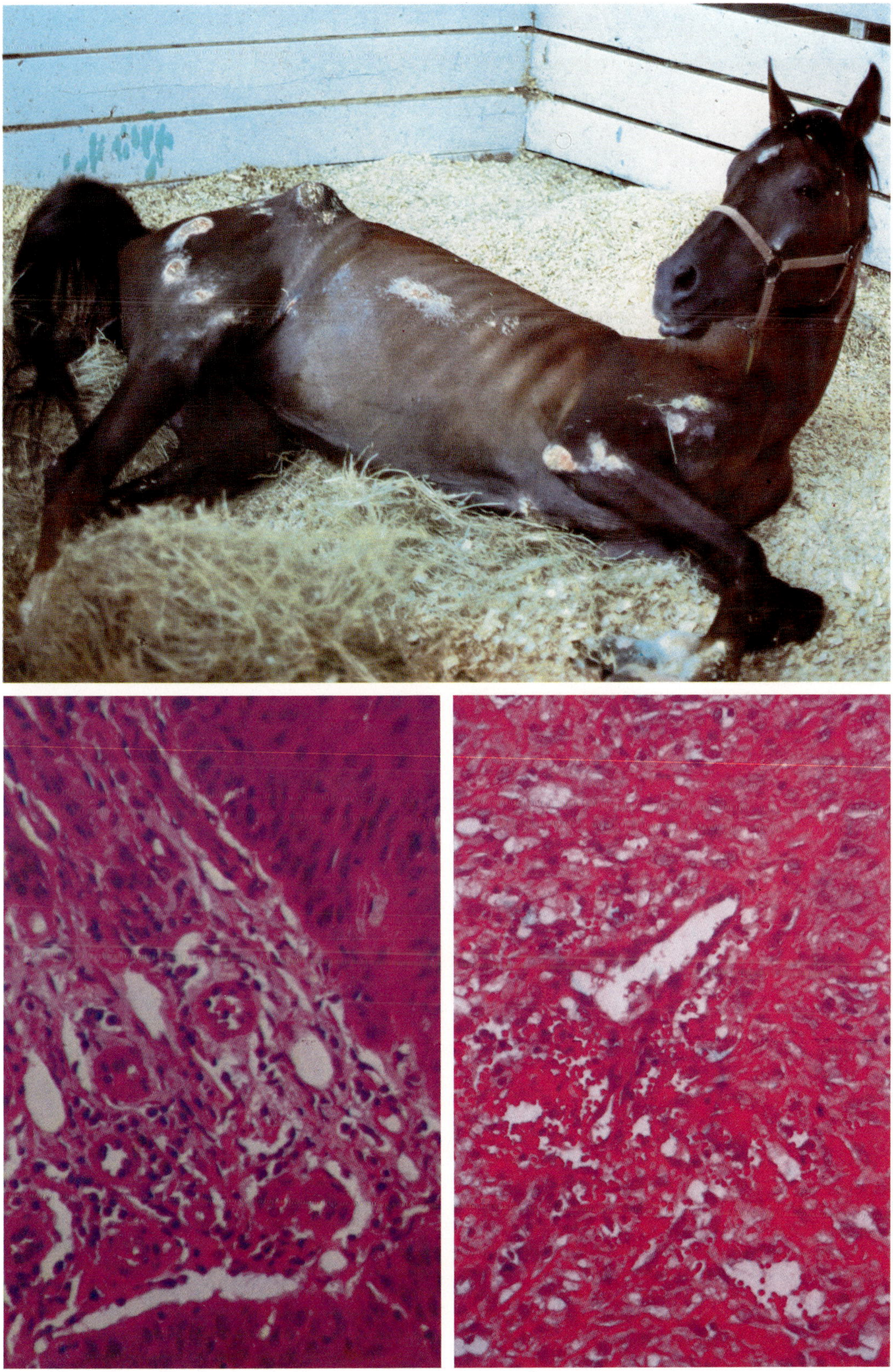

Decubitus Ulcers

An 11-year old Thoroughbred mare was hospitalized with complications of progressively severe chronic laminitis including multiple cutaneous ulcers that had increased in number and size over the past 5 months. The patient suffered from perforation of the soles and abscessed feet. She had great difficulty rising and spent most of the time lying down in the stall (Fig. A).

ADAMS, O.R.
Lameness in the Horse, p. 255. Lea & Febiger, Philadelphia, 1974.
COFFMAN, J.R.
Hoof Circulation in Equine Laminitis. Journal of the American Veterinary Medical Association 156:76, 1970.
MILLER, M. and SACHS, M.L.
About Bedsores. What You Need To Know To Help Prevent and Treat Them. J.P. Lippincott Company, Philadelphia, 1974.
PINKUS, H. and MEHREGAN, A.H.
A Guide to Dermatohistopathology, p. 198 Appleton Century Crofts, New York, 1981.
ROOK, A.J., WILKINSON, D.S. and EBLING, F.J.G.
Textbook of Dermatology, p. 431–433 Blackwell Scientific Publications, Oxford 1972.

D

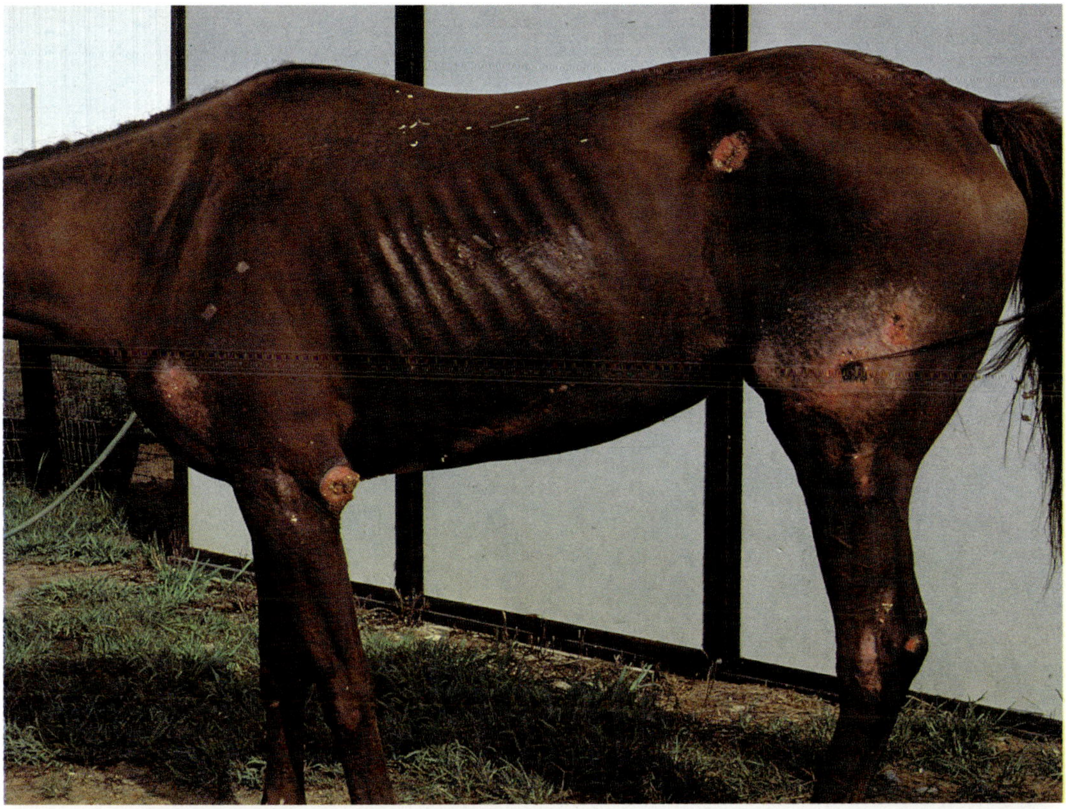

E

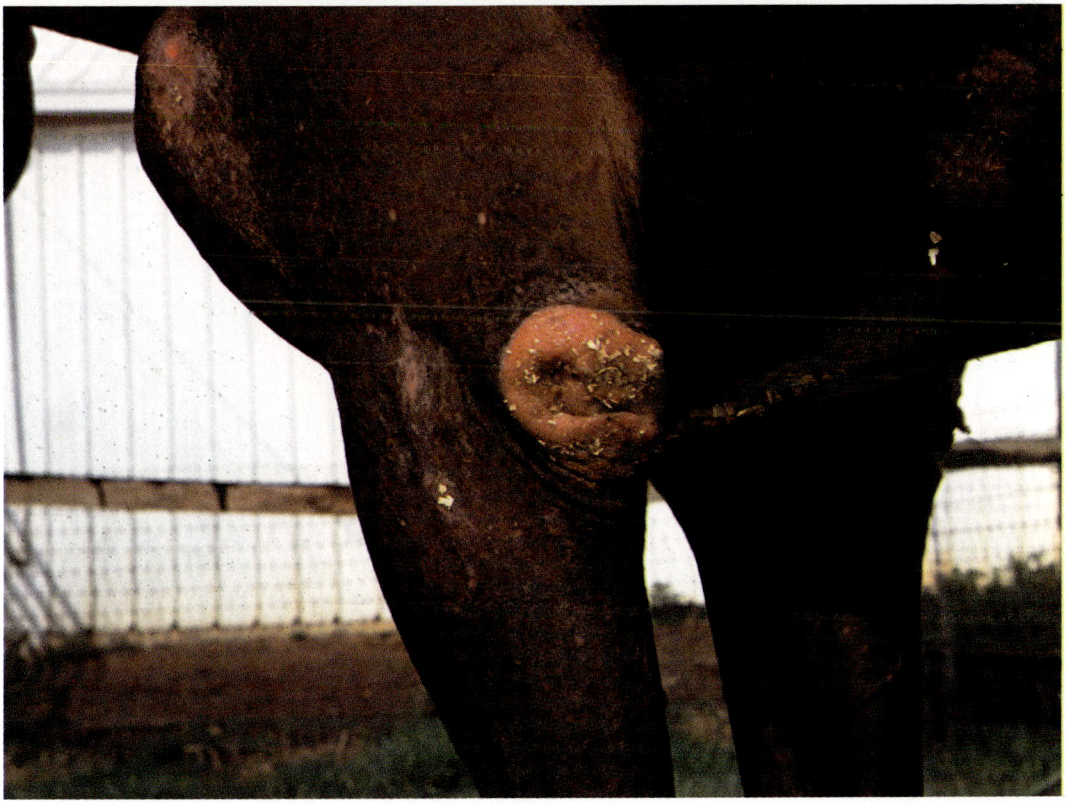

Systemic Treatment

Once the subject of treatment is divided into local and systemic, the simple lines of classification disappear, replaced by a tangled skein of causes and effects. Rational treatment must be directed both at the local disease and the systemic causes of locally manifested disease. Thus, the discussion immediately embarks upon a veritable sea of pathology, and all that this brief tract can do is to point a finger in the several directions the course of treatment may take.

In the broadest sense, skin diseases and cutaneous loci of general diseases may be developmental or acquired, spontaneous and naturally-occurring as well as induced, due to abuses of intent or of neglect, well-meaning or malicious, in company with intelligence or ignorance, and even, disconcertingly, iatrogenic. We scarcely need to be reminded that the web of pathogenesis may be spun as much from predisposing factors, such as skin color or lowered host resistance, as from direct causes.

Etiologic classification would include at least the following, listed alphabetically:

1. Endocrine
2. Genetic
3. Immunologic
4. Infectious
5. Metabolic
6. Neoplastic
7. Nutritional
8. Toxic
9. Traumatic

Anatomic consideration would, of course, be divided into the several organ systems, each affecting the common integument in its own peculiar way.

Any dermatosis that has a remote cause or effect or that is inaccessible and unresponsive to local methods may qualify for systemic treatment. Representative of such agents and regimes are:

1. Anthelmintics (including antifilarials)
2. Antimicrobials (including antimycotics)
3. Antimetabolites
4. Ataractics and anesthetics
5. Analgesics and nonsteroidal anti-inflammatories
6. Hormonals (including adrenocorticosteroids)
7. Immunotherapeutics (including antihistamines)
8. Diuretics
9. Vitamins, minerals and dietary supplements

Obvious overlaps exist. Adrenocorticosteroids may be used to modulate immune reactions, to combat inflammation, and to provide analgesia. Diethylcarbamazine (DEC) appears to counteract the slow-reacting substance of anaphylaxis similarly to antihistamine's effect on histamine; but in treatment of onchocerciasis, DEC is also used as a filaricide. Levamisole likewise holds membership in the immunotherapeutics as well as the anthelmintics. Certain antibiotics such as amphotericin-B are used primarily as antimycotic drugs.

Penicillin and streptomycin, widely-favored for their antibacterial activity, are also recognized therapeutics against the actinomycete causing dermatophilosis. Other antibiotics are also antimetabolites. Certain ataractics are analgesic. Any classification system, be it based on pharmacologic action or chemical structure, is doomed to such ambiguities.

Anthelmintics. Deserving special attention are 5 drugs or groups of drugs classified as anthelmintics or in a narrower sense as antinematodals; namely, 1) the benzimidazoles, 2) levamisole HCL, 3) the organophosphorus compounds, 4) diethylcarbamazine citrate, and 5) the avermectins.

For nearly 20 years, the benzimidazoles have dominated the large animal drug market for a safe, dependable, broad-spectrum anthelmintic with some ovicidal and larvicidal action. In addition, thiabendazole, the initial compound, has fungicidal or fungistatic activity in concentrations of 1:400,000 to 1:2 million, or when administered topically in a 4% ointment. This effect has been demonstrated against Aspergillus, Pithomyces, Trichophyton and Microsporum (Rossoff, 1974). Since the early 1960's, at least 5 other benzimidazoles have appeared on the market.

The first injectable large animal anthelmintic in modern times was levamisole, an imidazothiazole effective against nematodes of the lungs and gastrointestinal tract and given by either subcutaneous injection or the oral route. It has demonstrated microfilaricidal activity of interest in treatment of onchocerciasis. In the area of immunotherapeutics, levamisole has exhibited an effect on host defenses by modulating cell-mediated immune responses, including polymorphonuclear leucocyte, macrophage, or T cell functions. It is under further investigation and its clinical use for these purposes is still somewhat controversial (JONES, et al, 1977; MEYERS, et al, 1980).

Introduced as pesticides, the organophosphorus compounds have found use as anthelmintics, there being no fewer than 5 such agents available today. The two principally used in the horse are dichlorvos and trichlorfon. They have extended the range of action of the benzimidazoles to include both the migrating and sessile stages of gasterophilus (bot) larvae. To complement this activity, trichlorfon has been used with much success to treat the active parasitic granuloma of cutaneous habronemiasis. Using a single intravenous dose of 25 mg/kg body weight diluted in 1 l 5% dextrose or physiological saline solution, summer sores that were resistant to other treatments healed in approximately 30 days. Toxicity was prevented by premedication with half a grain (30 mg) atropine sulfate by subcutaneous injection 20 minutes prior to administration (BOYD and BULLARD, 1968; JONES et al, 1977). Trichlorfon has also been used successfully on small lesions as a topical paste. Ronnel, a third organophosphorus compound, has been used successfully to treat cutaneous habronemiasis by the oral route of administration (ROSSOFF, 1974).

Diethylcarbamazine citrate (DEC) in veterinary medicine has been most commonly associated with its use as a preventive for heartworm disease in dogs, and in conjunction with styrylpyridinium chloride, prevention of hookworms as well (JONES, et al, 1977). In humans, GOLDSMITH (1980) stated that DEC is the drug of first choice for the treatment of filariasis infections specifying that, in onchocerciasis (*0. volvulus*), the drug flushes microfilariae from the dermis into the epidermis, after which some microfilariae may be found in blood, urine, sputum, aqueous humor and cerebrospinal fluid. DEC was credited with killing adult worms of some genera but not of *O. volvulus* or *Dirofilaria immitis*. In the horse, SLOCOMBE et al (1980) pointed out similar limitations against the intestinal phase as well as migrating larvae of *Strongylus vulgaris*, but added that continuous low doses of DEC may be effective against third stage larvae, and if so would be useful to prevent the molt which releases the noxious antigens. In this regard, GOLDSMITH (1980) noted in the human that DEC was safe at therapeutic levels, but that mild to severe allergic symptoms ("Mazzotti reaction" in onchocerciasis) were frequent as a result of the release of foreign protein from dying microfilariae or adult worms. BELLO (1979) had reported use of DEC (6.6 mg/kg P.O. Q.D. for 4–6 months) to prevent recurrence of chronic colic on the theory that such distress was due to intestinal allergy, and that the DEC was inhibiting the Slow Reacting Substance-Anaphylaxis (SRS-A) as has been pointed out by FRICK (1980) in recognizing DEC as an immunomodulating drug. In controlling what might be defined as the animal parallel of the Mazzotti reaction, BELLO (1979) advocated the concommitant use of dexamethasone (total dose of 10, 10, 5, and 5 mg) on days 1–4 of DEC treatment.

The avermectins are a new class of anthelmintics belonging to the macrolides, a group of closely related compounds consisting mainly of antibiotics including erythromycin, carbomycin, oleandomycin, and spiramycin (BELLO, 1979; CATCHPOOL, 1980). They are administered by intramuscular injection of low volume (approximately 5 ml/454 kg) to achieve the effective concentration of 200 mcg/kg body weight. The spectrum of activity includes: Gasterophilus spp. (2nd and 3rd instars), Habronema spp., large strongyles, both the immature and adult forms of small strongyles and pinworms, *Onchocerca cervicalis* microfilariae in the skin, and larvacidal activity against migrating 4th stage *Strongylus vulgaris* (BELLO, 1979).

Antimicrobials. No area of systemic treatment has seen such a varied experience as the antimicrobials. From previous discussion, we know that the effects of certain antibiotics may be exerted against fungi and nematodes as well as bacteria. The pathogenicity of the infection as well as accessibility to systemic circulation will determine the minimum inhibitory concentration and thus the dosage rate and duration. Nor does this overlook the economic factors and alternative methods. Therefore, any formulary that attempts to tabulate recommended doses is certain to be misunderstood in some cases. In an effort to be helpful, however, and to abbreviate discussion, the following values are offered for consideration. It is presumed that selection is based on in vitro culture and sensitivity as well as the clinical judgement that comes with experience.

Daily Dosage Rates and Routes

Antimicrobial	Per Os	Intramuscular	Intravenous
Penicillins			
Penicillin G Potassium	–	10 to 50 thousand U/kg Q.I.D.	10 to 100 thousand U/kg Q.I.D.
Procaine	–	20 to 50 thousand U/kg B.I.D.	–
Benzathine	–	40 thousand U/kg Q. 5-10 days	–
Ampicillin, sodium	–	15 to 50 mg/kg, Q.I.D.	25 to 100 mg/kg Q.I.D.
Oxacillin	–	25 to 50 mg/kg, B.I.D.	Same
Aminoglycosides			
Dihydrostreptomycin sulfate	–	10 to 15 mg/kg B.I.D. or prorated T.I.D.	–
Kanamycin	–	5 mg/kg T.I.D.	–
Neomycin	15 mg/kg Q.D. (Mfgr's recc)	–	–
Gentamycin	–	1 to 2 mg/kg T.I.D.	Same. Concentration not to exceed 1 mg/ml over 1 to 2 hr infusion time.
Others			
Erythromycin	–	–	3.3 mg/kg T.I.D. or 2.5 mg/kg Q.I.D.
Chloramphenicol*	22 to 50 mg/kg T.I.D. to Q.I.D.	Same	Same
Oxytetracycline	–	–	5 to 7.5 mg/kg B.I.D.
Cephalosporins			
Cephalothin	–	Dosage not established for horses	–
Cephaloridine	–	Same as above	–
Isoniazid	5 to 15 mg/kg B.I.D. (or 5 mg/kg B.I.D. for 14 days, then 2.2 mg/kg B.I.D. for 42 days)	–	–
Antifungal Antibiotics			
Amphotericin B	–	–	Not established for horse
Griseofulvin	10 mg/kg in feed for 7 days or longer	–	–

* Efficacy of systemic blood levels from oral dosage has been contested.

Ataractics, Analgesics, and Nonsteroidal Anti-Inflammatories. When the animal patient's tolerance for pain and itching has been exceeded, treatment is necessary to control the scratching, rubbing, biting, pawing, and stamping that inevitably result in further aggravation and even mutilation of the affected part. If the vicious cycle is not broken, giving the tissues a chance to rest and heal, acute diseases become chronic and chronic ones intractable. Medical problems become surgical, and owners even dispair of the patient's life.

Although the subject heading is broad, a half-dozen, commonly-used drugs are sufficient for illustration. Acetylpromazine maleate (Acepromazine) and promazine hydrochloride (Sparine) are ataractics or tranquilizers safe for use in the horse. Promazine HCL is the older drug available in oral as well as parenteral forms. The dosage rate for intravenous or intramuscular injection is 0.44 to 1.10 mg/kg, and it is compatible with the barbiturates. Acetylpromazine is given only by intramuscular or intravenous injection at the rate of 4.4 to 8.8 mg/kg body weight. It has been found through clinical usage to be compatible with the nonnarcotic analgesics, xylazine hydrochloride (Rompun[R]) and pentazocine (Talwin[R]) as well as the ultrashort-acting barbiturates, thiamylal sodium and pentothal sodium, and the muscle relaxant, glyceryl guiaicolate. As psychotropic agents, they are helpful to control anxiety and suppress irritability.

Xylazine HCL is classified as an analgesic and a sedative. It is compatible with ketamine HCL, morphine, and diazepam (Valium[R]) as well as the drugs mentioned in the previous paragraph. However, Xylazine potentiates barbiturates, necessitating reduction of the dosage rates and careful monitoring of the patient. Dosage rates are 0.5 to 1.1 mg/kg intravenously or 1.0 to 2.2 mg/kg intramuscularly.

Pentazocine HCL has been hailed as a nonaddicting and effective analgesic (Schedule IV controlled drug) that enjoys compatibility with acetylpromazine, the two being often used in combination. Its principal effects are upon the CNS and smooth muscle, similar to the opiates, and its analgesic potency has been rated as one-half that of morphine. There remains some controversy, however, as to how well pentazocine compares with meperidine in analgesic qualities. The dosage rate varies somewhat from 15 to 30 mg/CWT (0.33 to 0.66 mg/kg) by injection intravenously or intramuscularly.

The nonsteroidal antiinflammatory drugs comprise a long list made longer by the attention paid them through their use and abuse in the performance horse, particularly in racing. Their action is attributed to the inhibition of enzymes that form prostaglandins. By reducing tissue prostaglandins, the pain hypersensitivity in inflamed tissues is reduced. The older member of the group was aspirin; and the newer, phenylbutazone (Butazolidin[R]). Since its introduction, interest has intensified and a recent listing by TOBIN (1981) showed 19 different generic compounds. Phenylbutazone is given intravenously at the daily rate of 2.2 to 4.4 mg/kg Q.D. or B.I.D. P.R.N., or per Os by tablet or suspended in syrup 4.4 to 8.8 mg/kg in one or two doses. The parenteral solution is quite irritating if given accidentally out of the vein.

Flunixin meglumine (Banamine[R]) appears to be more potent than other members of the group and can be given intramuscularly as well as intravenously and orally. The dosage rate is 1.0 mg/kg Q.D.

Adrenocorticosteroids. Of specific interest in this group are the glucocorticoids which suppress the connective tissue response to injury, whether traumatic, anaphylactic, or infective. Stabilization of lysosomes in damaged tissue, increased capillary tone and selective permeability that diminish plasma exudation are all desirable features of the anti-inflammatory effect. Use of the glucocorticoids in the treatment of skin diseases must be in awareness, however, of the potential disadvantages, namely, reduction of circulating eosinophils and lymphocytes, involution of lymph nodes, thymus, and spleen, lowered antibody production and immunosuppression. These considerations assume grave proportions in the face of consequential infection or when host resistance has been compromised by concurrent disease. Another concern in the horse is the apparent predisposing effect of certain glucocorticoids for laminitis, such as triamcinolone and dexamethasone. Although use of these agents will no doubt continue, indiscriminate use and larger than recommended doses are to be questioned.

It is understood that prolonged systemic use of glucocorticoids will result in adrenocortical atrophy and resultant hypoadrenocorticism reminiscent of Addison's Disease. This can be averted by the briefest systemic regimen possible with discontinuation in graded doses and in conjunction with administration of ACTH. In prolonged regimens, alternate day therapy is the commonly accepted preferred practice.

The analgesic effect of glucocorticoids may disadvantageously abolish the conscience of pain which causes the patient to rest the injured part. If this is perceived to be a problem, rest should be enforced by confinement or other means of protection.

Lastly, high doses of glucocorticoids may induce premature parturition. Their use systemically in pregnant animals is to be exercised with caution, even though the mare is not generally considered to be as sensitive as the cow or the ewe.

Diuretics. Furosemide is classified as a diuretic that exerts its action by affecting the reabsorption of sodium primarily in the ascending limb of the loop of Henle. Indications for its use include the treatment of edema or any pathological accumulation of noninflammatory fluid. Since inflammatory disease and wounds of the horse are so often attended by edema which interferes with arterial supply as well as venous and lymphatic drainage, the management of this complication becomes a major consideration in many clinical cases. Of course contraindications in certain diseases of heart, liver and kidney, as well as acid:base imbalance still apply. The dosage rate is 0.55 to 1.10 mg/kg (5 to 10 ml/1000 lb) Q. 12 to 24 hours, of a 5% solution injected intravenously or intramuscularly.

Conclusion. The influence of nutrition and the benefits of dietary management to the health of the skin and haircoat is a subject of such awesome dimensions as to defy discussion in this limited space. The use of supplements in the diet of horses finds precedent in antiquity from the time when arsenic was added to the feed to improve the coat and tobacco and chenopodium to rid the worms. Today, more's the likelihood that a horse suffers from overfeeding, the latter generations having forgotten the Arab admonition that fat and idleness are the enemies of the horse. Attention must be given to the subtraction of needless supplements and of dangerously superfluous supplements, such as 2 or 3 extra sources of Vitamin D added to a ration that wasn't deficient in the first place. Protein supplements and concentrates are fed in overabundance and roughage is neglected. Many horses live out their productive careers without access to decent pasture. Overcrowding is the rule and this prevents desirable rotation of land areas, increasing the incidence of parasitism. Thus, through errors of management, imposition of an artificial environment, and ignorance of the effects of evolution on the development of the horse and his peculiar requirements, it is safe to say that most of our patients' problems especially those related to diet are man-made.

BELLO, T.R.
Perspectives on Current Equine Anthelmintic Therapy: Misunderstanding and Clarification. Proceedings of the American Association of Equine Practitioners, 25:261, 1979.

BOYD, C.L. and BULLARD, T.L.
Journal of American Veterinary Medical Association, 153:324, 1968.

CATCHPOOL, J.F.
Chapter 54, Drugs with Specialized Indications. Review of Medical Pharmacology, 7th Ed., Lange Medical Publications, Los Altos, California, 1980.

FRICK, O.L.
Immediate Hypersensitivity Basic and Clinical Immunology, 3rd Ed. Lange Medical Publications, Los Altos, California, 1980.

FUNDENBERG, H.H.; STITES, D.P.; CALDWELL, J.L. and WELLS, J.V.
Basic and Clinical Immunology, 3rd Ed., Lange Medical Publications, Los Altos, California, 1980.

GOLDSMITH, R.S.
Chapter 13, Anthelmintic Drugs. Review of Medical Pharmacology, 7th Ed. Lange Medical Publications, Los Altos, California, 1980.

HUBER, W.G.
Section 13, Chemotherapy of Microbial, Fungal, and Viral Diseases. Veterinary Pharmacology and Therapeutics, 4th Ed. The Iowa State University Press, Ames, 1977.

JONES, L.M.; BOOTH, N.H.; and MACDONALD, L.E.
Veterinary Pharmacology and Therapeutics, 4th Ed. The Iowa State University Press, Ames, 1977.

KINSELL, R. and SWICK, C.L.
Formulary, Purdue University School of Veterinary Medicine Pharmacy, 1981. (Unpublished)

KNIGHT, H.D.
Antimicrobial Agents Used in the Horse. Proceedings of the American Association of Equine Practitioners, 21:131, 1975.

KNIGHT, H.D.:
Antimicrobic Susceptibility Patterns in Horses. Equine Pharmacology – Second Symposium. Edited by Powers, J.D. and T.E. Published by American Association of Equine Practitioners, 1978.

McMULLAN, W.C.
Equine Dermatology. Proceedings of American Association of Equine Practitioners, 22:293, 1976.

MEYERS, F.H.; JAWETZ, E. and GOLDFIEN, A.
Review of Medical Pharmacology, 7th Ed. Lange Medical Publications, Los Altos, California, 1980.

ROBERSON, E.L.
Chapter 52, Antinematodal Drugs. Veterinary Pharmacology and Therapeutics, 4th Ed. The Iowa State University Press, Ames. 1977.

ROSSOFF, I.S.
Handbook of Veterinary Drugs. Springer Publishing Co., New York, 1974.

SLOCOMBE, J.O.D.; McGRAW, B.M.; PENNOCK, P.W.; and LLEWELLYN, H.R.
Anthelmintic Treatment of Migrating Stages of *Strongylus vulgaris*. Proceedings of the American Association of Equine Practitioners, 26:37, 1980.

TOBIN, T.
Drugs and the Performance Horse. Charles C. Thomas, Publisher, Springfield, Illinois, 1981.

Local Treatment

Diseases of the skin are unique because they are accessible to the direct application of drugs on a definite place, namely to local or topical treatment.

The person handling this type of treatment is in an advantageous situation due to several reasons. First, treatment can usually be started early in the course of the disease because cutaneous problems become quickly apparent. Second, effectiveness (or lack of it) can be readily evaluated through close clinical inspection of the lesions to ascertain whether they involute or not. Third, good tolerance is easily appreciated by the lack or presence of signs of irritation so when the latter occurs, prevention of undesirable effects can be achieved by immediate withdrawal of the treatment.

Several equally important aspects of every local treatment must always be considered by the therapist. They are: 1) the vehicle; 2) the concentration of the active agent; 3) the amount of treatment; 4) the frequency of application; 5) the method of application; and 6) the area of treatment.

1. **Vehicle.** The vehicle is the material, usually without specific pharmacological action, employed as the carrier for the drug that one wishes to administer to the patient. As pointed out by WILKINSON (1972) although penetration of an active agent is a predominant requirement, other considerations should be taken into account when selecting a vehicle. Some of these are: the use of pure ingredients; the avoidance of incompatibilities; the possible degradation of the original vehicle by storage; and the physical effects of a vehicle in its own right.

In dermatology, three broad categories of vehicles are used: liquid vehicles (applied as soaks or wet dressings); semiliquid vehicles (applied as lotions or liniments) and solid vehicles (applied as gels, creams, ointments, or pastes).

Lerner and Lerner (1960) presented in a schematic form, the rationale for the indication of each type of vehicle according to the stage of the dermatoses. The following is a modification of that diagram.

Indications for Topical Treatment

Decreasing acuteness of lesions →

SOLUTIONS →	LOTIONS LINIMENTS →	GELS CREAMS OINTMENTS PASTES
weeping	edema	scaling
heat	heat	lichenification
edema	chapping	pruritus
crusting	pruritus	infection
pruritus	infection	erythema
infection	erythema	
erythema		

In addition to the physical characteristics of the vehicle it is important to remember that certain vehicles have a particular ability to penetrate the stratum corneum and become systemically absorbed. The classical example of penetration because of its rapidity is dimethyl sulfoxide (DMSO) which profoundly alters the cutaneous barrier as it was shown in guinea pig skin by electron microscopy (MONTES et al 1967). When one needs to deliver antimicrobial therapy onto the stratum corneum, such as in the case of superficial fungal infections, vehicles like polyethylene glycol 400 are useful because they can carry into the stratum corneum broad spectrum imidazole derivatives like clotrimazole (KIRKPATRICK and MONTES 1974).

2. **Concentration of the Active Agent.** This is the quantity of the active substance per unit volume or weight. When dealing with dermatological preparations, the concentration is usually expressed on a percentage basis in relation to one hundred grams of vehicle. Prior to any treatment, it is always important to verify the concentration of the preparation to be applied, particularly now adays that the combination of very active agents and highly penetrative vehicles is constantly enhancing the power of the preparations thus changing the status of topical pharmacology. For example, twenty years ago hydrocortisone acetate in an ointment base was commonly used at regular

concentrations of 1% – 2%. In contrast, today, the powerful fluorinated steroids such as fluocinonide, fluocinolone acetonide, or betamethasone benzoate in gel bases at much lower concentrations (0.01% – 0.025%) are widely employed.

When a water-containing vehicle is used, the preparation will be more reliable if contained in a tightly-closed tube. A jar, on the other hand, will allow frequent evaporation of the water, thus gradually increasing the original concentration of the active agent. This must be remembered when handling such preparations because one will be easily delivering larger amounts of active drug than indicated by the label.

3. **Amount of Treatment.** In the case of systemic treatments, the basic principle is to administer precisely determined amounts of a drug. When dealing with local treatments, although this is also desirable, it is not practically feasible for the obvious reason that the quantity of a preparation is not usually measured by the therapist. However, if an effort is made to do this one can fairly well estimate the amount of drug that is being delivered each time a topical preparation is applied. Prior to the initiation of a treatment program, we like to project its duration and to establish the amount of the preparation to be used over the same length of time. Thus we can tell, since we know the concentration of the active agent, how much of the latter will be received by the patient as a total dose. If adopted as a rule, this policy can be very useful to prevent not only local overtreatment but also unwarranted systemic absorption leading to side effects. For example, in patients with extensive burns (Case 18), when the cutaneous barrier has become widely open the patient may easily experience an undesirable concentration of drug in the blood and in tissues other than the treated skin.

4. **Frequency of Application.** This is usually specified as the number of applications over a 24-hour period. In general, two applications a day are the most common schedule for areas that are treated in an open fashion without a covering dressing. When a dressing is used, like in many of the pododermatoses, one application a day is sufficient. However, it should be remembered that the occlusion produced by the dressing may lead to microbial proliferation, thus it is of paramount importance to clean the treated area to remove contaminants each time the dressing is changed. Vehicles containing significant proportions of paraffin such as those used to deliver the antimitotic agent dithranol (GAY et al 1972) sometimes are very occlusive themselves and their action rather prolonged so the preparations are applied once daily.

5. **Method of Application.** An essential requirement of any topical treatment is the use of gentleness when applying the medication. Even minor rubbing or scratching may lead to the aggravation of what one is trying to cure. Perhaps better than in any other dermatological condition this was shown in human psoriasis when it became apparent that mechanical removal of the scales leads to excoriations (BRODY 1975). Scanning electron microscopy demonstrated later (MONTES et al 1979) that these excoriations, although clinically minor, should not be regarded as insignificant because even the small ones show prominent accumulation of blood cells and fibrin.

When dealing with an infectious process, care must be taken not to introduce a secondary invader or to spread the infection by unnecessary rubbing beyond the affected area. We like to use a sterile cotton swab or surgical sponge which are discarded each time after an application is made. If large amounts of a preparation have to be applied over a sizeable area, sterile disposable polyethylene gloves can also be very useful.

6. **Area of Treatment.** Not all the areas of the skin are identical in their absorption of local treatments, in their tolerance to the various agents and in their response to topical therapy. Consequently, one must always remember the importance of regional dermatology as explained before. Areas where skin surfaces are in close and almost continuous contact will provide a natural occlusion so if topical steroids are used, the fluorinated ones should be avoided to prevent atrophy of the skin, teleangiectasiae or systemic absorption. The latter will occur easily in the same regions with some preparations, for example, those which contain estrogens. Places near the mucous membranes (the periorbital skin being a noteworthy example) must be very carefully treated using the minimum necessary amount of preparation and protecting the edges of the mucous membrane.

BRODY, I.
Do excoriations in psoriasis delay or prevent the effect of topical treatment? Journal of Cutaneous Pathology 2:163–169 (1975)

GAY, M., MOORE, W.J., MORGAN, J.M., MONTES, L.F.
Anthralin Toxicity. Archives of Dermatology 105: 213–215 (1972)

KIRKPATRICK, C. H., and MONTES, L. F.
Chronic Mucocutaneous Candidiasis Journal of Cutaneous Pathology 1:211–229 (1974)
LERNER, M. R. and LERNER, A. B.
Dermatologic Medications. The Year Book Publishers, Chicago 1960.
MONTES, L. F., DAY, J. L., WAND, C. J., KENNEDY, L.
Ultrastructural changes in the horny layer following local application of dimethyl sulfoxide. Journal of Investigative Dermatology 48:184–196 (1967).
MONTES, L. F., WILBORN, W. H., and BRODY, I.
Low strength anthralin in psoriasis. Journal of Cutaneous Pathology 6:445–456 (1979).
WILKINSON, D. S.
Topical Therapy in Textbook of Dermatology. Edited by Rook, A., Wilkinson, D. S. and Ebling, F. J. G. Blackwell Scientific Publishers. Oxford 1972.

Surgery

Dermatologic surgery differs not in principle from that for any other discipline. The foundations are:

1. Asepsis
2. Hemostasis
3. Dissection
4. Reconstruction
5. Rehabilitation

Skin Biopsy. Much attention is paid to the biopsy for reliable diagnosis and prognosis. In BAKER and LEYLAND's histological survey of tumors of the skin of the horse (1975), 72 of 157 horses (46%) had skin tumors, but 31 horses or nearly 20% of all the cases had granulomas. In describing carcinomas of the penis and prepuce, JUBB and KENNEDY (1970) stated the characteristics that may be appreciated on gross inspection, but quickly added that the tumors require microscopic differentiation from the granulomas caused by larvae of Habronema spp. The similarity of gross lesions in so many skin diseases necessitates the use of biopsy technique as a routine.

Space-Occupying Lesions. Superficial tumefactions and deformities occurring in or displacing the skin include an interesting list of possibilities:

1. Neoplasms (e.g., sarcoid, melanoma, squamous cell carcinoma, fibroma)
2. Granulomas (e.g., habronemiasis, botryomycosis, phycomycosis, exuberant)
3. Hematomas
4. Seromas
5. Cysts and nodules (e.g., dermoid, sebaceous, parasitic)
6. Abscesses
7. Sinuses, fistulas, ulcers and eschars
8. Herniations (e.g., synovial sheaths, muscle, viscera)
9. Scars (e.g., keloids, calluses, prurigo nodularis)
10. Congenital anomalies (e.g., atresia, hypoplasia, agenesis)

Applications. The applications of surgery to dermatology as it is practiced in equine medicine are innumerable even if restricted to the minor procedures. Add to the above wounds of every description and all of the consequences of infection which may require local management at the skin level, and the list taxes the imagination.

Wounds must be explored and debrided, cleansed, closed, and protected. Spreading infections must be arrested and allowed to localize before they are incised and drained. Atresias are opened and fissures closed. Redundant tissue that interferes with function is removed and scars revised. Hernias are repaired and fistulas excised. Abscesses are opened and sterilized, and cyst walls dissected free. Seromas and hematomas are carefully evacuated and packed for further control. Neoplasms and granulomas are treated by antimetabolite and antibiotic, antimycotic and anthelmintic, by knife dissection and cryosurgery, by ionizing radiation and immunotherapeutics. Newer techniques of grafting such as the mesh graft (HANSELKA, 1975, and BOOTH, 1982) promise better days for management of skin loss on the lower leg.

Electrosurgery for coagulation, fulguration and desiccation, as well as cutting, has been widely used but newer electronics has greatly sophisticated the modality, and it has a broad range of applications from major to minor.

The introduction of laser radiation has found many uses in skin surgery. Dependent upon the energy source, a selective spectrum of colors of tissue is possible. For example, the argon laser beam can be so controlled that it coagulates but does not vaporize red tissue. Laser energy can be so designed that it is absorbed by only pigmented tissue, which explains its ability to pass through the cornea and lens of the eye to be absorbed by a lesion on the retina. The carbon dioxide laser wavelengths are absorbed entirely by water and development of this discovery is making possible nearly bloodless surgery.

Cryosurgery has established itself as a method of choice for many in the management of neoplasms and granulomas in veterinary surgery. Its efficacy on sarcoids and certain infectious granulomas such as resistant phycomycosis has been impressive to say the least. As with any new technique, use and abuse have exceeded intent. Careful attention to detail including proper use of thermocouples in the tissues and the double freeze-thaw treatment regime as well as sensible selection of cases and vigilant followup for recurrence should realize the highest potential expected from the method.

BAKER, J.R. and LEYLAND, A.
Histological Survey of Tumours of the Horse with particular reference to those of the skin. The Veterinary Record 96:419, 1975.
BOOTH, LARRY C.
Split-Thickness Autogenous Skin Transplantation in the Horse. Journal of the American Veterinary Medical Association 180:754, 1982.
DOMONKOS, A.N.; ARNOLD, H.L.; and ODOM, R.B.
Andrews' Diseases of the Skin. Seventh Edition, W.B. Saunders Co., Philadelphia, 1982.
HANSELKA, D.V.
Inexpensive Mesh Grafting Technique in the Horse Proceedings of the American Association of Equine Practitioners 21:191, 1975.
JUBB, K.V.F. and KENNEDY, P.C.
Pathology of Domestic Animals. V.1, Academic Press, New York, 1970.
TWIDALE, J.D.
Cryosurgery of Equine Skin Lesions Using Solid Metal Probes. Proceedings of the American Association of Equine Practitioners 23:317, 1977.

Index